Clinical Management of Movement Disorders

Clinical Management of Movement Disorders

Editor

Lazzaro di Biase

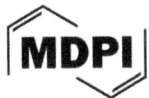

Basel • Beijing • Wuhan • Barcelona • Belgrade • Novi Sad • Cluj • Manchester

Editor
Lazzaro di Biase
Campus Bio-Medico
University Hospital
Foundation
Rome, Italy

Editorial Office
MDPI
St. Alban-Anlage 66
4052 Basel, Switzerland

This is a reprint of articles from the Special Issue published online in the open access journal *Journal of Clinical Medicine* (ISSN 2077-0383) (available at: https://www.mdpi.com/journal/jcm/special_issues/movement_disorders_clinical).

For citation purposes, cite each article independently as indicated on the article page online and as indicated below:

Lastname, A.A.; Lastname, B.B. Article Title. *Journal Name* **Year**, *Volume Number*, Page Range.

ISBN 978-3-0365-9903-8 (Hbk)
ISBN 978-3-0365-9904-5 (PDF)
doi.org/10.3390/books978-3-0365-9904-5

© 2024 by the authors. Articles in this book are Open Access and distributed under the Creative Commons Attribution (CC BY) license. The book as a whole is distributed by MDPI under the terms and conditions of the Creative Commons Attribution-NonCommercial-NoDerivs (CC BY-NC-ND) license.

Contents

About the Editor vii

Lazzaro di Biase
Clinical Management of Movement Disorders
Reprinted from: *J. Clin. Med.* **2024**, *13*, 43, doi:10.3390/jcm13010043 1

Lazzaro di Biase, Alessandro Di Santo, Maria Letizia Caminiti, Pasquale Maria Pecoraro, Simona Paola Carbone and Vincenzo Di Lazzaro
Dystonia Diagnosis: Clinical Neurophysiology and Genetics
Reprinted from: *J. Clin. Med.* **2022**, *11*, 4184, doi:10.3390/jcm11144184 5

Maja Rogić Vidaković, Ivana Gunjača, Josipa Bukić, Vana Košta, Joško Šoda, Ivan Konstantinović, et al.
The Patho-Neurophysiological Basis and Treatment of Focal Laryngeal Dystonia: A Narrative Review and Two Case Reports Applying TMS over the Laryngeal Motor Cortex
Reprinted from: *J. Clin. Med.* **2022**, *11*, 3453, doi:10.3390/jcm11123453 23

Elena Pinero-Pinto, Rita Pilar Romero-Galisteo, María Carmen Sánchez-González, Isabel Escobio-Prieto, Carlos Luque-Moreno and Rocío Palomo-Carrión
Motor Skills and Visual Deficits in Developmental Coordination Disorder: A Narrative Review
Reprinted from: *J. Clin. Med.* **2022**, *11*, 7447, doi:10.3390/jcm11247447 45

Konstantin G. Heimrich, Aline Schönenberg, Diego Santos-García, Pablo Mir, COPPADIS Study Group and Tino Prell
The Impact of Nonmotor Symptoms on Health-Related Quality of Life in Parkinson's Disease: A Network Analysis Approach
Reprinted from: *J. Clin. Med.* **2023**, *12*, 2573, doi:10.3390/jcm12072573 59

Lazzaro di Biase, Lorenzo Ricci, Maria Letizia Caminiti, Pasquale Maria Pecoraro, Simona Paola Carbone and Vincenzo Di Lazzaro
Quantitative High Density EEG Brain Connectivity Evaluation in Parkinson's Disease: The Phase Locking Value (PLV)
Reprinted from: *J. Clin. Med.* **2023**, *12*, 1450, doi:10.3390/jcm12041450 73

Maria do Carmo Vilas-Boas, Pedro Filipe Pereira Fonseca, Inês Martins Sousa, Márcio Neves Cardoso, João Paulo Silva Cunha and Teresa Coelho
Gait Characterization and Analysis of Hereditary Amyloidosis Associated with Transthyretin Patients: A Case Series
Reprinted from: *J. Clin. Med.* **2022**, *11*, 3967, doi:10.3390/jcm11143967 83

Harald Hefter, Theodor S. Kruschel, Max Novak, Dietmar Rosenthal, Tom Luedde, Sven G. Meuth, et al.
Differences in the Time Course of Recovery from Brain and Liver Dysfunction in Conventional Long-Term Treatment of Wilson Disease
Reprinted from: *J. Clin. Med.* **2023**, *12*, 4861, doi:10.3390/jcm12144861 111

France Woimant, Dominique Debray, Erwan Morvan, Mickael Alexandre Obadia and Aurélia Poujois
Efficacy and Safety of Two Salts of Trientine in the Treatment of Wilson's Disease
Reprinted from: *J. Clin. Med.* **2022**, *121*, 3975, doi:10.3390/jcm11143975 127

Belén González-Herrero, Ilaria Antonella Di Vico, Erlick Pereira, Mark Edwards and Francesca Morgante
Treatment of Dystonic Tremor of the Upper Limbs: A Single-Center Retrospective Study
Reprinted from: *J. Clin. Med.* **2023**, *12*, 1427, doi:10.3390/jcm12041427 . . . . **139**

Adrianna Szczakowska, Agata Gabryelska, Oliwia Gawlik-Kotelnicka and Dominik Strzelecki
Deep Brain Stimulation in the Treatment of Tardive Dyskinesia
Reprinted from: *J. Clin. Med.* **2023**, *12*, 1868, doi:10.3390/jcm12051868 . . . . **149**

Siin Kim and Hae Sun Suh
Treatment Changes and Prognoses in Patients with Incident Drug-Induced Parkinsonism Using a Korean Nationwide Healthcare Claims Database
Reprinted from: *J. Clin. Med.* **2023**, *12*, 2860, doi:10.3390/jcm12082860 . . . . **165**

About the Editor

Lazzaro di Biase

Dr Lazzaro di Biase, Md, PhD is a Clinical Neurologist with a PhD in Science of Aging and Tissue Regeneration at the Campus Bio-Medico University Hospital Foundation of Rome. He has clinical and international research experience in the field of neurodegenerative disease and movement disorders. Dr di Biase has worked as a clinical researcher in the Nuffield Department of Clinical Neurosciences at Oxford University and University College London, UK, and as a visiting doctor in the Movement Disorders Clinic at the Toronto Western Hospital, Canada. His expertise and innovative research in clinical neurology and neurophysiology and expertise in developing novel technologies have led to advances in the differential diagnosis of tremor syndromes, and the diagnosis, monitoring and adaptive closed-loop therapy of Parkinson's Syndrome, with four patents filed as inventor and an innovative startup founded (spinoff of Campus Bio-Medico University). Throughout his career, Dr di Biase has received honours and awards from a number of scientific societies in the field of neurology. Dr. Di Biase is also the national coordinator of the Study Group on Telemedicine for the Italian Society of Clinical Neurophysiology. He is the author of several scientific articles in peer-reviewed journals and book chapters in the field of neurology; he is also the editor for the Neurology section of the scientific journal *Annals of Medicine* and is an invited reviewer of several peer-reviewed journals in the field of neuroscience.

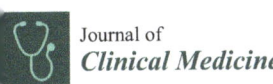 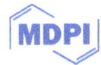

Editorial

Clinical Management of Movement Disorders

Lazzaro di Biase

Neurology Unit, Campus Bio-Medico University Hospital Foundation, Via Álvaro del Portillo 200, 00128 Rome, Italy; l.dibiase@policlinicocampus.it

Citation: di Biase, L. Clinical Management of Movement Disorders. *J. Clin. Med.* **2024**, *13*, 43. https://doi.org/10.3390/jcm13010043

Received: 15 December 2023
Accepted: 19 December 2023
Published: 21 December 2023

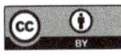

Copyright: © 2023 by the author. Licensee MDPI, Basel, Switzerland. This article is an open access article distributed under the terms and conditions of the Creative Commons Attribution (CC BY) license (https://creativecommons.org/licenses/by/4.0/).

1. Introduction

Movement disorders include a wide and heterogeneous variety of signs and syndromes, which are classified as hyperkinetic [1] and hypokinetic disorders [2]. Diagnoses of both hyperkinetic and hypokinetic movement disorders are still based on clinical evaluation [1,3]. Indeed, hyperkinetic movement disorders should be classified according to their time features (rhythmicity, speed, and duration of the muscular contraction), space characteristics (body distribution, muscular pattern, and amplitude of the movement), and body state (action/rest, eventual suppressibility, and wakefulness) [4]. Conversely, bradykinesia, rest tremors, and rigidity represent the cardinal motor symptoms for the diagnosis of the parkinsonian syndrome [3]. However, especially for Parkinson's disease (PD), diagnostic accuracy is notably influenced by a significant error rate [5], which is related to the lack of objective biomarkers for the in vivo diagnosis of PD. A quantitative and objective analysis of motor performances appears to be a necessary approach [6–8]. For this purpose, the integration of Artificial Intelligence (AI) to smart devices has shown potential for improving diagnostic accuracy, facilitating both in-clinic and at-home assessments of motor performances of movement disorders [9,10]. Pertaining to diagnoses, smart devices have demonstrated the possibility of identifying a whole variety of motor symptoms, such as bradykinesia [11,12], rigidity [13,14], tremors [15–18], gait, balance and posture [12,19–21], and motor complications [22], even at home [23,24]. Nevertheless, the therapeutic side can also be frustrating due to a lack of information related to the whole-day motor state fluctuation, since the clinical visit can last from 30 min to 1 h and therefore can only evaluate a small piece of the day. However, a significant effort is still required to produce solid normative data for a clinical validation on a large scale.

In this Special Issue, we embark on a journey through the multifaceted world of movement disorders, capturing the various contributions of studies that focus on improving both the diagnostic and the therapeutic aspects of movement disorders. This Special Issue contains seven articles and four reviews, which are briefly discussed in the next paragraph.

2. Overview of Published Articles

Clinical neurophysiology and genetics could help in the diagnostic process of one of the most studied hyperkinetic disorders, namely dystonia (Contributor 1). On this topic, Rogić Vidaković et al. (Contributor 2) propose a narrative review and case reports on focal laryngeal dystonia, highlighting innovative treatment approaches such as transcranial magnetic stimulation (TMS). Pinero-Pinto et al. (Contributor 3) present a narrative review, and discuss the interplay between motor skills and visual deficits in developmental coordination disorder, broadening our understanding of this complex condition. Regarding hypokinetic movement disorders, Heimrich et al. (Contributor 4) propose an innovative network analysis, which delves into the often-overlooked non-motor symptoms in Parkinson's disease (PD) and their profound impact on patients' quality of life. Adding a technological dimension to the diagnosis of Parkinson's disease, di Biase et al. (Contributor 5) utilize a high-density EEG to explore brain connectivity in these patients, offering a novel diagnostic perspective. In light of objective symptom evaluations, Vilas-Boas et al.

(Contributor 6) provide a fascinating case series on gait analysis using an optical system and force platforms in hereditary amyloidosis patients, a study that underscores the importance of comprehensive and quantitative symptom assessment. During recent decades, different advanced therapeutic techniques have been developed in order to also face motor problems, not only in terms of hyperkinetic movement disorders, but also of hypokinetic disorders like PD [25–31]. A well-established and innovative treatment for movement disorders is Deep Brain Stimulation (DBS), which has been found to be a successful application for the treatment of both various hyperkinetic movement disorders [32] and PD [33]. In terms of the treatment aspect of movement disorders, Hefter et al. (Contributor 7), shed light on the differential recovery timelines of brain and liver dysfunctions in Wilson's Disease, a well-known cause of secondary dystonia, highlighting the complexities of treatment responses. On the same topic, Woimant et al. (Contributor 8) examine Trientine salts in the treatment of Wilson's Disease, offering hope for management strategies. In a similar vein to addressing treatment challenges, González-Herrero et al. (Contributor 9) retrospectively study and critically evaluate the treatment options for dystonic tremors of the upper limbs, a condition that often puzzles clinicians. In a shift towards treatment innovations, Szczakowska et al. (Contributor 10) review the role of Deep Brain Stimulation (DBS) in managing tardive dyskinesia, a challenging and often distressing condition. Finally, Kim et al. (Contributor 11) provide valuable insights into the treatment changes and prognoses of drug-induced parkinsonism, a pressing concern in clinical practice, especially in South Korea.

3. Future Directions

Together, these papers not only advance our understanding of movement disorders, but also open new avenues for research and clinical practice. Different strategies have been proposed by the authors, ranging from neurophysiological to machine learning approaches. However, new therapeutic insights for movement disorders will probably arise from the evidence of sensibility of the neurons to not only pharmacological stimulation, but also to electrical [34], magnetic [35], or ultrasound stimulations [36]. Beyond the objective analyses, the possibility of real-time monitoring of a patient affected by a movement disorder (especially PD) throughout the course of the whole day could also increase the reliability of clinical assistance. Knowledge of the motor state variability of such a complex patient during the day could lead to tailored therapy, avoiding motor complications such as levodopa-induced dyskinesias or underdosed levodopa regimens [37,38]. Biochemical, neurophysiological, and wearable sensor data could be part of a multiparametric modular sensing system that regulates therapy according to the motor state [39,40].

Conflicts of Interest: The author declares no conflict of interest.

List of Contributors

1. di Biase, L.; Di Santo, A.; Caminiti, M.L.; Pecoraro, P.M.; Carbone, S.P.; Di Lazzaro, V. Dystonia diagnosis: clinical neurophysiology and genetics. *J. Clin. Med.* **2022**, *11*, 4184. https://doi.org/10.3390/jcm11144184.
2. Rogić Vidaković, M.; Gunjača, I.; Bukić, J.; Košta, V.; Šoda, J.; Konstantinović, I.; Bošković, B.; Bilić, I.; Režić Mužinić, N. The patho-neurophysiological basis and treatment of focal laryngeal dystonia: a narrative review and two case reports applying TMS over the laryngeal motor cortex. *J. Clin. Med.* **2022**, *11*, 3453. https://doi.org/10.3390/jcm11123453.
3. Pinero-Pinto, E.; Romero-Galisteo, R.P.; Sánchez-González, M.C.; Escobio-Prieto, I.; Luque-Moreno, C.; Palomo-Carrión, R. Motor Skills and Visual Deficits in Developmental Coordination Disorder: A Narrative Review. *J. Clin. Med.* **2022**, *11*, 7447. https://doi.org/10.3390/jcm11247447.
4. Heimrich, K.G.; Schönenberg, A.; Santos-García, D.; Mir, P.; COPPADIS Study Group; Prell, T. The Impact of Nonmotor Symptoms on Health-Related Quality of Life in Parkinson's Disease: A Network Analysis Approach. *J. Clin. Med.* **2023**, *12*, 2573. https://doi.org/10.3390/jcm12072573.

5. di Biase, L.; Ricci, L.; Caminiti, M.L.; Pecoraro, P.M.; Carbone, S.P.; Di Lazzaro, V. Quantitative High Density EEG Brain Connectivity Evaluation in Parkinson's Disease: The Phase Locking Value (PLV). *J. Clin. Med.* **2023**, *12*, 1450. https://doi.org/10.3390/jcm12041450
6. Vilas-Boas, M.D.C.; Fonseca, P.F.P.; Sousa, I.M.; Cardoso, M.N.; Cunha, J.P.S.; Coelho, T. Gait Characterization and Analysis of Hereditary Amyloidosis Associated with Transthyretin Patients: A Case Series. *J. Clin. Med.* **2022**, *11*, 3967. https://doi.org/10.3390/jcm11143967.
7. Hefter, H.; Kruschel, T.S.; Novak, M.; Rosenthal, D.; Luedde, T.; Meuth, S.G.; Albrecht, P.; Hartmann, C.J.; Samadzadeh, S. Differences in the time course of recovery from brain and liver dysfunction in conventional long-term treatment of Wilson disease. *J. Clin. Med.* **2023**, *12*, 4861.
8. Woimant, F.; Debray, D.; Morvan, E.; Obadia, M.A.; Poujois, A. Efficacy and Safety of Two Salts of Trientine in the Treatment of Wilson's Disease. *J. Clin. Med.* **2022**, *11*, 3975.
9. González-Herrero, B.; Di Vico, I.A.; Pereira, E.; Edwards, M.; Morgante, F. Treatment of Dystonic Tremor of the Upper Limbs: A Single-Center Retrospective Study. *J. Clin. Med.* **2023**, *12*, 1427.
10. Szczakowska, A.; Gabryelska, A.; Gawlik-Kotelnicka, O.; Strzelecki, D. Deep brain stimulation in the treatment of tardive dyskinesia. *J. Clin. Med.* **2023**, *12*, 1868.
11. Kim, S.; Suh, H.S. Treatment Changes and Prognoses in Patients with Incident Drug-Induced Parkinsonism Using a Korean Nationwide Healthcare Claims Database. *J. Clin. Med.* **2023**, *12*, 2860.

References

1. Weiner, W.J.; Tolosa, E. *Hyperkinetic Movement Disorders*; Elsevier: Amsterdam, The Netherlands, 2012.
2. Kalia, L.V.; Lang, A.E. Parkinson's disease. *Lancet* **2015**, *386*, 896–912. [CrossRef] [PubMed]
3. Poewe, W.; Seppi, K.; Tanner, C.M.; Halliday, G.M.; Brundin, P.; Volkmann, J.; Schrag, A.-E.; Lang, A.E. Parkinson disease. *Nat. Rev. Dis. Primers* **2017**, *3*, 17013. [CrossRef] [PubMed]
4. di Biase, L.; Di Santo, A.; Caminiti, M.L.; Pecoraro, P.M.; Di Lazzaro, V. Classification of dystonia. *Life* **2022**, *12*, 206. [CrossRef] [PubMed]
5. Rizzo, G.; Copetti, M.; Arcuti, S.; Martino, D.; Fontana, A.; Logroscino, G. Accuracy of clinical diagnosis of Parkinson disease: A systematic review and meta-analysis. *Neurology* **2016**, *86*, 566–576. [CrossRef] [PubMed]
6. Matias, R.; Paixão, V.; Bouça, R.; Ferreira, J.J. A perspective on wearable sensor measurements and data science for Parkinson's disease. *Front. Neurol.* **2017**, *8*, 677. [CrossRef] [PubMed]
7. Maetzler, W.; Klucken, J.; Horne, M. A clinical view on the development of technology-based tools in managing Parkinson's disease. *Mov. Disord.* **2016**, *31*, 1263–1271. [CrossRef] [PubMed]
8. Mei, J.; Desrosiers, C.; Frasnelli, J. Machine learning for the diagnosis of Parkinson's disease: A review of literature. *Front. Aging Neurosci.* **2021**, *13*, 633752. [CrossRef] [PubMed]
9. Cavallo, F.; Moschetti, A.; Esposito, D.; Maremmani, C.; Rovini, E. Upper limb motor pre-clinical assessment in Parkinson's disease using machine learning. *Park. Relat. Disord.* **2019**, *63*, 111–116. [CrossRef]
10. Xu, S.; Pan, Z. A novel ensemble of random forest for assisting diagnosis of Parkinson's disease on small handwritten dynamics dataset. *Int. J. Med. Inform.* **2020**, *144*, 104283. [CrossRef]
11. Stamatakis, J.; Ambroise, J.; Crémers, J.; Sharei, H.; Delvaux, V.; Macq, B.; Garraux, G. Finger tapping clinimetric score prediction in Parkinson's disease using low-cost accelerometers. *Comput. Intell. Neurosci.* **2013**, *2013*, 717853. [CrossRef]
12. Tosi, J.; Summa, S.; Taffoni, F.; di Biase, L.; Marano, M.; Rizzo, A.C.; Tombini, M.; Schena, E.; Formica, D.; Di Pino, G. Feature Extraction in Sit-to-Stand Task Using M-IMU Sensors and Evaluatiton in Parkinson's Disease. In Proceedings of the 2018 IEEE International Symposium on Medical Measurements and Applications (MeMeA), Rome, Italy, 11–13 June 2018; pp. 1–6.
13. Endo, T.; Okuno, R.; Yokoe, M.; Akazawa, K.; Sakoda, S. A novel method for systematic analysis of rigidity in Parkinson's disease. *Mov. Disord. Off. J. Mov. Disord. Soc.* **2009**, *24*, 2218–2224. [CrossRef] [PubMed]
14. Kwon, Y.; Park, S.-H.; Kim, J.-W.; Ho, Y.; Jeon, H.-M.; Bang, M.-J.; Koh, S.-B.; Kim, J.-H.; Eom, G.-M. Quantitative evaluation of parkinsonian rigidity during intra-operative deep brain stimulation. *Bio-Med. Mater. Eng.* **2014**, *24*, 2273–2281. [CrossRef]
15. Deuschl, G.; Krack, P.; Lauk, M.; Timmer, J. Clinical neurophysiology of tremor. *J. Clin. Neurophysiol.* **1996**, *13*, 110–121. [CrossRef] [PubMed]
16. Cole, B.T.; Roy, S.H.; De Luca, C.J.; Nawab, S. Dynamic neural network detection of tremor and dyskinesia from wearable sensor data. In Proceedings of the 2010 Annual International Conference of the IEEE Engineering in Medicine and Biology, Buenos Aires, Argentina, 31 August–4 September 2010; Volume 2010, pp. 6062–6065. [CrossRef]
17. Fraiwan, L.; Khnouf, R.; Mashagbeh, A.R. Parkinson's disease hand tremor detection system for mobile application. *J. Med. Eng. Technol.* **2016**, *40*, 127–134. [CrossRef] [PubMed]
18. Erro, R.; Pilotto, A.; Esposito, M.; Olivola, E.; Nicoletti, A.; Lazzeri, G.; Magistrelli, L.; Dallocchio, C.; Marchese, R.; Bologna, M. The Italian tremor Network (TITAN): Rationale, design and preliminary findings. *Neurol. Sci.* **2022**, *43*, 5369–5376. [CrossRef] [PubMed]
19. Garg, A.; Munia, T.T.K.; Fazel-Rezai, R.; Tavakolian, K.; Zeng, W.; Liu, F.; Wang, Q.; Wang, Y.; Ma, L.; Zhang, Y. Parkinson's disease classification using gait analysis via deterministic learning. *PLoS ONE* **2016**, *633*, 268–278. [CrossRef]

20. Schlachetzki, J.C.; Barth, J.; Marxreiter, F.; Gossler, J.; Kohl, Z.; Reinfelder, S.; Gassner, H.; Aminian, K.; Eskofier, B.M.; Winkler, J. Wearable sensors objectively measure gait parameters in Parkinson's disease. *PLoS ONE* **2017**, *12*, e0183989. [CrossRef] [PubMed]
21. Suppa, A.; Kita, A.; Leodori, G.; Zampogna, A.; Nicolini, E.; Lorenzi, P.; Rao, R.; Irrera, F. L-DOPA and freezing of gait in Parkinson's disease: Objective assessment through a wearable wireless system. *Front. Neurol.* **2017**, *8*, 406. [CrossRef]
22. Luis-Martínez, R.; Monje, M.H.; Antonini, A.; Sánchez-Ferro, Á.; Mestre, T.A. Technology-enabled care: Integrating multidisciplinary care in Parkinson's disease through digital technology. *Front. Neurol.* **2020**, *11*, 575975. [CrossRef]
23. Fisher, J.M.; Hammerla, N.Y.; Ploetz, T.; Andras, P.; Rochester, L.; Walker, R.W. Unsupervised home monitoring of Parkinson's disease motor symptoms using body-worn accelerometers. *Park. Relat. Disord.* **2016**, *33*, 44–50. [CrossRef]
24. Sica, M.; Tedesco, S.; Crowe, C.; Kenny, L.; Moore, K.; Timmons, S.; Barton, J.; O'Flynn, B.; Komaris, D.-S. Continuous home monitoring of Parkinson's disease using inertial sensors: A systematic review. *PLoS ONE* **2021**, *16*, e0246528. [CrossRef] [PubMed]
25. Del Sorbo, F.; Albanese, A. Levodopa-induced dyskinesias and their management. *J. Neurol.* **2008**, *255*, 32–41. [CrossRef] [PubMed]
26. Stocchi, F.; Tagliati, M.; Olanow, C.W. Treatment of levodopa-induced motor complications. *Mov. Disord. Off. J. Mov. Disord. Soc.* **2008**, *23*, S599–S612. [CrossRef] [PubMed]
27. Olanow, C.W.; Kieburtz, K.; Odin, P.; Espay, A.J.; Standaert, D.G.; Fernandez, H.H.; Vanagunas, A.; Othman, A.A.; Widnell, K.L.; Robieson, W.Z. Continuous intrajejunal infusion of levodopa-carbidopa intestinal gel for patients with advanced Parkinson's disease: A randomised, controlled, double-blind, double-dummy study. *Lancet Neurol.* **2014**, *13*, 141–149. [CrossRef] [PubMed]
28. Manson, A.J.; Turner, K.; Lees, A.J. Apomorphine monotherapy in the treatment of refractory motor complications of Parkinson's disease: Long-term follow-up study of 64 patients. *Mov. Disord. Off. J. Mov. Disord. Soc.* **2002**, *17*, 1235–1241. [CrossRef] [PubMed]
29. Obeso, J.A.; Olanow, C.W.; Nutt, J.G. Levodopa motor complications in Parkinson's disease. *Trends Neurosci.* **2000**, *23*, S2–S7. [CrossRef] [PubMed]
30. Melgari, J.-M.; Salomone, G.; di Biase, L.; Marano, M.; Scrascia, F.; Di Lazzaro, V. Dyskinesias during levodopa–carbidopa intestinal gel (LCIG) infusion: Management inclinical practice. *Park. Relat. Disord.* **2015**, *21*, 327–328. [CrossRef]
31. Salomone, G.; Marano, M.; di Biase, L.; Melgari, J.-M.; Di Lazzaro, V. Dopamine dysregulation syndrome and punding in levodopa-carbidopa intestinal gel (LCIG) infusion: A serious but preventable complication. *Park. Relat. Disord.* **2015**, *21*, 1124–1125. [CrossRef]
32. Krack, P.; Volkmann, J.; Tinkhauser, G.; Deuschl, G. Deep brain stimulation in movement disorders: From experimental surgery to evidence-based therapy. *Mov. Disord.* **2019**, *34*, 1795–1810. [CrossRef]
33. Rizzone, M.G.; Fasano, A.; Daniele, A.; Zibetti, M.; Merola, A.; Rizzi, L.; Piano, C.; Piccininni, C.; Romito, L.; Lopiano, L. Long-term outcome of subthalamic nucleus DBS in Parkinson's disease: From the advanced phase towards the late stage of the disease? *Park. Relat. Disord.* **2014**, *20*, 376–381. [CrossRef]
34. Di Lazzaro, V.; Rothwell, J.C. Corticospinal activity evoked and modulated by non-invasive stimulation of the intact human motor cortex. *J. Physiol.* **2014**, *592*, 4115–4128. [CrossRef] [PubMed]
35. Lefaucheur, J.-P.; André-Obadia, N.; Antal, A.; Ayache, S.S.; Baeken, C.; Benninger, D.H.; Cantello, R.M.; Cincotta, M.; de Carvalho, M.; De Ridder, D. Evidence-based guidelines on the therapeutic use of repetitive transcranial magnetic stimulation (rTMS). *Clin. Neurophysiol.* **2014**, *125*, 2150–2206. [CrossRef] [PubMed]
36. Zhang, T.; Pan, N.; Wang, Y.; Liu, C.; Hu, S. Transcranial focused ultrasound neuromodulation: A review of the excitatory and inhibitory effects on brain activity in human and animals. *Front. Hum. Neurosci.* **2021**, *15*, 749162. [CrossRef] [PubMed]
37. Grandas, F.; Galiano, M.L.; Tabernero, C. Risk factors for levodopa-induced dyskinesias in Parkinson's disease. *J. Neurol.* **1999**, *246*, 1127–1133. [CrossRef] [PubMed]
38. Bastide, M.F.; Meissner, W.G.; Picconi, B.; Fasano, S.; Fernagut, P.-O.; Feyder, M.; Francardo, V.; Alcacer, C.; Ding, Y.; Brambilla, R. Pathophysiology of L-dopa-induced motor and non-motor complications in Parkinson's disease. *Prog. Neurobiol.* **2015**, *132*, 96–168. [CrossRef] [PubMed]
39. Little, S.; Pogosyan, A.; Neal, S.; Zavala, B.; Zrinzo, L.; Hariz, M.; Foltynie, T.; Limousin, P.; Ashkan, K.; FitzGerald, J. Adaptive deep brain stimulation in advanced Parkinson disease. *Ann. Neurol.* **2013**, *74*, 449–457. [CrossRef]
40. di Biase, L.; Tinkhauser, G.; Martin Moraud, E.; Caminiti, M.L.; Pecoraro, P.M.; Di Lazzaro, V. Adaptive, personalized closed-loop therapy for Parkinson's disease: Biochemical, neurophysiological, and wearable sensing systems. *Expert Rev. Neurother.* **2021**, *21*, 1371–1388. [CrossRef]

Disclaimer/Publisher's Note: The statements, opinions and data contained in all publications are solely those of the individual author(s) and contributor(s) and not of MDPI and/or the editor(s). MDPI and/or the editor(s) disclaim responsibility for any injury to people or property resulting from any ideas, methods, instructions or products referred to in the content.

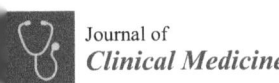

Review

Dystonia Diagnosis: Clinical Neurophysiology and Genetics

Lazzaro di Biase [1,2,3,*], Alessandro Di Santo [1,2], Maria Letizia Caminiti [1,2], Pasquale Maria Pecoraro [1,2], Simona Paola Carbone [1,2] and Vincenzo Di Lazzaro [1,2]

1. Neurology Unit, Campus Bio-Medico University Hospital Foundation, Via Álvaro del Portillo 200, 00128 Rome, Italy; a.disanto@unicampus.it (A.D.S.); m.caminiti@unicampus.it (M.L.C.); p.pecoraro@unicampus.it (P.M.P.); simonapaola.carbone@unicampus.it (S.P.C.); v.dilazzaro@policlinicocampus.it (V.D.L.)
2. Unit of Neurology, Neurophysiology, Neurobiology, Department of Medicine, Campus Bio-Medico University of Rome, Via Álvaro del Portillo 21, 00128 Rome, Italy
3. Brain Innovations Lab., Campus Bio-Medico University of Rome, Via Álvaro del Portillo 21, 00128 Rome, Italy
* Correspondence: l.dibiase@policlinicocampus.it or lazzaro.dibiase@gmail.com; Tel.: +39-062-2541-1220

Abstract: Dystonia diagnosis is based on clinical examination performed by a neurologist with expertise in movement disorders. Clues that indicate the diagnosis of a movement disorder such as dystonia are dystonic movements, dystonic postures, and three additional physical signs (mirror dystonia, overflow dystonia, and geste antagonists/sensory tricks). Despite advances in research, there is no diagnostic test with a high level of accuracy for the dystonia diagnosis. Clinical neurophysiology and genetics might support the clinician in the diagnostic process. Neurophysiology played a role in untangling dystonia pathophysiology, demonstrating characteristic reduction in inhibition of central motor circuits and alterations in the somatosensory system. The neurophysiologic measure with the greatest evidence in identifying patients affected by dystonia is the somatosensory temporal discrimination threshold (STDT). Other parameters need further confirmations and more solid evidence to be considered as support for the dystonia diagnosis. Genetic testing should be guided by characteristics such as age at onset, body distribution, associated features, and coexistence of other movement disorders (parkinsonism, myoclonus, and other hyperkinesia). The aim of the present review is to summarize the state of the art regarding dystonia diagnosis focusing on the role of neurophysiology and genetic testing.

Keywords: dystonia; clinical diagnosis; neurophysiology; genetics

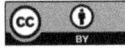

1. Introduction

Dystonia is a term used to identify hyperkinetic movement disorders in which dystonia is the prominent feature. However, dystonia can also be present in other conditions. According to the etiology, dystonia can be distinguished as acquired, inherited, or idiopathic. The diagnosis of dystonia is based on clinical examination conducted by physicians with expertise in movement disorders through a careful examination of the phenomenology of the condition that allows for a classification of dystonia. For the diagnosis of dystonia syndrome, the examiner should follow the definition of dystonia approved in the last expert consensus [1], articulated in three subdefinitions:

1. Dystonia is a movement disorder characterized by sustained or intermittent muscle contractions causing abnormal, often repetitive, movements, postures, or both.
2. Dystonic movements are typically patterned, twisting, and may be tremulous.
3. Dystonia is often initiated or worsened by voluntary action and associated with overflow muscle activation.

The examiner should focus on the classic five physical signs of dystonia syndromes: two main physical signs (dystonic movements and dystonic posture) and three additional physical signs (mirror dystonia, overflow dystonia and geste antagonists/sensory tricks) [2,3].

The role of laboratory analysis, neuroimaging studies, neurophysiology, and genetic tests is to support the etiology definition of the disease, according to the Axis II of Dystonia classification [1,4].

The aim of the present review is to summarize the state of the art regarding dystonia diagnosis focusing on the role of neurophysiology and genetic testing.

2. Clinical Neurophysiology

Clinical neurophysiology techniques such as EMG mapping [2,5] allow clinicians to support the diagnosis of dystonia and to explore the activity of individual muscles which is not always easy to achieve with a clinical inspection alone. In addition, clinical neurophysiology with different techniques, such as transcranial magnetic stimulation (TMS) [6,7], transcranial direct current stimulation (tDCS) [8,9], or the newest transcranial focused ultrasound stimulation (tFUS) [10–12], allow clinicians to explore in a non-invasive way the brain functions In recent years, these techniques have been widely used as tools to characterize distinctive features and improve diagnostic accuracy for different movement disorders [13], particularly parkinsonian syndromes [14–16], tremor syndromes [17–19], myoclonus [20], and dystonia [21]. The literature includes several studies that use different neurophysiological tests to assess dystonia [22] (Table 1). Despite the amount of evidence, most of the studies on dystonia neurophysiology have a small sample size and focus on specific forms of dystonia (e.g., DYT-TOR1A); therefore, results are not always generalizable to all forms of dystonia. Neurophysiology assessment is not formally included in the diagnostic process [1]; however, neurophysiological tests can support the diagnosis.

Since the early 1980s, neurophysiology has been used to characterize dystonia pathophysiology. Most studies were performed in focal hand dystonia (FHD) [22]. At first, dystonia was classified as a basal ganglia (BG) disorder; however, in recent years, evidence points to a disorder arising from a complex network system involving the cerebral cortex (motor and sensory area), the basal ganglia, the brainstem, and the cerebellum [43,44], suggesting that is it possible that several structures could be simultaneously involved in the pathogenesis of dystonia subtypes [43,44].

The electromyographic (EMG) pattern observed in dystonia patients records simultaneous activation of agonist and antagonist muscles (co-contraction), prolonged duration of EMG bursts, and involuntary overflow activation of muscles not directly involved in the movement [3,23].

The most relevant neurophysiological feature shared by all dystonia subtypes is the reduced inhibition of central motor circuits [22]. This is demonstrated by characteristics in several structures: (1) at the subcortical level, a reduction of presynaptic inhibition in the spinal cord has been reported in patients with FHD [24]; (2) at the brainstem level, - a reduced inhibition in the blink reflex recovery cycle in blepharospasm patients [25] and an impairment of the trigeminocervical reflex produced by infraorbital nerve stimulation in torticollis patients was noted [26]; and (3) at the motor cortex level, a loss of inhibition was demonstrated with several transcranial magnetic stimulation (TMS) protocols. Several studies reported abnormalities in dystonic patients of paired pulse protocol as short intracortical inhibitions (SICI), that is, an inhibition of motor cortex response produced by a subthreshold conditioning stimulus followed by a supra-threshold stimulus. SICI is reduced in different subtypes of dystonia [27–29]. Reduced transcallosal inhibition was also demonstrated in FHD patients with mirror dystonia. In these patients, stimulation of one hemisphere does not suppress motor responses evoked by a stimulus delivered about 10 ms later over the contralateral hemisphere, as observed in normal subjects [30]. Finally, the duration of the cortical silent period (SP), the inhibition of ongoing muscular activity produced by a TMS pulse during muscle contraction, is reduced in dystonic patients [31], and the lack of suppression could be related to some specific tasks [32].

In recent years, the relevance of the cerebellum in dystonia's pathophysiology has been investigated [45]. The eye blink classic conditioning (EBCC) protocols consist of electric stimulation of the supraorbital nerve. This protocol that involves cerebellar circuits shows impairment in focal dystonia patients [33], while it is normal in inherited dystonia caused by the DYT-TOR1A and DYT-THAP1 gene mutation [34]. A further test evaluates the motor cortex inhibition produced by cerebellar stimulation. In control subjects, stimulation of one cerebellar hemisphere produces a suppression of the contralateral motor cortex at intervals between 5 and 10 ms [46]. Cerebellar inhibition is impaired in dystonic patients [35].

Table 1. Main neurophysiological findings in dystonia.

	Neurophysiological Test	Results	Accuracy	Ref.
Loss inhibition	EMG	Prolonged bursts Co-contraction agonist and antagonist muscles Overflow to other muscles	NA	[23]
	Spinal cord reciprocal inhibition	Reduced reciprocal inhibition	NA	[24]
	Blink reflex recovery cycle	Reduced inhibition of R2 component	NA	[25]
	Short latency trigemino-sternocleidomastoid response	Impairment of the trigemino-cervical reflex	NA	[26]
	SICI	Reduced in most studies	NA	[27–29]
	IHI	Loss of suppression	NA	[30]
	SP	Reduced	NA	[31,32]
Cerebellum	EBCC	Impaired in primary focal dystonia Normal in DYT-TOR1A and DYT-THAP1 dystonia	NA	[33,34]
	CBI	Absent	NA	[35]
Sensory Abnormalities	GOT	Increased SD threshold in blepharospasm, CD, FHD Normal in DYT-TOR1A	NA	[36]
	STDT	Abnormally increased STDT (higher in CD patients with tremor). No statistical differences between CD and PD	CD compared to ET: • ≤67 ms: 100% Sens 100% NPV • ≥120 ms 100% Spec, 100% PPV	[37]
	TVR	Abnormally increased	NA	[38]
Maladaptive Plasticity	PAS	Abnormally increased in dystonic patients Normal in functional dystonia and DYT-TOR1A carrier	NA	[39]
	HF-RSS	Reduced inhibition	NA	[40]
Basal Ganglia	LFP recordings (GPi)	Synchronized activities in 4–10 Hz band	NA	[41,42]

Legend: CBI: cerebellar brain inhibition; CD: cervical dystonia; EBCC: eyeblink classic conditioning; EMG: electromyography; ET: essential tremor; GOT: grating orientation task; HF-RSS: high-frequency repetitive somatosensory stimulation; IHI: inter-hemispheric inhibition; NA: not available. NPV: negative predictive value; PAS: paired associative stimulation; PD: Parkinson's disease; PPV: positive predictive value; Sens: sensitivity; SD: spatial discrimination; SICI: short intra-cortical inhibition; SP: silent period; Spec: specificity; STDT: somatosensory temporal discrimination threshold; TVR: tonic vibration reflex.

Traditionally, dystonia was referred to as a motor disorder; however, several recent studies have provided evidence on the role of the somatosensory system in dystonia pathogenesis. Several studies suggested that abnormalities in the somatosensory system are present in almost all dystonic patients, and several neurophysiology tests investigated these findings. The most relevant discovery is the abnormality in the somatosensory temporal discrimination threshold (STDT) [37]. STDT represents the shorter interval at which two different stimuli are perceived as separate. Cervical dystonia (CD) patients have abnormally increased STDT, and the effect seems higher in CD patients with tremor. In a validation study, 51 CD were compared to essential tremor (ET) patients and Parkinson's disease (PD) patients. The authors found that compared to ET patients, if STDT is ≤67 ms, it has 100% sensitivity and 100% negative predictive value, while if STDT is ≥120 ms, it has 100% specificity and 100% positive predictive value to differentiate ET from CD. However, no statistically significant differences were found between the PD and CD groups even though evidence suggests that STDT is normal in the early PD phase and becomes abnormal in later stages, while STDT is abnormally increased from the first stages of dystonia disease. Another important feature in dystonic patients is the somatosensory discrimination threshold tested with a grating orientation task (GOT) that is a measure of spatial tactile discrimination. These parameters results increased in all idiopathic forms of dystonia, while they are normal in inherited disease cases [36]. Proprioception is also altered in dystonic patients as demonstrated by an abnormally increased tonic vibration reflex (TVR) [38]. Moreover, a study demonstrated that dystonic patients have kinanesthesia impairment seen as abnormal perception of the Aristotle's illusion, suggesting cortical impairment of somatosensory processes [47]. One possible cause of all these abnormalities could be a deficit in the lateral (or surround) inhibition process, as demonstrated by a somatosensory-evoked potential (SEPs) study [48].

Finally, another possible contribution to dystonic pathophysiology is represented by maladaptive plasticity. Abnormal sensory-motor plasticity was demonstrated using a paradigm termed paired associative stimulation (PAS) In this TMS protocol, cortical stimulation is paired with peripheral nerve stimulation at an interstimulus interval of 25 ms resulting in long-term potentiation-like phenomenon (LTP). This form of LTP is pathologically enhanced in FHD [39]. Maladaptive plasticity could be a key factor in the development of dystonic symptoms and a peculiar feature of dystonic patients as suggested by other studies that did not find the same increased plasticity in DYT-TOR1A carrier subjects [49] and in psychogenic dystonia patients [50]. A pronounced increase of PAS-related plasticity was also reported in Costello syndrome, a genetic syndrome characterized by pronounced dystonia [51,52]. Furthermore, evidence of abnormal plasticity in dystonic patients was highlighted with the use of high-frequency repetitive somatosensory stimulation (HF-RSS) [40]. HF-RSS is a repetitive electric stimulation delivered though surface electrodes on the skin that enhances inhibitory sensorimotor processes. In HS, it usually increases inhibition, while in CD patients inhibition is reduced.

Although all this evidence suggests that dystonia is a complex network disorder involving the brainstem, the basal ganglia, the thalamus, the cortex, and the cerebellum [44], originally dystonia was referred to as basal ganglia disease. Several trials point out that electrical modulation of the basal ganglia network through continuous deep brain stimulation (DBS) in internal globus pallidus (GPi) could improve generalized dystonia symptoms [53]. DBS electrodes were also used to invasively record synchronized neuronal activities, pointing out that in line with other movement disorders, pathological basal ganglia oscillatory activities [54] can be found in dystonic patients [41,42]. This invasive recording of local field potentials (LFP) of basal ganglia revealed that GPi and external globus pallidus (GPe) have a decreased discharge rate and irregular firing in dystonic patients [55,56]. In addition, LFP studies demonstrated that pallidus nuclei of dystonic patients show excessive synchronized activities in the 4–10 Hz frequency band [42].

The study of oscillatory activities in neurological disorders [54] revealed new pathological biomarkers in recent years. Several authors suggested that these abnormalities could be used as biomarkers to deliver electrical DBS only in response to pathological neuronal oscillation (adaptative DBS-aDBS). This technique was mainly evaluated in Parkinson's disease patients [57–59] in which LFP monitoring could be supported by multiparametric [60] motor symptoms monitoring [61–63] with the assistance of artificial intelligence algorithms [64]. It has been suggested that this protocol could be translated to dystonic patients with specific biomarkers, such as GPi LFPs theta-alpha band activity [41,42,53], in combination with dystonic muscle activity monitoring through subcutaneous EMG or wearable accelerometer devices [53].

3. Dystonia Genetics

Dystonia genetics is a wide field with continuous updates. After the first description of DYT-TOR1A, several other genes have been proposed as linked with the dystonia phenotype [65]. As in other fields of genetics, after the first years focused on the genetic marker, the focus is moving on to proteomics, searching the causal link between the protein produced by these genes and the phenotype of dystonia. Camargos and Cardoso [66] proposed a model of the "dystonia cell" linking the dystonic genes to the proteins function (Figure 1), based mainly on the classic DYT nomenclature.

The classic DYT nomenclature is based on locus symbols (e.g., DYT 1) and has been used for several years. It is still used in literature and clinical practice [67]. However, the system of locus symbols has been challenged by advances in techniques of genetics research that allow us to define the causative gene, as explained by Marras et al. [68], and the need to renovate the nomenclature system has arisen. The MDS Task Force for the Nomenclature of Genetic Movement Disorders proposed new recommendations, whose use in research and clinical practice is strongly encouraged [69]. This new nomenclature strictly connects the prefix to the predominant phenotype and considers the causative gene rather than the locus symbols (e.g., DYT 1 is now named DYT-TOR1A) [4]. The prefix DYT is used only if dystonia is the prominent disease feature due to a pathogenetic mutation [69]. Otherwise, if another movement disorder is a prominent feature along with dystonia, a double prefix would be assigned (e.g., DYT/PARK-ATP1A3). Indeed, genetic dystonia can be isolated or combined with other movement disorders such as parkinsonism, myoclonus, or other hyperkinesia (Figure 2).

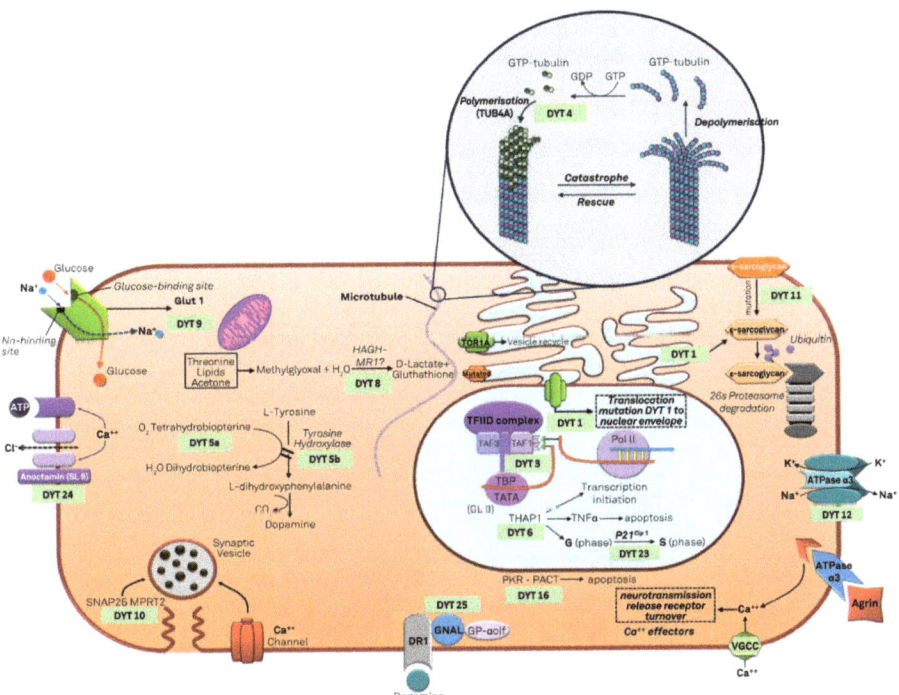

Figure 1. The "dystonia cell" describe the cellular pathway involved in genetic dystonias (modified under the terms and conditions of the Creative Commons Attribution (CC BY) license from [66]).

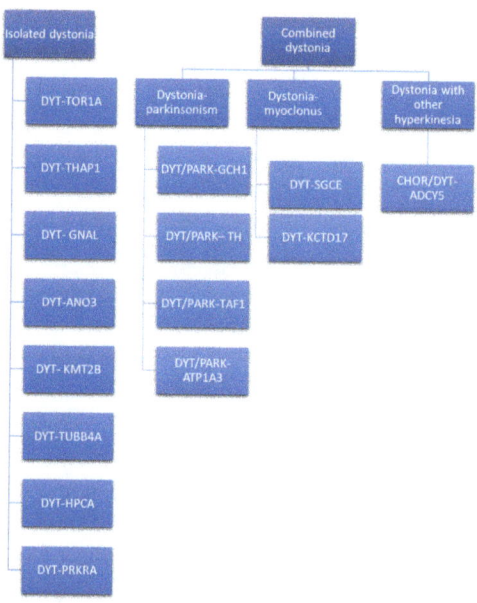

Figure 2. Isolated and combined genetic forms of dystonia [69].

Moreover, in the proposed nomenclature and in the last consensus update on dystonia, the term complex dystonia is used, referring to conditions in which dystonia predominates the clinical phenotype but occurs in the context of a complex disease including symptoms other than movement disorders [1,69]. For example, Wilson disease is named according to the proposed nomenclature with a DYT prefix (DYT-ATP7B), and the same happens for Lesch–Nyhan syndrome and other infantile and childhood onset disease [69]. Given that most of isolated hereditary dystonia is recognized as an autosomal dominant inheritance, the mode of transmission cannot be used as the only criterion to make a differential diagnosis. To guide the clinician towards a genetic diagnosis of dystonia, at least clinical phenotype and age of onset should be considered (Table 2). If dystonia dominates the clinical picture, one of the isolated dystonias may be considered, and the gene mutations involved may be DYT-TOR1A, DYT-THAP1, DYT-GNAL, DYT-ANO3, DYT-KMT2B, DYT-TUBB4A, DYT-HPCA, and DYT-PRKRA [70]. The last-mentioned dystonia is a controversial classification, as it is considered as combined dystonia by some authors [71] and as isolated dystonia by others [70]. Indeed, despite parkinsonism being described in about half the patients, it seemed to be caused not by true parkinsonian features, but by slow movements of dystonic body parts [70]. The isolated form of dystonia could be distinguished according to the age of onset, body distribution, temporal pattern, associated features, responses to drugs, response to DBS, and brain imaging. Regarding age of onset, in infancy, childhood, and adolescence DYT-TOR1A, DYT-THAP1, DYT-KMT2B, DYT-TUBB4A, DYT-PRKRA, and DYT-HPCA are more probable, while DYT-ANO3 and DYT-GNAL begin in early adulthood. In particular, DYT-ANO3 recognizes two peaks of the age of onset: one in infancy/childhood and one in early-late adulthood [70]. Age at onset may by modified by several aspects, e.g., penetrance as is the case of DYT-TOR1A [72]. Hence, age of onset alone cannot be used as the only criteria to orient the diagnosis. According to body distribution, generalized forms of isolated dystonia are mainly due to DYT-TOR1A, DYT-THAP1, DYT-KMT2B, DYT-HPCA, and DYT-PRKRA. Among these, DYT-TOR1A, DYT-HPCA, and DYT-KMT2B usually begin in the lower limbs asymmetrically with secondary generalization. In contrast, DYT-THAP1 may initiate in the upper part of the body, involving cranio–cervical districts, speech difficulties, and the upper limbs, with successive generalizations [73]. If DYT-TOR1A begins in the upper limbs, it tends to be focal.

Focal and segmental isolated dystonia are more likely caused by DYT-GNAL and DYT-ANO3. These two forms of dystonia typically begin at the cervical level and may cause head tremor [70]. DYT-GNAL may be suspected if age at onset is in early-late adulthood. In case of early involvement of craniofacial muscles with laryngeal dystonia and speech difficulties, with secondary generalization involving the arms at younger ages, DYT-ANO3 becomes more probable [70]. Another peculiar form of isolated dystonia with focal distribution involving the cervical district and causing spasmodic dysphonia is caused by DYT-TUBB4A. This focal form may successively evolve into a generalized dystonia [74]. Regarding the temporal pattern, except for the last-mentioned dystonia, all the other isolated dystonia follows a persistent temporal pattern. Associated features may guide the clinician in the differential diagnosis. The presence of additional phenotypic characteristic, such as microcephaly, short stature, intellectual disability, abnormal eye movements, myoclonus, dysmorphisms, and psychiatric symptoms, may be suggestive of DYT-KMT2B [70]. Thin face, body habitus, and hobby horse gait are described in the DYT-TUBB4A [75]. None of the isolated forms of dystonia respond to L-Dopa; DYT-TOR1A, DYT-THAP1, DYT-ANO3, DYT-KMT2B, and DYT-HPCA may respond to anticholinergics [70]. Response to alcohol is described in DYT-GNAL and DYT-TUBB4A. It is important to define the genetic etiology of the dystonia because response to DBS varies according to the genetic conditions, and this is an important prognostic factor to be considered when selecting patients for advanced therapy. Indeed, is well known that DYT-TOR1A, DYT-THAP1, DYT-ANO3, DYT-GNAL, and DYT-KMT2B show a good response to DBS with a target in the GPi, unlike the other forms of isolated dystonia [76–79]. Brain imaging is not conclusive in distinguishing between the several forms of isolated dystonia, as the sole characteristic described is pallidal hypointensity in DYT-KMT2B [70].

Combined dystonia is characterized by the coexistence of another movement disorder in addition to dystonia. The association of dystonia with parkinsonism defines dystonia–parkinsonism. The monogenic forms of dystonia–parkinsonism are DYT/PARK-GCH1, DYT/PARK-TH, DYT/PARK-TAF1, and DYT/PARK-ATP1A3 [71]. Contrary to what has been observed for isolated dystonia, combined dystonia recognizes a different mode of inheritance: autosomal dominant inheritance is characteristic of DYT/PARK-GCH1 and DYT/PARK-ATP1A3, while autosomal recessive inheritance is typical of DYT/PARK-TH. X-linked transmission characterizes DYT/PARK-TAF1 (also known as Lubag syndrome). Among this, it is of paramount importance to diagnose the dopa-responsive dystonia, DYT/PARK-GCH1. Indeed, patients have excellent and sustained response to L-Dopa [80]. Another form of combined dystonia with response to L-Dopa is DYT/PARK-TH. These two forms of dystonia–parkinsonism may be differentiated according to age of onset, as DYT/PARK-GCH1 begins in infancy/childhood, while DYT/PARK-TH may initiate in infancy. Moreover, diurnal fluctuations of parkinsonian symptoms due to circadian variations in dopamine concentration are more pronounced in DYT/PARK-GCH1 than in DYT/PARK-TH [80]. An adjunctive feature may help in differential diagnosis among the two forms: the presence of hypotonia is suggestive of DYT/PARK-TH, while in DYT/PARK-GCH1 hyperreflexia has been described [81]. The coexistence of non-motor features orients towards the diagnosis of DYT/PARK-GCH1, while a more complex clinical picture, with autonomic disturbances, ptosis, and oculogyric crisis is suggestive of DYT/PARK-TH. In both forms, dystonia begins as focal with subsequent generalization [82–85].

Table 2. Isolated and combined genetic types of dystonia.

Phenotype	Gene/Locus	Inheritance/Penetrance	OMIM	Age of Onset	Body Distribution	Temporal Pattern	Associated Features	Drugs Response Dopa	Drugs Response Other Drugs	Alcohol	DBS Response	Brain Imaging Findings	References
Isolated	TOR1A/DYT 1	AD/Reduced	128100	Childhood-Adolescence-Early adulthood	Generalized	Persistent	none	No	Anticholinergics	No	Good	None	[70]
	THAP1/DYT 6	AD/48%	602629	Childhood-Adolescence	Segmental-generalized	Persistent	Laryngeal dystonia/dysarthria/dysphonia	No	Anticholinergics	No	Variable	None	[70,73]
	ANO3/DYT 24	AD/NA	615034	Infancy/childhood, early and late adulthood	Focal-Segmental	Persistent	Tremor	Yes	Anticholinergics/Antiepileptics	No	Good	None	[70,78]
	GNAL/DYT 25	AD/High	615073	Early adulthood-Late adulthood	Focal-segmental, occasionally generalized	Persistent	none	No	No	Yes	Good	None	[70]
	KMT2B/DYT 28	AD/Incomplete	617284	Infancy-Childhood-Adolescence	Generalized	Persistent	Nonmotor signs, neurodevelopmental disorders, Dysmorphisms, Psychiatric symptoms,	No	Anticholinergics	No	Good	Pallidal hypointensity	[70]
	HPCA/DYT 2	AR	224500	Infancy/childhood	Generalized	Persistent	Psychiatric features, cognitive impairment, dystonic tremor	No	Anticholinergics	No	Not know	None	[70]
	TUBB4A/DYT 4	AD/High	128101	Childhood-Adolescence	Focal-generalized	Spasmodic dysphonia	Thin face-body habitus-hobby horse gait	No	No	Yes	Not known	None	[74,75]
	PRKRA/DYT 16	AR/NA	612067	Infancy-Childhood-Adolescence	Generalized	Persistent	Parkinsonism, Hyperreflexia	No	No	No	Not known	None	[70]

Table 2. Cont.

Phenotype	Gene/Locus	Inheritance/Penetrance	OMIM	Age of Onset	Body Distribution	Temporal Pattern	Associated Features	Dopa	Other Drugs	Alcohol	DBS Response	Brain Imaging Findings	References
Parkinsonism	GCH1/DYT 5a	AD/90%	128230	Infancy-Childhood	Mostly generalized	Diurnal fluctuations	Parkinsonism-spasticity-non motor features	Yes	None	No	Not known	None	[80,81]
Parkinsonism	TH/DYT 5b	AR/NA	605407	Infancy	Mostly generalized	Diurnal fluctuations	Parkinsonism-ptosis-hypotonia-autonomic disturbances, oculogyric crises, developmental delay	Yes	None	No	Not known	None	[82–85]
Combined KC	TAF1/DYT 3	XL/Full	314250	Early adulthood-Late adulthood	Generalized	Persistent	Parkinsonism, jaw opening dystonia, bulbar involvement, striatal toe	No	None	No	Variable	Striatal atrophy and pallidum volume loss in pallidum	[86–89]
Combined KC	ATP1A3/DYT12	AD/Incomplete	128235	Adolescence-Early adulthood	Generalized-Segmental	Persistent	Abrupt onset, Fluctuating course, Parkinsonism, Postural instability, Psychiatric features	No	None	No	Not known	None	[85,90,91]
Myoclonus	SGCE/DYT11	AD/Reduced (maternal imprinting)	159900	Childhood-Adolescence	Focal-segmental	Persistent	Myoclonic jerks mainly of the neck, prominent psychiatric features	No	None	Yes	Variable	None	[71]
Myoclonus	KCTD17/DYT26	AD/NA	616398	Childhood-Adolescence	Focal-segmental	Persistent	Myoclonus of upper limbs, psychiatric features	No	None	No	Good	None	[92]
Hyperkinesia	ADCY5	AD/NA	600293	Childhood	Focal-segmental-generalized	Paroxysmal worsening	Generalized choreoathetosis, Facial dyskinesia, myoclonus, learning difficulties, behavioral abnormalities	No	Caffeine	No	Variable	None	[76,93,94]

Legend: AD autosomic dominant, AR autosomic recessive, XL X Linked, NA not available.

DYT/PARK TAF1 differs from the previous mentioned strains for the age of onset, body distribution of dystonia, and neuroimaging. This form of combined dystonia begins in early to late adulthood and, contrary to DYT/PARK-GCH1 that begins with foot dystonia and then progress cranially, DYT/PARK TAF1 involves mainly the upper body, with characteristic jaw opening dystonia and bulbar involvement. Another difference with respect to the dopa-responsive dystonia is the absence of diurnal fluctuation. Brain imaging shows striatal atrophy and pallidum volume loss, considered an expression of the neurodegenerative nature of the disease. This form recognizes an X-linked transmission, hence is more frequent in males [86–89]. Abrupt onset, fluctuating course, psychiatric features, and postural instability may raise suspicion of DYT/PARK-ATP1A3. This disease begins with dystonic spasms, usually following a provoking event (fever, infection, childbirth, alcohol binging, fall, excessive exercise, heat exposure, and psychological stress), with a plateau within 30–60 days of disease onset, with no significant improvement [90]. Dystonia begins in limbs and develops with a characteristic rostrocaudal gradient, cranial symptoms being more severe than upper limbs and lower limbs [91].

Combined dystonia also encompasses dystonia associated with myoclonus and other hyperkinetic disorders. To date, two forms of dystonia–myoclonus have received confirmations: DYT-SGCE and DYT-KCTD17. These diseases have several features in common: age of onset is in the first or second decade of life, myoclonic jerks involve the upper body, and in DYT-SGCE also the neck may be involved. In both diseases, dystonia affects the upper part of the body, with involvement of upper limbs and the cranio-cervical region. If in DYT-SGCE myoclonic jerks dominates the clinical picture, in DYT-KCTD17 dystonia seems to be the prominent feature. Interestingly, DYT-SGCE myoclonic symptoms respond to alcohol, while in DYT-KCTD17 this response is absent [71,92].

Dystonia may coexist with other hyperkinetic disorders, such as chorea, as observed in several forms of complex dystonia. Marras et al. [69] also classify CHOR/DYT-ADCY5 as combined dystonia. This disease is characterized by a plethora of hyperkinetic disorders, such as chorea, dystonia, and myoclonus, beginning in early childhood and with a characteristic fluctuating or paroxysmal course. Interestingly, symptoms do not disappear during sleep, resulting in significant disturbances, and may respond to caffeine [93,94]. Response to DBS is lower than in other form of monogenic dystonia [76].

Genetic Testing and Genetic Counseling

According to the EFNS dystonia guidelines, genetic testing is not sufficient to make a diagnosis of dystonia in the absence of clinical features suggestive of dystonia [95]. Therefore, the clinical picture should orient the decision to carry out genetic testing [96–98].

The previously mentioned guidelines recommend, with a level B of evidence, the DYT-TOR1A testing for patients with limb-onset, primary dystonia with onset before age 30 [98], and in those with onset after age 30 if they have an affected relative with early-onset dystonia [98]. Guidelines do not recommend DYT-TOR1A testing in asymptomatic individuals in dystonia families as a good practice point. After exclusion of DYT-TOR1A, in early-onset dystonia or familial dystonia with cranio-cervical predominance, DYT-THAP1 testing is recommended [73]. It is considered a good practice point to conduct a diagnostic levodopa trial in every patient with early-onset dystonia without an alternative diagnosis [99]. Individuals with early-onset myoclonus affecting the arms or neck, particularly if positive for autosomal-dominant inheritance and if triggered by action, should be tested for the DYT-SGCE gene [100].

In clinical practice, genetic testing consists of of using predefined panels for dystonia. The whole-exome sequencing (WES) is also a resource to consider; however, it is expensive and requires a long time. Zech et al. [101] proposed an algorithm to predict diagnostic success rate of WES in individuals with dystonia. This algorithm assigns a score to three clinical characteristics:

- Age at onset (0–20 years: score 2; >21 years: score 0),
- Body distribution (generalized or segmental: score 1; focal: score 0),

- Dystonia category (complex dystonia: score 2; combined dystonia: score 1; isolated dystonia: score 0).

Summary scores range from 0 to 5 and predict the diagnostic success rate of WES in individuals with dystonia. If the score is three, the sensitivity is 96% and the specificity is 62%; if the score is five, the sensitivity is 62% and the specificity is 86%. Hence, if the score is equal to or higher than three, whole-exome sequencing is recommended [101].

An extensive discussion about genetic counseling goes beyond the scope of this review. The main concept to underscore is that genetic counseling depends largely on the determination of the mode of inheritance of a specific cause of an inherited dystonia in an individual (i.e., autosomal dominant, autosomal recessive, mitochondrial, X-linked inheritance). According to the inheritance, Table 3 describes all the possible diseases [4].

Moreover, penetrance must be considered because of the influence of the phenotypic expression of dystonia [102]. For example, for two hereditary forms of dystonia, mechanisms affecting penetrance have been identified:

- DYT-SGCE dystonia has maternal imprinting of the gene, meaning that the dystonia-myoclonus only manifests when SGCE pathogenic variants are paternally inherited [103].
- DYT-TOR1A has a reduced penetrance of the GAG deletion in TOR1A, from about 35% to 3% in individuals who also have a heterozygous NM_000113.2:646G>C (p.Asp216His) variant in TOR1A on the other allele [72].

Genetic counseling should be offered to the patients and the family by qualified personnel and, according to the EFNS dystonia guideline, is recommended [95].

Table 3. Inherited causes of dystonia.

Autosomal Dominant	
Disease	OMIM Code
- Oppenheim dystonia (DYT-TOR1A)	#128100
- Childhood and adult onset-familial cranial limb dystonia (DYT-THAP1)	#602629
- Dopa-responsive dystonia (DYT/PARK-GCH1)	#128230
- Rapid-onset dystonia–parkinsonism (DYT/PARK-ATP1A3)	#128235
- Myoclonus–dystonia (DYT-SGCE)	#159900
- Neuroferritinopathy (NBIA/CHOREA-FTL)	#606159
- Dentatorubral-pallidoluysian atrophy	#125370
- Huntington's disease	#143100
- Machado–Joseph disease (SCA-ATXN3)	#109150
- Creutzfeldt–Jakob disease	#123400
- Primary Familial Brain Calcification	#213600
- Myclonic-dystonia 26 (DYT-26)	#616398
- Dystonia-28 (DYT-KMT2B)	#617284
- Dystonia-30 (DYT-30)	#619291
- Dystonia-33 (DYT-33)	#619687
- Dystonia-25 (DYT-GNAL)	#615073

Table 3. *Cont.*

Disease	OMIM Code
Autosomal Dominant	
- Dystonia-24 (DYT-ANO3)	#615034
- Dystonia-4 (DYT-TUBB4A)	#129101
- Dystonia-26 (DYT-KCTD17)	#616398
- Dyskinesia with orofacial involvement (CHOR/DYT-ADCY5)	#606703
Autosomal recessive:	
- Wilson disease	#277900
- Neurodegeneration with brain iron accumulation type 1 (NBIA/DYT-PANK2)	#234200
- Neurodegeneration with brain iron accumulation type 2, infantile neuroaxonal dystrophy (NBIA/DYT/PARK-PLA2G6)	#610217
- Aceruloplasminemia (NBIA/DYT/PARK-C)	#604290
- Fatty acid hydroxylase-associated neurodegeneration (FAHN) (HSP/NBIA-FA2H)	#612319
- Early-onset parkinsonism (PARK-Parkin) (PARK-PINK1)	#608309
- Aromatic-L-amino acid decarboxylase (DYT-DDC)	#608643
- Early-onset dystonia with parkinsonism (DYT-PRKRA)	#612067
- Niemann–Pick type C	#257220
- Juvenile neuronal ceroid-lipofuscinosis (Batten disease)	#204200
- GM1 gangliosidosis (DYT/PARK-GLB1) type III, chronic/adult form	#230500
- GM2 gangliosidosis	#272750
- Metachromatic leukodystrophy	#250100
- Homocystinuria	#277400
- Glutaric acidemia (DYT/CHOR-GCDH)	#231670
- Methylmalonic aciduria (DYT/CHOR-MUT)	#251000
- Hartnup disease	#234500
- Ataxia telangiectasia	#208900
- Friedreich ataxia	#229300
- Neuroacanthocytosis	#200150
- Dopa-responsive dystonia (DYT/PARK-TH)	#605407
- Neuronal intranuclear hyaline inclusion disease	#603472
- Hereditary spastic paraplegia (HSP-SPG7)	#607259
- Sjögren–Larsson syndrome (ichthyosis, spasticity, intellectual disability)	#270200

Table 3. *Cont.*

Autosomal recessive:	
- Biotin-responsive basal ganglia disease (DYT-SLC19A3)	#607483
- Dystonia musculorum deformans 2 (DYT-HPCA)	#224500
- Zech-boesch syndrom (DYT-31)	#619565
X-linked recessive:	
- Dystonia-parkinsonism or Lubag syndrome (DYT/PARK-TAF1)	#314250
- Lesch-Nyhan syndrome (DYT/CHOR-HPRT)	#300322
- Mohr-Tranebjaerg syndrome (Deafness–dystonia syndrome) (DYT-TIMM8A)	#304700
X-linked dominant	
- Rett syndrome	#312750
Mitochondrial	
- Leigh syndrome	#256000
- Leber's hereditary ocular neuropathy plus dystonia (DYT-mt-ND6)	#500001

Legend: OMIM code = Online Mendelian Inheritance in Man code (reproduced under the terms and conditions of the Creative Commons Attribution (CC BY) license from [4]).

4. Discussion

The present review summarized the possible contribution of clinical neurophysiology and genetic testing to clinical examination for dystonia diagnosis (Figure 3).

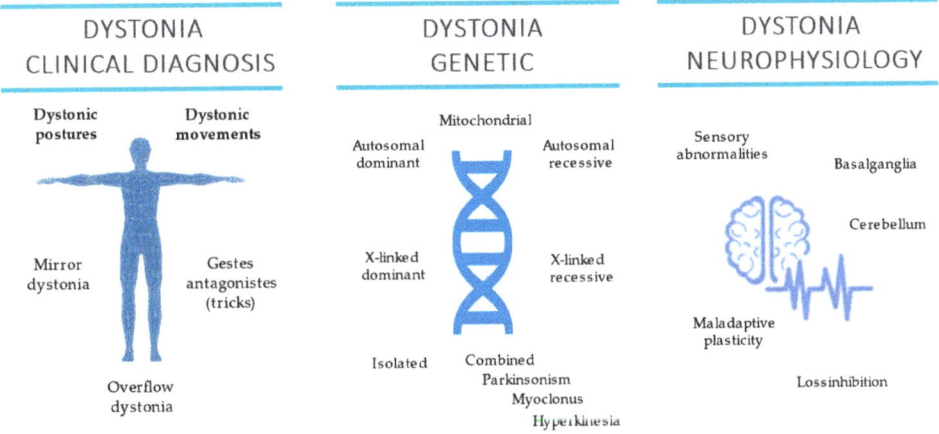

Figure 3. Dystonia clinical diagnosis and genetic and clinical neurophysiology features.

However, dystonia diagnosis is still based on clinical examination conducted by physicians with expertise in movement disorders. The clinical diagnosis should be based on the observations of two core characteristics and of adjunctive features [1]. According to the EFNS dystonia guidelines, a neurophysiological test may help diagnosis despite low evidence (class IV), hence further and proper studies are needed [95]. However, the role of neurophysiology is not marginal, being an important resource to enlighten the pathophysiology of dystonia (Table 1). Among neurophysiological alterations observed in dystonia, sensitivity, specificity, and positive predictive value have been evaluated only for

STDT. That is pathologically increased in patients affected by cervical dystonia compared to patients affected by essential tremor [37]. Neurophysiology also represents an excellent support for the therapy of dystonia in the case of EMG-guided botulinum toxin injection. In future applications, neurophysiology could guide adaptive DBS. Indeed, LFP recorded in GPi could be used as input signals to modulate stimulation parameters as currently used for Parkinson's disease [104].

Once dystonia has been clinically diagnosed, the definition of the etiology is needed [1]. The etiological diagnosis of dystonia cannot ignore the role of genetics testing. Several genes have been described as causes of isolated, combined, or complex forms of dystonia (see Table 2). Regarding isolated dystonia, age at onset, body distribution (focal, segmental or generalized), and associated features may orient the clinicians towards a specific form of monogenic dystonia. In combined dystonia, the second most represented movement disorder, the clinical picture guides the clinician in the direction of dystonia associated with parkinsonism, myoclonus, or other hyperkinesia. The choice to request WES to reach a diagnosis should be carefully considered when panels for dystonia fail to detect causative mutations. Zech et al. proposed an interesting and feasible algorithm to predict diagnostic success rate of WES, according to dystonia characteristics [101]. The algorithm considers tree items (age at onset, body distribution, dystonia category) and assigns a score to each one. If the summary score is equal or higher than three, WES is recommended because of a high probability to identify causative mutations.

Considering the inheritance mode and the risk of transmission of the disease in the context of the same family, genetic counseling should be offered to the patients and a multidisciplinary approach involving geneticists, psychologist is desirable.

Author Contributions: Conceptualization, L.d.B.; writing—original draft preparation, L.d.B., A.D.S., M.L.C., P.M.P. and S.P.C.; writing—review and editing, L.d.B. and V.D.L.; supervision, V.D.L. All authors have read and agreed to the published version of the manuscript.

Funding: This research received no external funding.

Institutional Review Board Statement: Not applicable.

Informed Consent Statement: Not applicable.

Conflicts of Interest: The authors declare no conflict of interest.

References

1. Albanese, A.; Bhatia, K.; Bressman, S.B.; DeLong, M.R.; Fahn, S.; Fung, V.S.; Hallett, M.; Jankovic, J.; Jinnah, H.A.; Klein, C.; et al. Phenomenology and classification of dystonia: A consensus update. *Mov. Disord.* **2013**, *28*, 863–873. [CrossRef]
2. Albanese, A.; Lalli, S. Is this dystonia? *Mov. Disord.* **2009**, *24*, 1725–1731. [CrossRef]
3. Albanese, A.; Di Giovanni, M.; Lalli, S. Dystonia: Diagnosis and management. *Eur. J. Neurol.* **2018**, *26*, 5–17. [CrossRef]
4. Di Biase, L.; Di Santo, A.; Caminiti, M.L.; Pecoraro, P.M.; Di Lazzaro, V. Classification of Dystonia. *Life* **2022**, *12*, 206. [CrossRef]
5. Van Gerpen, J.A.; Matsumoto, J.Y.; Ahlskog, J.E.; Maraganore, D.M.; McManis, P.G. Utility of an EMG mapping study in treating cervical dystonia. *Muscle Nerve* **2000**, *23*, 1752–1756. [CrossRef]
6. Edwards, M.J.; Talelli, P.; Rothwell, J.C. Clinical applications of transcranial magnetic stimulation in patients with movement disorders. *Lancet Neurol.* **2008**, *7*, 827–840. [CrossRef]
7. Chen, R.; Cros, D.; Curra, A.; Di Lazzaro, V.; Lefaucheur, J.-P.; Magistris, M.R.; Mills, K.; Rösler, K.M.; Triggs, W.J.; Ugawa, Y.; et al. The clinical diagnostic utility of transcranial magnetic stimulation: Report of an IFCN committee. *Clin. Neurophysiol.* **2008**, *119*, 504–532. [CrossRef]
8. Fregni, F.; Boggio, P.S.; Santos, M.C.; Lima, M.; Vieira, A.L.; Rigonatti, S.P.; Silva, M.T.A.; Barbosa, E.R.; Nitsche, M.A.; Pascual-Leone, A. Noninvasive cortical stimulation with transcranial direct current stimulation in Parkinson's disease. *Mov. Disord.* **2006**, *21*, 1693–1702. [CrossRef]
9. Ferrucci, R.; Mameli, F.; Ruggiero, F.; Priori, A. Transcranial direct current stimulation as treatment for Parkinson's disease and other movement disorders. *Basal Ganglia* **2015**, *6*, 53–61. [CrossRef]
10. Darrow, D.P. Focused Ultrasound for Neuromodulation. *Neurotherapeutics* **2019**, *16*, 88–99. [CrossRef]
11. Di Biase, L.; Falato, E.; Di Lazzaro, V. Transcranial Focused Ultrasound (tFUS) and Transcranial Unfocused Ultrasound (tUS) Neuromodulation: From Theoretical Principles to Stimulation Practices. *Front. Neurol.* **2019**, *10*, 549. [CrossRef]
12. Di Biase, L.; Falato, E.; Caminiti, M.L.; Pecoraro, P.M.; Narducci, F.; Di Lazzaro, V. Focused Ultrasound (FUS) for Chronic Pain Management: Approved and Potential Applications. *Neurol. Res. Int.* **2021**, *2021*, 1–16. [CrossRef]

3. Hallett, M. Chapter 1 Movement disorders: Overview. In *Handbook of Clinical Neurophysiology*; Elsevier: Amsterdam, The Netherlands, 2003; pp. 3–4.
4. Bologna, M.; Suppa, A.; Di Stasio, F.; Conte, A.; Fabbrini, G.; Berardelli, A. Neurophysiological studies on atypical parkinsonian syndromes. *Park. Relat. Disord.* **2017**, *42*, 12–21. [CrossRef]
5. Valls-Solé, J. Neurophysiological characterization of parkinsonian syndromes. *Neurophysiol. Clin. Neurophysiol.* **2000**, *30*, 352–367. [CrossRef]
6. Valls-Solé, J.; Valldeoriola, F. Neurophysiological correlate of clinical signs in Parkinson's disease. *Clin. Neurophysiol.* **2002**, *113*, 792–805. [CrossRef]
7. Di Biase, L.; Brittain, J.-S.; Shah, S.A.; Pedrosa, D.; Cagnan, H.; Mathy, A.; Chen, C.C.; Martín-Rodríguez, J.F.; Mir, P.; Timmerman, L.; et al. Tremor stability index: A new tool for differential diagnosis in tremor syndromes. *Brain* **2017**, *140*, 1977–1986. [CrossRef]
8. Di Pino, G.; Formica, D.; Melgari, J.M.; Taffoni, F.; Salomone, G.; di Biase, L.; Caimo, E.; Vernieri, F.; Guglielmelli, E. Neurophysiological bases of tremors and accelerometric parameters analysis. In Proceedings of the 2012 4th IEEE RAS & EMBS International Conference on Biomedical Robotics and Biomechatronics (BioRob), Rome, Italy, 24–27 June 2012; pp. 1820–1825.
9. Deuschl, G.; Krack, P.; Lauk, M.; Timmer, J. Clinical Neurophysiology of Tremor. *J. Clin. Neurophysiol.* **1996**, *13*, 110–121. [CrossRef]
10. Caviness, J.N. Chapter 32 The clinical neurophysiology of myoclonus. In *Handbook of Clinical Neurophysiology*; Hallett, M., Ed.; Elsevier: Amsterdam, The Netherlands, 2003; pp. 521–548.
11. Kaji, R. Chapter 28 Dystonia. In *Handbook of Clinical Neurophysiology*; Hallett, M., Ed.; Elsevier: Amsterdam, The Netherlands, 2003; pp. 451–461.
12. Hallett, M. Neurophysiology of dystonia: The role of inhibition. *Neurobiol. Dis.* **2011**, *42*, 177–184. [CrossRef]
13. Rothwell, J.C.; Obeso, J.A.; Day, B.L.; Marsden, C.D. Pathophysiology of dystonias. *Adv. Neurol.* **1983**, *39*, 851–863.
14. Nakashima, K.; Rothwell, J.C.; Day, B.L.; Thompson, P.D.; Shannon, K.; Marsden, C.D. Reciprocal inhibition between forearm muscles in patients with writer's cramp and other occupational cramps, symptomatic hemidystonia and hemiparesis due to stroke. *Brain* **1989**, *112*, 681–697. [CrossRef]
15. Berardelli, A.; Rothwell, J.; Day, B.L.; Marsden, C.D. Pathophysiology of blepharospasm and oromandibular dystonia. *Brain* **1985**, *108*, 593–608. [CrossRef]
16. Quartarone, A.; Girlanda, P.; Di Lazzaro, V.; Majorana, G.; Battaglia, F.; Messina, C. Short latency trigemi-no-sternocleidomastoid response in muscles in patients with spasmodic torticollis and blepharospasm. *Clin. Neurophysiol.* **2000**, *111*, 1672–1677. [CrossRef]
17. Huang, Y.-Z.; Rothwell, J.; Lu, C.-S.; Wang, J.-J.; Chen, R.-S. Restoration of motor inhibition through an abnormal premotor-motor connection in dystonia. *Mov. Disord.* **2010**, *25*, 696–703. [CrossRef]
18. Espay, A.; Morgante, F.; Purzner, J.; Gunraj, C.A.; Lang, A.; Chen, R. Cortical and spinal abnormalities in psychogenic dystonia. *Ann. Neurol.* **2006**, *59*, 825–834. [CrossRef]
19. Di Lazzaro, V.; Oliviero, A.; Profice, P.; Dileone, M.; Pilato, F.; Insola, A.; Della Marca, G.; Tonali, P.; Mazzone, P. Reduced cerebral cortex inhibition in dystonia: Direct evidence in humans. *Clin. Neurophysiol.* **2009**, *120*, 834–839. [CrossRef]
20. Beck, S.; Shamim, E.A.; Richardson, S.P.; Schubert, M.; Hallett, M. Inter-hemispheric inhibition is impaired in mirror dystonia. *Eur. J. Neurosci.* **2009**, *29*, 1634–1640. [CrossRef]
21. Chen, R.; Wassermann, E.M.; Caños, M.; Hallett, M. Impaired inhibition in writer's cramp during voluntary muscle activation. *Neurology* **1997**, *49*, 1054–1059. [CrossRef]
22. Tinazzi, M.; Farina, S.; Edwards, M.; Moretto, G.; Restivo, D.; Fiaschi, A.; Berardelli, A. Task–specific impairment of motor cortical excitation and inhibition in patients with writer's cramp. *Neurosci. Lett.* **2005**, *378*, 55–58. [CrossRef]
23. Kojovic, M.; Pareés, I.; Kassavetis, P.; Palomar, F.J.; Mir, P.; Teo, J.; Cordivari, C.; Rothwell, J.; Bhatia, K.; Edwards, M.J. Secondary and primary dystonia: Pathophysiological differences. *Brain* **2013**, *136*, 2038–2049. [CrossRef]
24. Sadnicka, A.; Teo, J.; Kojovic, M.; Pareés, I.; Saifee, T.A.; Kassavetis, P.; Schwingenschuh, P.; Katschnig–Winter, P.; Stamelou, M.; Mencacci, N.E.; et al. All in the blink of an eye: New insight into cerebellar and brainstem function in DYT1 and DYT6 dystonia. *Eur. J. Neurol.* **2014**, *22*, 762–767. [CrossRef]
25. Brighina, F.; Romano, M.; Giglia, G.; Saia, V.; Puma, A.; Giglia, F.; Fierro, B. Effects of cerebellar TMS on motor cortex of patients with focal dystonia: A preliminary report. *Exp. Brain Res.* **2008**, *192*, 651–656. [CrossRef]
26. Molloy, F.M.; Zeuner, K.E.; Dambrosia, J.M.; Carr, T.D.; Hallett, M. Abnormalities of spatial discrimination in focal and generalized dystonia. *Brain* **2003**, *126*, 2175–2182. [CrossRef]
27. Conte, A.; Ferrazzano, G.; Belvisi, D.; Manzo, N.; Battista, E.; Voti, P.L.; Nardella, A.; Fabbrini, G.; Berardelli, A. Somatosensory temporal discrimination in Parkinson's disease, dystonia and essential tremor: Pathophysiological and clinical implications. *Clin. Neurophysiol.* **2018**, *129*, 1849–1853. [CrossRef]
28. Grünewald, R.A.; Shipman, J.M.; Sagar, H.J.; Yoneda, Y. Idiopathic focal dystonia: A disorder of muscle spindle afferent processing? *Brain* **1997**, *120*, 2179–2185. [CrossRef]
29. Quartarone, A.; Bagnato, S.; Rizzo, V.; Siebner, H.R.; Dattola, V.; Scalfari, A.; Morgante, F.; Battaglia, F.; Romano, M.; Girlanda, P. Abnormal associative plasticity of the human motor cortex in writer's cramp. *Brain* **2003**, *126*, 2586–2596. [CrossRef]
30. Erro, R.; Rocchi, L.; Antelmi, E.; Liguori, R.; Tinazzi, M.; Berardelli, A.; Rothwell, J.; Bhatia, K.P. High frequency somatosensory stimulation in dystonia: Evidence for defective inhibitory plasticity. *Mov. Disord.* **2018**, *33*, 1902–1909. [CrossRef]

41. Silberstein, P.; Kühn, A.A.; Kupsch, A.; Trottenberg, T.; Krauss, J.K.; Wöhrle, J.C.; Mazzone, P.; Insola, A.; Di Lazzaro, V.; Oliviero, A.; et al. Patterning of globus pallidus local field potentials differs between Parkinson's disease and dystonia. *Brain* **2003**, *126*, 2597–2608. [CrossRef]
42. Chen, C.C.; Kühn, A.A.; Trottenberg, T.; Kupsch, A.; Schneider, G.-H.; Brown, P. Neuronal activity in globus pallidus interna can be synchronized to local field potential activity over 3–12 Hz in patients with dystonia. *Exp. Neurol.* **2006**, *202*, 480–486. [CrossRef]
43. Conte, A.; Rocchi, L.; Latorre, A.; Belvisi, D.; Rothwell, J.C.; Berardelli, A. Ten-Year Reflections on the Neurophysiological Abnormalities of Focal Dystonias in Humans. *Mov. Disord.* **2019**, *34*, 1616–1628. [CrossRef]
44. Latorre, A.; Rocchi, L.; Bhatia, K.P. Delineating the electrophysiological signature of dystonia. *Exp. Brain Res.* **2020**, *238*, 1685–1692. [CrossRef]
45. Bologna, M.; Berardelli, A. The cerebellum and dystonia. *Handb. Clin. Neurol.* **2018**, *155*, 259–272. [CrossRef]
46. Di Lazzaro, V.; Molinari, M.; Restuccia, D.; Leggio, M.; Nardone, R.; Fogli, D.; Tonali, P. Cerebro-cerebellar interactions in man: Neurophysiological studies in patients with focal cerebellar lesions. *Electroencephalogr. Clin. Neurophysiol. Potentials Sect.* **1994**, *93*, 27–34. [CrossRef]
47. Tinazzi, M.; Marotta, A.; Fasano, A.; Bove, F.; Bentivoglio, A.R.; Squintani, G.; Pozzer, L.; Fiorio, M. Aristotle's illusion reveals interdigit functional somatosensory alterations in focal hand dystonia. *Brain* **2013**, *136*, 782–789. [CrossRef]
48. Tinazzi, M.; Priori, A.; Bertolasi, L.; Frasson, E.; Mauguière, F.; Fiaschi, A. Abnormal central integration of a dual somatosensory input in dystonia Evidence for sensory overflow. *Brain* **2000**, *123*, 42–50. [CrossRef]
49. Edwards, M.J.; Huang, Y.-Z.; Mir, P.; Rothwell, J.; Bhatia, K.P. Abnormalities in motor cortical plasticity differentiate manifesting and nonmanifesting DYT1 carriers. *Mov. Disord.* **2006**, *21*, 2181–2186. [CrossRef]
50. Quartarone, A.; Rizzo, V.; Terranova, C.; Morgante, F.; Schneider, S.; Ibrahim, N.; Girlanda, P.; Bhatia, K.P.; Rothwell, J.C. Abnormal sensorimotor plasticity in organic but not in psychogenic dystonia. *Brain* **2009**, *132*, 2871–2877. [CrossRef]
51. Dileone, M.; Profice, P.; Pilato, F.; Alfieri, P.; Cesarini, L.; Mercuri, E.; Leoni, C.; Tartaglia, M.; Di Iorio, R.; Zampino, G.; et al. Enhanced human brain associative plasticity in Costello syndrome. *J. Physiol.* **2010**, *588*, 3445–3456. [CrossRef]
52. Dileone, M.; Zampino, G.; Profice, P.; Pilato, F.; Leoni, C.; Ranieri, F.; Capone, F.; Tartaglia, M.; Brown, P.; Di Lazzaro, V. Dystonia in Costello syndrome. *Park. Relat. Disord.* **2012**, *18*, 798–800. [CrossRef]
53. Piña-Fuentes, D.; Beudel, M.; Little, S.; van Zijl, J.; Elting, J.W.; Oterdoom, D.L.M.; van Egmond, M.E.; van Dijk, J.M.C.; Tijssen, M.A.J. Toward adaptive deep brain stimulation for dystonia. *Neurosurg. Focus* **2018**, *45*, E3. [CrossRef]
54. Assenza, G.; Capone, F.; di Biase, L.; Ferreri, F.; Florio, L.; Guerra, A.; Marano, M.; Paolucci, M.; Ranieri, F.; Salomone, G. Oscillatory activities in neurological disorders of elderly: Biomarkers to target for neuromodulation. *Front. Aging Neurosci.* **2017**, *9*, 189. [CrossRef]
55. Starr, P.A.; Rau, G.M.; Davis, V.; Marks, W.J.; Ostrem, J.L.; Simmons, D.; Lindsey, N.; Turner, R. Spontaneous Pallidal Neuronal Activity in Human Dystonia: Comparison With Parkinson's Disease and Normal Macaque. *J. Neurophysiol.* **2005**, *93*, 3165–3176. [CrossRef]
56. Vitek, J.L.; Delong, M.R.; Starr, P.A.; Hariz, M.I.; Metman, L.V. Intraoperative neurophysiology in DBS for dystonia. *Mov. Disord.* **2011**, *26*, S31–S36. [CrossRef]
57. Little, S.; Pogosyan, A.; Neal, S.; Ba, B.Z.; Zrinzo, L.; Hariz, M.; Foltynie, T.; Limousin, P.; Ashkan, K.; FitzGerald, J.; et al. Adaptive deep brain stimulation in advanced Parkinson disease. *Ann. Neurol.* **2013**, *74*, 449–457. [CrossRef]
58. Little, S.; Pogosyan, A.; Neal, S.; Zrinzo, L.; Hariz, M.; Foltynie, T.; Limousin, P.; Brown, P. Controlling Parkinson's Disease With Adaptive Deep Brain Stimulation. *J. Vis. Exp.* **2014**, *89*, e51403. [CrossRef]
59. Tinkhauser, G.; Pogosyan, A.; Debove, I.; Nowacki, A.; Shah, S.A.; Seidel, K.; Tan, H.; Brittain, J.-S.; Petermann, K.; Di Biase, L.; et al. Directional local field potentials: A tool to optimize deep brain stimulation. *Mov. Disord.* **2017**, *33*, 159–164. [CrossRef]
60. Di Biase, L.; Tinkhauser, G.; Martin Moraud, E.; Caminiti, M.L.; Pecoraro, P.M.; Di Lazzaro, V. Adaptive, personalized closed-loop therapy for Parkinson's disease: Biochemical, neurophysiological, and wearable sensing systems. *Expert Rev. Neurother.* **2021**, *21*, 1371–1388. [CrossRef]
61. Di Biase, L.; Di Santo, A.; Caminiti, M.L.; De Liso, A.; Shah, S.A.; Ricci, L.; Di Lazzaro, V. Gait Analysis in Parkinson's Disease: An Overview of the Most Accurate Markers for Diagnosis and Symptoms Monitoring. *Sensors* **2020**, *20*, 3529. [CrossRef]
62. Di Biase, L.; Summa, S.; Tosi, J.; Taffoni, F.; Marano, M.; Cascio Rizzo, A.; Vecchio, F.; Formica, D.; Di Lazzaro, V.; Di Pino, G.; et al. Quantitative Analysis of Bradykinesia and Rigidity in Parkinson's Disease. *Front. Neurol.* **2018**, *9*, 121. [CrossRef]
63. Raiano, L.; di Pino, G.; di Biase, L.; Tombini, M.; Tagliamonte, N.L.; Formica, D. PDMeter: A Wrist Wearable Device for an at-Home Assessment of the Parkinson's Disease Rigidity. *IEEE Trans. Neural Syst. Rehabil. Eng.* **2020**, *28*, 1325–1333. [CrossRef]
64. Di Biase, L.; Raiano, L.; Caminiti, M.L.; Pecoraro, P.M.; Di Lazzaro, V. Artificial intelligence in Parkinson's disease-symptoms identification and monitoring. In *Augmenting Neurological Disorder Prediction and Rehabilitation Using Artifi-cial Intelligence*; Elsevier: Amsterdam, The Netherlands, 2022; pp. 35–52.
65. Bressman, S.B. Dystonia genotypes, phenotypes, and classification. *Adv. Neurol.* **2004**, *94*, 101–107.
66. Camargos, S.; Cardoso, F. Understanding dystonia: Diagnostic issues and how to overcome them. *Arq. Neuropsiquiatr.* **2016**, *74*, 921–936. [CrossRef] [PubMed]
67. Kramer, P.L.; De Leon, D.; Ozelius, L.; Risch, N.; Bressman, S.B.; Brin, M.F.; Schuback, D.E.; Burke, R.E.; Kwiatkowski, D.J.; Shale, H.; et al. Dystonia gene in Ashkenazi Jewish population is located on chromosome 9q32-34. *Ann. Neurol.* **1990**, *27*, 114–120. [CrossRef] [PubMed]

68. Marras, C.; Lohmann, K.; Lang, A.; Klein, C. Fixing the broken system of genetic locus symbols: Parkinson disease and dystonia as examples. *Neurology* **2012**, *78*, 1016–1024. [CrossRef] [PubMed]
69. Marras, C.; Lang, A.; Van De Warrenburg, B.P.; Sue, C.M.; Tabrizi, S.J.; Bertram, L.; Mercimek-Mahmutoglu, S.; Ebrahimi-Fakhari, D.; Warner, T.; Durr, A.; et al. Nomenclature of genetic movement disorders: Recommendations of the international Parkinson and movement disorder society task force. *Mov. Disord.* **2016**, *31*, 436–457. [CrossRef]
70. Lange, L.M.; Junker, J.; Loens, S.; Baumann, H.; Olschewski, L.; Schaake, S.; Madoev, H.; Petkovic, S.; Kuhnke, N.; Kasten, M.; et al. Genotype–Phenotype Relations for Isolated Dystonia Genes: MDSGene Systematic Review. *Mov. Disord.* **2021**, *36*, 1086–1103. [CrossRef]
71. Weissbach, A.; Saranza, G.; Domingo, A. Combined dystonias: Clinical and genetic updates. *J. Neural Transm.* **2020**, *128*, 417–429. [CrossRef]
72. Risch, N.J.; Bressman, S.B.; Senthil, G.; Ozelius, L.J. Intragenic Cis and Trans Modification of Genetic Susceptibility in DYT1 Torsion Dystonia. *Am. J. Hum. Genet.* **2007**, *80*, 1188–1193. [CrossRef]
73. Djarmati, A.; A Schneider, S.; Lohmann, K.; Winkler, S.; Pawlack, H.; Hagenah, J.; Brüggemann, N.; Zittel, S.; Fuchs, T.; Raković, A.; et al. Mutations in THAP1 (DYT6) and generalised dystonia with prominent spasmodic dysphonia: A genetic screening study. *Lancet Neurol.* **2009**, *8*, 447–452. [CrossRef]
74. Hersheson, J.; Mencacci, N.E.; Davis, M.; Macdonald, N.; Trabzuni, D.; Ryten, M.; Pittman, A.; Paudel, R.; Kara, E.; Fawcett, K.; et al. Mutations in the autoregulatory domain of β-tubulin 4a cause hereditary dystonia. *Ann. Neurol.* **2012**, *73*, 546–553. [CrossRef]
75. Wilcox, R.A.; Winkler, S.; Lohmann, K.; Klein, C. Whispering dysphonia in an Australian family (DYT4): A clinical and genetic reappraisal. *Mov. Disord.* **2011**, *26*, 2404–2408. [CrossRef]
76. Artusi, C.A.; Dwivedi, A.; Romagnolo, A.; Bortolani, S.; Marsili, L.; Imbalzano, G.; Sturchio, A.; Keeling, E.G.; Zibetti, M.; Contarino, M.F.; et al. Differential response to pallidal deep brain stimulation among monogenic dystonias: Systematic review and meta-analysis. *J. Neurol. Neurosurg. Psychiatry* **2020**, *91*, 426–433. [CrossRef] [PubMed]
77. Rajan, R.; Garg, K.; Saini, A.; Radhakrishnan, D.M.; Careccio, M.; Bk, B.; Singh, M.; Srivastava, A.K. GPi-DBS for *KMT2B*-Associated Dystonia: Systematic Review and Meta-Analysis. *Mov. Disord. Clin. Pract.* **2021**, *9*, 31–37. [CrossRef] [PubMed]
78. Jiang, L.-T.; Li, L.-X.; Liu, Y.; Zhang, X.-L.; Pan, Y.-G.; Wang, L.; Wan, X.-H.; Jin, L.-J. The expanding clinical and genetic spectrum of ANO3 dystonia. *Neurosci. Lett.* **2020**, *746*, 135590. [CrossRef] [PubMed]
79. Sarva, H.; Trosch, R.; Kiss, Z.H.; Furtado, S.; Luciano, M.S.; Glickman, A.; Ms, D.R.; Ozelius, L.J.; Bressman, S.B.; Saunders-Pullman, R. Deep Brain Stimulation in Isolated Dystonia With a *GNAL* Mutation. *Mov. Disord.* **2018**, *34*, 301–303. [CrossRef] [PubMed]
80. Ichinose, H.; Ohye, T.; Takahashi, E.-I.; Seki, N.; Hori, T.-A.; Segawa, M.; Nomura, Y.; Endo, K.; Tanaka, H.; Tsuji, S.; et al. Hereditary progressive dystonia with marked diurnal fluctuation caused by mutations in the GTP cyclohydrolase I gene. *Nat. Genet.* **1994**, *8*, 236–242. [CrossRef]
81. Salles, P.A.; Terán-Jimenez, M.; Vidal-Santoro, A.; Chaná-Cuevas, P.; Kauffman, M.; Espay, A.J. Recognizing Atypical Dopa–Responsive Dystonia and Its Mimics. *Neurol. Clin. Pract.* **2021**, *11*, e876–e884. [CrossRef]
82. Dworniczak, B.; Lüdecke, B.; Bartholomé, K. A point mutation in the tyrosine hydroxylase gene associated with Segawa's syndrome. *Qual. Life Res.* **1995**, *95*, 123–125. [CrossRef]
83. Wevers, R.A.; Andel, J.F.D.R.-V.; Bräutigam, C.; Geurtz, B.; Heuvel, L.P.W.J.V.D.; Steenbergen-Spanjers, G.C.H.; Smeitink, J.A.M.; Hoffmann, G.F.; Gabreëls, F.J.M. A review of biochemical and molecular genetic aspects of tyrosine hydroxylase deficiency including a novel mutation (291delC). *J. Inherit. Metab. Dis.* **1999**, *22*, 364–373. [CrossRef]
84. Stamelou, M.; Mencacci, N.E.; Cordivari, C.; Batla, A.; Wood, N.W.; Houlden, H.; Hardy, J.; Bhatia, K.P. Myoclonus–dystonia syndrome due to tyrosine hydroxylase deficiency. *Neurology* **2012**, *79*, 435–441. [CrossRef]
85. Weissbach, A.; Pauly, M.G.; Herzog, R.; Hahn, L.; Halmans, S.; Hamami, F.; Bolte, C.; Camargos, S.; Jeon, B.; Kurian, M.A.; et al. Relationship of Genotype, Phenotype, and Treatment in Dopa-Responsive Dystonia: MDSGene Review. *Mov. Disord.* **2021**, *37*, 237–252. [CrossRef]
86. Makino, S.; Kaji, R.; Ando, S.; Tomizawa, M.; Yasuno, K.; Goto, S.; Matsumoto, S.; Tabuena, M.D.; Maranon, E.; Dantes, M.; et al. Reduced Neuron-Specific Expression of the TAF1 Gene Is Associated with X-Linked Dystonia-Parkinsonism. *Am. J. Hum. Genet.* **2007**, *80*, 393–406. [CrossRef] [PubMed]
87. Lee, L.V.; Pascasio, F.M.; Fuentes, F.D.; Viterbo, G.H. Torsion dystonia in Panay, Philippines. *Adv. Neurol.* **1976**, *14*, 137–151.
88. Brüggemann, N.; Heldmann, M.; Klein, C.; Domingo, A.; Rasche, D.; Tronnier, V.; Rosales, R.L.; Jamora, R.D.G.; Lee, L.V.; Münte, T.F. Neuroanatomical changes extend beyond striatal atrophy in X-linked dystonia parkinsonism. *Park. Relat. Disord.* **2016**, *31*, 91–97. [CrossRef] [PubMed]
89. Song, P.C.; Le Bs, H.; Acuna, P.; De Guzman, J.K.P.; Sharma, N.; Ba, T.N.F.; Dy, M.E.; Go, C.L. Voice and swallowing dysfunction in X-linked dystonia parkinsonism. *Laryngoscope* **2019**, *130*, 171–177. [CrossRef] [PubMed]
90. Brashear, A.; Dobyns, W.; Aguiar, P.D.C.; Borg, M.; Frijns, C.J.M.; Gollamudi, S.; Green, A.; Guimaraes, J.; Haake, B.C.; Klein, C.; et al. The phenotypic spectrum of rapid–onset dystonia–parkinsonism (RDP) and mutations in the ATP1A3 gene. *Brain* **2007**, *130*, 828–835. [CrossRef] [PubMed]

91. Aguiar, P.D.C.; Sweadner, K.J.; Penniston, J.T.; Zaremba, J.; Liu, L.; Caton, M.; Linazasoro, G.; Borg, M.; Tijssen, M.A.; Bressman, S.B.; et al. Mutations in the Na$^+$/K$^+$−ATPase α3 Gene ATP1A3 Are Associated with Rapid−Onset Dystonia Parkinsonism. *Neuron* **2004**, *43*, 169–175. [CrossRef]
92. Mencacci, N.E.; Rubio-Agusti, I.; Zdebik, A.; Asmus, F.; Ludtmann, M.H.; Ryten, M.; Plagnol, V.; Hauser, A.-K.; Bandres-Ciga, S.; Bettencourt, C.; et al. A Missense Mutation in KCTD17 Causes Autosomal Dominant Myoclonus−Dystonia. *Am. J. Hum. Genet.* **2015**, *96*, 938–947. [CrossRef]
93. Ferrini, A.; Steel, D.; Barwick, K.; Kurian, M.A. An Update on the Phenotype, Genotype and Neurobiology of ADCY5-Related Disease. *Mov. Disord.* **2021**, *36*, 1104–1114. [CrossRef]
94. Méneret, A.; Gras, D.; McGovern, E.; Roze, E. Caffeine and the Dyskinesia Related to Mutations in the *ADCY5* Gene. *Ann. Intern. Med.* **2019**, *171*, 439. [CrossRef]
95. Albanese, A.; Asmus, F.; Bhatia, K.; Elia, A.E.; Elibol, B.; Filippini, G.; Gasser, T.; Krauss, J.K.; Nardocci, N.; Newton, A.; et al. EFNS guidelines on diagnosis and treatment of primary dystonias. *Eur. J. Neurol.* **2010**, *18*, 5–18. [CrossRef]
96. Bressman, S.B.; Sabatti, C.; Raymond, D.; de Leon, D.; Klein, C.; Kramer, P.L.; Brin, M.F.; Fahn, S.; Breakefield, X.; Ozelius, L.J.; et al. The DYT1 phenotype and guidelines for diagnostic testing. *Neurology* **2000**, *54*, 1746–1753. [CrossRef] [PubMed]
97. American Society of Human Genetics Board of Directors. Points to consider: Ethical, legal, and psychosocial implications of genetic testing in children and adolescents. *Am. J. Hum. Genet.* **1995**, *57*, 1233–1241.
98. Klein, C.; Friedman, J.; Bressman, S.; Vieregge, P.; Brin, M.F.; Pramstaller, P.P.; de Leon, D.; Hagenah, J.; Sieberer, M.; Fleet, C.; et al. Genetic Testing for Early-Onset Torsion Dystonia (DYT1): Introduction of a Simple Screening Method, Experiences from Testing of a Large Patient Cohort, and Ethical Aspects. *Genet. Test.* **1999**, *3*, 323–328. [CrossRef] [PubMed]
99. Robinson, R.; McCarthy, G.T.; Bandmann, O.; Dobbie, M.; Surtees, R.; Wood, N. GTP cyclohydrolase deficiency; intrafamilial variation in clinical phenotype, including levodopa responsiveness. *J. Neurol. Neurosurg. Psychiatry* **1999**, *66*, 86–89. [CrossRef]
100. Valente, E.M.; Edwards, M.J.; Mir, P.; DiGiorgio, A.; Salvi, S.; Davis, M.; Russo, N.; Bozi, M.; Kim, H.-T.; Pennisi, G.; et al. The epsilon−sarcoglycan gene in myoclonic syndromes. *Neurology* **2005**, *64*, 737–739. [CrossRef]
101. Zech, M.; Jech, R.; Boesch, S.; Škorvánek, M.; Weber, S.; Wagner, M.; Zhao, C.; Jochim, A.; Necpál, J.; Dincer, Y.; et al. Monogenic variants in dystonia: An exome−wide sequencing study. *Lancet Neurol.* **2020**, *19*, 908–918. [CrossRef]
102. Klein, C.; Lohmann, K.; Marras, C.; Münchau, A. Hereditary Dystonia Overview. In *GeneReviews(®)*; Adam, M.P., Ardinger, H.H., Pagon, R.A., Wallace, S.E., Bean, L.J.H., Stephens, K., Amemiya, A., Eds.; University of Washington: Seattle, WA, USA, 1993.
103. Müller, B.; Hedrich, K.; Kock, N.; Dragasevic, N.; Svetel, M.; Garrels, J.; Landt, O.; Nitschke, M.; Pramstaller, P.P.; Reik, W.; et al. Evidence That Paternal Expression of the ε-Sarcoglycan Gene Accounts for Reduced Penetrance in Myoclonus-Dystonia. *Am. J. Hum. Genet.* **2002**, *71*, 1303–1311. [CrossRef]
104. Arlotti, M.; Colombo, M.; Bonfanti, A.; Mandat, T.; Lanotte, M.M.; Pirola, E.; Borellini, L.; Rampini, P.; Eleopra, R.; Rinaldo, S.; et al. A New Implantable Closed−Loop Clinical Neural Interface: First Application in Parkinson's Disease. *Front. Neurosci.* **2021**, *15*, 763235. [CrossRef]

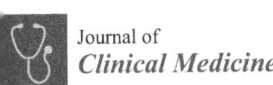

Review

The Patho-Neurophysiological Basis and Treatment of Focal Laryngeal Dystonia: A Narrative Review and Two Case Reports Applying TMS over the Laryngeal Motor Cortex

Maja Rogić Vidaković [1,*], Ivana Gunjača [2], Josipa Bukić [3], Vana Košta [4], Joško Šoda [5], Ivan Konstantinović [6], Braco Bošković [7], Irena Bilić [7] and Nikolina Režić Mužinić [8,*]

1. Laboratory for Human and Experimental Neurophysiology, Department of Neuroscience, University of Split School of Medicine, 21000 Split, Croatia
2. Department of Medical Biology, University of Split School of Medicine, 21000 Split, Croatia; igunjaca@mefst.hr
3. Department of Pharmacy, University of Split School of Medicine, 21000 Split, Croatia; jbukic@mefst.hr
4. Department of Neurology, University Hospital Split, 21000 Split, Croatia; vanakosta@gmail.com
5. Signal Processing, Analysis, and Advanced Diagnostics Research and Education Laboratory (SPAADREL), Faculty of Maritime Studies, University of Split, 21000 Split, Croatia; jsoda@pfst.hr
6. Department of Neurosurgery, University Hospital of Split, 21000 Split, Croatia; ivan.konstan@gmail.com
7. Department of Otorhinolaryngology, University Hospital of Split, 21000 Split, Croatia; bboskovic01@gmail.com (B.B.); ire.bilic@gmail.com (I.B.)
8. Department of Medical Chemistry and Biochemistry, University of Split School of Medicine, 21000 Split, Croatia
* Correspondence: maja.rogic@mefst.hr (M.R.V.); nikolina.rezic@mefst.hr (N.R.M.)

Abstract: Focal laryngeal dystonia (LD) is a rare, idiopathic disease affecting the laryngeal musculature with an unknown cause and clinically presented as adductor LD or rarely as abductor LD. The most effective treatment options include the injection of botulinum toxin (BoNT) into the affected laryngeal muscle. The aim of this narrative review is to summarize the patho-neuro-physiological and genetic background of LD, as well as the standard recommended therapy (BoNT) and pharmacological treatment options, and to discuss possible treatment perspectives using neuro-modulation techniques such as repetitive transcranial magnetic stimulation (rTMS) and vibrotactile stimulation. The review will present two LD cases, patients with adductor and abductor LD, standard diagnostic procedure, treatments and achievement, and the results of cortical excitability mapping the primary motor cortex for the representation of the laryngeal muscles in the assessment of corticospinal and corticobulbar excitability.

Keywords: spasmodic dysphonia; laryngeal dystonia; dystonia; focal dystonia; focal laryngeal dystonia

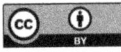

1. Introduction

The laryngeal motor cortex (LMC) plays a vital role in human voice and speech production. The functional organization of LMC and its interactions with other cortical (such as Broca's area) and subcortical brain regions warrants further investigation due to still as of yet unsuccessful treatments of neurological voice disorders such as laryngeal dystonia (LD). To date, methodologies for mapping LMC with TMS [1–6] and intraoperatively by electrical stimulation (ES) techniques [5–7] have been previously developed to record corticobulbar motor evoked potentials (MEPs) from laryngeal muscles. Except for estimating the amplitude and latency of MEPs recorded from laryngeal muscles, the cortical silent period (cSP) was investigated from the thyroarytenoid muscle as a measure of LMC excitability in the TMS study [8]. Currently, it is thought that the cSP reflects an intracortical inhibitory process mediated by $GABA_A$ and $GABA_B$ receptors [9,10]. Previous work using TMS has indicated reduced inhibition to be characteristic of focal laryngeal dystonia (LD), hand dystonia, cervical dystonia, and spasmodic dysphonia (focal laryngeal dystonia) [11].

Focal LD is a rare, idiopathic disease affecting the intrinsic muscles of the larynx with a prevalence of 14–35 per 100,000 people, predominantly affecting women (4:1 ratio) [12,13], with average onset at around 40 years of age [14,15]. Vocal symptoms range from sporadic difficulty to sustained inability to phonate, with vocal tremors (voice breaks) or strained or choked speech. LD presents with two phenotypes, the more common adductor LD (adLD) and the relatively rare abductor LD (abLD). Although symptoms of these two types of LD differ, both are characterized by the loss of voluntary control of voice/speech production. Currently, there is no cure for LD, and the disease is often treated with botulinum toxin (BoNT), speech, and supportive voice therapy, and not frequently by using medication due to side effects [16–19]. Reliably good responses can be expected for the adductor LD with BoNT, with a reduction in voice breaks, reduction in speaking effort, and increased quality of life. However, BoNT therapy requires regular injections every three or several months to ensure the continuity of benefits. Patients often experience bothersome side effects, including pain from injections, breathiness, dysphagia, and hypophonia. A less common side effect of BoNT is dysphagia which can be severe [17].

This narrative review aims to summarize the knowledge on the patho-neurophysiological and genetic background of LD, standard recommended therapies, pharmacological treatment options, and the knowledge and promises of using neuro-modulation techniques such as repetitive transcranial magnetic stimulation (rTMS) and vibrotactile stimulation in the treatment of focal LD. The review will present two LD cases, patients with adLD and abLD, diagnostic procedure, and treatment achievement.

2. LD Terminology, Speech Task Specificity, and Clinical Assessment

The group of multidisciplinary experts of the NIH/NIDCD Workshop on Research Priorities in Spasmodic Dysphonia/Laryngeal Dystonia (August 2019) adopted the term laryngeal dystonia (LD) instead of "spasmodic dysphonia", and LD was recognized as a multifactorial, phenotypical heterogeneous form of isolated dystonia [13]. The isolated, focal LD is a rare neurological disorder of the laryngeal muscles affecting speech production while leaving whispering and innate and/or upper respiratory vocal behaviors such as crying, coughing, yawing, or laughing unaffected. The clinical assessment is challenging due to the lack of diagnostic biomarkers, and very often, the establishment of the diagnosis is delayed by approximately 4–5 years [13]. LD is frequently diagnosed by standard procedures, including: (a) endo-video-stroboscopic examination to evaluate vocal fold anatomy and movements during speech and other vocal activities of the larynx; (b) speech-language pathological examination assessing voice symptoms (including acoustic analysis); and (c) neurological evaluation for signs of regional dystonia, other movement disorders or any other neurological deficit (lesion). LD symptomatology is differentiated from dystonic vocal tremor, essential tremor, and muscle tension dysphonia based on LD task specificity [13]. Multidisciplinary experts from neurology, otolaryngology, speech-language pathology, neurosurgery, genetics, and neuroscience might be involved in establishing LD diagnosis or conducting research.

3. LD Risk Factors

3.1. Genetic Risk Factors

The LD etiology remains unknown and is considered characteristically multifactorial. According to reported findings, up to 25.3% of LD patients have a family history of dystonia [13]. Hereditary dystonias are genetically and clinically heterogeneous. To date, genetic variants that have been studied among LD patients include mutations in the *TOR1A, TUBB4A, THAP1, ANO3, GNAL, SGCE, PRKRA, COL6A3*, and *KMT2B* genes [13,20,21] (Supplementary Table S1, [22–44]). The known genetic forms of LD include the mostly autosomal dominant mode of inheritance.

3.2. Extrinsic Risk Factors

Although there is no established link between focal LD to occur due to the causative influence of extrinsic factors, some health conditions and environmental agents might have a role as a trigger for LD [13]. Family history of dystonia and a history of psychological disturbances such as depression, anxiety, and stress might lead to a potential risk factor in developing LD [13]. Further, white females, as well as professionals using their voice more pronouncedly as teachers, speech and language pathologists, and singers, have been identified as having a higher risk of developing LD [13]. Underlying LD risk factors also include infections of the respiratory system, gastrointestinal diseases, and neck injuries [45].

4. Patho- Neurophysiology of LD

4.1. Neural Structures and Function

Although the pathophysiology of LD is not fully known, it has been suggested that LD is a functional and structural disorder involving a complex neuronal network comprising basal ganglia structures, the thalamus, and their connections with cortical areas, the cerebellum, and sensorimotor cortex [46–52]. Alterations in activity of speech-related areas mediating motor preparation and execution were reported in the primary motor cortex for oro-laryngeal muscle representation, the middle frontal gyrus, the inferior frontal gyrus (i.e., Broca's area) [48,50,53–57], and the temporal [48] and parietal brain areas [58]. Further, the adductor and abductor laryngeal muscle movements are under the voluntary control of the corticobulbar tract projecting to the nucleus ambiguous of the brainstem. Alterations in the microstructural and functional integrity of the corticobulbar tract descending pathway from the primary motor cortex for representation of laryngeal musculature to the brain stem nuclei involved in voice/speech production might also be implicated in the pathophysiology of LD [51]. Processing of auditory and visual information during speech might also have a role in the pathophysiology of LD [55,56].

4.2. Knowledge of the Neurophysiological Basis of LD

Neurophysiological studies indicate altered inhibitory mechanisms in LD, as with cervical dystonia and focal dystonia of the hand. More precisely, cSP has been reported to be shortened in laryngeal thyroarytenoid muscle patients with adLD [8,11]. The cSP is measured as the duration of the electrical silence in the laryngeal muscle during vocalization and the simultaneous application of a single magnetic pulse with TMS at an intensity greater than the resting motor threshold (RMT) for the upper extremity hand muscle [8]. The cSP duration is a measure of $GABA_B$-mediated inhibition of the motor cells of the primary motor cortex through the activity of inhibitory interneurons located within the superficial cortical layers of the primary motor cortex [8]. Decreased inhibition in the primary motor cortex may be due to dysfunction that may also occur in other cortical or subcortical areas that send projections to the primary motor $GABA_B$ inhibitory interneurons [8]. Thus, decreased inhibition of $GABA_B$ within the primary motor cortex may result from the dysregulation of neural circuits that consequently affect the balance of excitation and inhibition in the primary motor cortex [8]. There is no convincing and reliable evidence of changes in other neurophysiological measures such as the RMT or the active motor threshold in LD [8,11]. There are insufficient studies using TMS in patients with LD that could provide information on neurophysiological measures other than cSP, such as inhibitory measures of long-interval intracortical inhibition (LICI), short-interval intracortical inhibition (SICI), and short and long afferent latency inhibition (SAI, LAI). LICI is a paired-pulse technique with a conditioned magnetic pulse on intensity above the threshold and test stimuli (intensity below the threshold) applied in intervals between 50–200 ms leading to the suppression of cortical activity (suppression of motor evoked potential amplitude). SICI is a paired-pulse technique with a conditioned pulse below the threshold and test stimuli (above the threshold) applied in intervals between 1.5–2.1 ms leading to the suppression of cortical activity (suppression of motor evoked potential amplitude) [59,60]. There are no data for LICI and SICI in LD. SAI and LAI are techniques that can induce the suppression of motor evoked potential amplitude by applying an electrical pulse to the periphery (median nerve) followed by a magnetic pulse over the primary motor cortex (usually induced at an interstimulus interval of N20 ms + 2 for SAI and LAI is induced at an interstimulus interval of about 200 ms). SAI and LAI measures relate to $GABA_A$ transmission [59–61]. So far, there is evidence of reduced afferent inhibition in focal dystonia of the arm or cervical dystonia [62–65].

Decreased afferent-induced inhibition indicates abnormal sensorimotor integration within the primary motor cortices, which is not surprising as it is known that the processing of sensory (sensorimotor) information in dystonia is altered. The presence of a sensory gesture (in cervical dystonia) also suggests abnormal reliance on sensorimotor networks and a potential mechanism for alleviating dystonic contraction. Understanding the mechanisms leading to reduced afferent-induced inhibition in isolated dystonia may provide new therapeutic goals that could be explored in future research to alleviate sensorimotor symptoms. Future neurophysiological studies with transcranial magnetic stimulation (TMS) should use more homogenous cohorts of adLd and abLD subjects and publish raw data values of corticobulbar motor evoked potentials from affected and non-affected laryngeal muscles, cSP, SICI, and SAI measures.

5. Focal LD Treatment Options

5.1. Standard Treatment with Botulinum Toxin (BoNT)

Botulinum toxin is a natural neurotoxin produced by the bacteria Clostridium botulinum that causes muscular paralysis. The primary mechanism of action of the toxin is via the inhibition of calcium-dependent exocytosis and the release of acetylcholine at the neuromuscular junction [66]. The effect of botulinum toxin is reversible because the nerve terminals recover the ability to release acetylcholine into the neuromuscular junction. Two types have been developed for clinical use in humans: type A has the longest duration of effect and diffuses less from the injection point compared with type B. The dosing differs significantly between type A and type B preparations. The most common type of botulinum toxin used in LD therapy is type A (Botox, Allergan, Irvine, CA, USA; Dysport, Ipsen, Ltd., Slough, UK). Adverse effects of botulinum toxin treatment may result from over-weakening of the intended target muscle and unintended weakening of the surrounding muscles. Therefore, both appropriate dosing and the tissue distribution of the toxin are crucial. In general, the dose is proportional to the targeted muscle mass, although the range of therapeutic dosing is typically highly variable [67]. Some patients get the best results from a unilateral dose and others from bilateral treatment. For example, in bilateral injections for adLD, therapeutic doses range from 0.3–15 U per thyroarytenoid muscle, although most adLD is well controlled with doses of 0.625–2.5 U [44]. The American Academy of Otolaryngology-Head and Neck Surgery ("AAO-HNS") considers botulinum toxin a safe and effective modality for the treatment of LD, and it may be offered as primary therapy for this disorder. The goal of treatment is to give an injection that will provide just enough weakness to relieve spasm in the target muscles for as long as possible without causing unnecessary weakness in neighboring muscles resulting in dysphagia, and prolonged breathiness (adductor), or airway compromise (abductor) [68]. There are a variety of injection approaches to deliver botulinum toxin to the larynx: percutaneous injection with EMG guidance (most traditional), percutaneous with laryngoscopic guidance, and supraglottic botulinum toxin injection with laryngoscopic guidance. For adLD, the intrinsic laryngeal injection muscles are the thyroarytenoid, lateral cricoarytenoid, and interarytenoid muscles. These muscles can all be accessed through the cricothyroid membrane. For the thyroarytenoid muscle, it is helpful to bend the needle upward to 30–45°. The needle is inserted through the skin either at or just off the midline. The needle tip is then directed superiorly and laterally, advancing towards the ipsilateral thyroarytenoid muscle. The cricothyroid membrane is palpated to inject into the lateral cricoarytenoid muscle, and the needle is placed through the cricothyroid membrane in this location and is angled superiorly. Further, the lateral cricoarytenoid muscle is more lateral than the thyroarytenoid muscle and is encountered more superficially. For abLD, the posterior cricoarytenoid muscle can be accessed anteriorly by piercing through the cricoid rostrum or laterally by rotating the larynx. The lateral approach to the cricoarytenoid muscle requires a relaxed patient, preferably with a relatively thin neck. The patient must tolerate the clinician applying moderate pressure/force on their larynx to rotate the posterior aspect of the cricoid into a position to allow access. The needle is inserted traversing the pyriform sinus and inferior constrictor, then it is further advanced until it stops abruptly against the cricoid cartilage's rostrum [69,70].

5.2. The Long Term Effects of BoNT

Although botulinum toxin is generally considered safe, its widespread use and the constantly expanded indications raise safety issues. In February 2008 and April 2009, the Food and Drug Administration (FDA) published an early communication regarding botulinum toxin type A and botulinum toxin type B, informing physicians that these drugs have been associated with systemic adverse reactions, including respiratory compromise and death resembling those seen with botulism, in which botulinum toxin spreads to the body beyond the injection site [71]. In 2005, the FDA raised safety issues regarding botulinum toxin in a published analysis of adverse events covering the period from 1989 to 2003. According to that publication, there were 407 adverse event reports related to the therapeutic use of botulinum toxin (median dose of 100 units), 217 of which met the FDA's definition of serious adverse events. Few data on the long-term adverse events of botulinum toxin were identified. Most of them concern the therapeutic use of botulinum toxin. Long-term safety data indicate that toxic effects of botulinum toxin can appear at the 10th or 11th injection after prior uncomplicated injections. The longest follow-up study of 45 patients continuously treated with botulinum toxin for 12 years identified 20 adverse events in 16 patients, including dysphagia, ptosis, neck weakness, nausea/vomiting, blurred vision, marked weakness, chewing difficulties, hoarseness, edema, dysarthria, palpitations, and general weakness [72]. Diffusion of botulinum toxin to contralateral muscles has also been reported. Animal studies have shown that botulinum toxin can spread to a distance of 30–45 mm from the injection site [72]. However, generalized diffusion of botulinum toxin is possible, especially after long-term therapeutic or cosmetic use. The effects of generalized diffusion are not well studied. The mechanism responsible for the generalized diffusion of botulinum toxin is not known. Proposed hypotheses concern either a systemic spread or a retrograde axonal spread of the toxin. Systemic toxin spread can lead to adverse events suggesting botulism, including muscle weakness or paralysis, dysarthria, dysphonia, dysphagia, and respiratory arrest.

Additionally, experimental studies in rodents have shown that botulinum toxin receptors exist in the central nervous system, and a small amount of botulinum toxin crosses the blood-brain barrier [73]. This raises the possibility that botulinum toxin is transported in a retrograde manner, similar to tetanus toxin, and may cause centrally mediated side effects [74]. Davidson and Ludlow [75] studied whether physiological changes can be found in laryngeal muscles following repeated treatment with botulinum toxin injections in spasmodic dysphonia. Seven patients whose treatment consisted of multiple unilateral thyroarytenoid injections were examined more than six months following their most recent botulinum toxin injection by fiberoptic laryngoscopy and electromyography. Comparisons were made between injected and contralateral noninjected muscles' motor unit characteristics, muscle activation patterns, and vocal fold movement characteristics. The results demonstrated that motor unit characteristics differed between injected and noninjected muscles and that these differences were more significant in patients less than 12 months since the last injection. Motor unit duration differences were reduced, and motor unit amplitude and numbers of turns were increased in muscles sampled over one year after injection. These results suggest that while the physiologic effects of botulinum toxin are reversible, the re-innervation process continues past 12 months following injection [75]. Repeated injections may eventually enhance the pathological innervation, leading to tolerance and even exacerbation of local symptoms.

Moreover, they cause muscle fibrosis after several years, though such an effect has not been shown in shorter follow-ups so far [76] Resistance to botulinum toxin due to the development of antibodies to the toxin has also been reported as a long-term adverse event of the therapeutic use of botulinum toxin [76]. Immunoresistance develops within the first years of therapy. It is unlikely to develop if immunoresistance to botulinum toxin is not noted within the first four years.

5.3. Review of the Literature on BoNT and Deep Brain Stimulation (DBS) Treatment

Table 1 presents findings of BoNT treatments of LD and an overview of the literature on invasive brain modulation with deep brain stimulation (DBS) [77–81]. The efficacy and safety of BoNT were established for the treatment of LD, and this approach is considered by most to be the treatment of choice for spasmodic dysphonia/LD, particularly adLD [16]. Most studies report about 75–95% improvement in voice symptoms after BoNT [81,82]. Invasive brain stimulation with the DBS of unilateral or bilateral globus pallidus internus (GPi) or subthalamic nucleus (STN) has been approved by the FDA for the treatment of drug-refractory generalized, segmental, and cervical dystonias and hemidystonia [13,83,84], as well as for the treatment of essential tremor in adult patients whose tremor is not adequately controlled with medication. Table 1 presents patients with essential tremor and LD treated with DBS [78–80]. Generally, it is agreed that LD may show a poorer response to DBS [85,86].

Table 1. Literature overview on standard BoNT therapy and invasive brain modulation treatment effects.

Literature	No Subjects	Age	Sex (M/F)	Laryngeal Dystonia (Adductor/Abductor)	Clinical Presentation	Medical Treatment	Medical Treatment Outcome
Santos et al. [77]	1	61	F	Adductor	Tense voice, vocal tiredness, breathy voice, laryngeal pain, loss of voice extension, lack of frequency control	5U of type A Botulin Toxin (Botox) in the left thyroarytenoid muscle	Increased respiratory capacity and maximum speech time
Evidente et al. [78]	3	74 71 65	F F M	Adductor	Essential hand tremor with laryngeal dystonia	Bilateral ventralis intermedius (VIM) DBS	Could easily phonate with no vocal tremor, improvement of USDRS scores post-DBS compared to pre-DBS, and with stimulator on compared to stimulator off
Krüger et al. [79]	2	85 73	F	Adductor	Essential limb tremor with laryngeal dystonia	Bilateral ventrointermediate (VIM) nucleus DBS of the thalamus	Unanticipated improvement of their SD symptom; powerful unilateral benefit in both patients; hand dominant related probably
Poologaindran et al. [80]	1	79	F	Adductor	Right upper limb tremor with laryngeal dystonia	Left ventral intermediate (VIM) nucleus of the thalamus	Significantly improved SD vocal dysfunction compared with no stimulation (DBS off), as measured by the USDRS and VRQOL
Stewart et al. [81]	60	6078	42 F 18 M	Adductor	Roughness, strain-strangled voice quality, and increased expiratory effort	BoNT	Subjects reported benefit from BoNT injections, and had self-selected to return for continuing BoNT management of their voice symptoms when the benefits of the BoNT injections had diminished

Abbreviations: Unified Spasmodic Dysphonia Rating Scale (USDRS); voice-related quality of life (VRQOL).

5.4. Pharmacological Treatment Possibilities and Effectiveness in Dystonia Treatment

The most commonly used dystonia treatment, BoNT, has some limitations, e.g., it is painful for patients and can cause swallowing difficulties. Therefore, there is still an unmet need for effective dystonia pharmacological treatment [62]. The currently available pharmacological treatment involves medicines that act on gamma-aminobutyric acid (GABA), dopamine, or acetylcholine neurotransmitter pathways. Furthermore, novel treatments are also mainly focused on the same neurotransmitter pathways central in dystonia pathophysiology. However, most of the widely used drugs among dystonia patients still have low levels of efficacy evidence [87,88].

Trihexyphenidyl, one of the most commonly used anticholinergic drugs, is the treatment of choice for childhood-onset dystonia, as it has been usually well tolerated in this patient group. It could also be used in adults. The daily dose should be determined empirically but it most commonly ranges between 5–15 mg, though, if tolerated, dosages could be much higher (100 mg is the maximal daily dose recommended). The initial dosage is usually 1 mg, and then it should be increased by 2 mg every 3–7 days divided into three daily doses. The major concern regarding its use is the possibility of trihexyphenidyl to increase intraocular pressure which leads to vision blurring and possibly narrow-angle glaucoma. Other not so uncommon adverse reactions are sedation, memory impairment, psychosis, chorea, blurred vision, urinary retention, constipation, and dry mouth. Levodopa, in combination with carbidopa, an inhibitor of aromatic amino acid decarboxylation, is a widely used dopaminergic drug in dystonia patients. The dose and titration are similar to their use in mild Parkinson's disease (slow titration till daily doses of 300–400 mg of levodopa divided in three doses, starting with 50 mg of levodopa). The most common side effects are low blood pressure, nausea, confusion, and dyskinesia. Lastly, as adjunctive therapy, GABA agonists are used to relaxing muscles in dystonia patients. The most commonly used benzodiazepines in LD patients are clonazepam, diazepam and lorazepam [87]. A maximal recommended daily dose of clonazepam is 4 mg divided into 2–3 doses. The start is usually with 0.25–0.5 mg 2–3 times a day, and then the dosage is slowly increased every 3–5 days to 0.5 mg. The most common side effects are sedation, depression, nocturnal drooling, and behavioral disinhibition. Caution must be taken because abrupt discontinuation can trigger seizures. There are several other potential dystonia treatment alternatives described in the literature. The first one would be a medication that acts as vesicular monoamine transporter 2 inhibitors (VMAT2). The well-known representative of this medication group is tetrabenazine. Furthermore, the other medication groups are as follows: sodium oxybate; antihypertensive medication clonidine; antiepileptic's gabapentin; zonisamide; antidepressant escitalopram, a selective serotonin reuptake inhibitor; and hypnotic medication zolpidem. Future therapies of dystonia should involve gene therapy aimed at the specific genes of dystonia patients [88,89].

Sodium oxybate is a sodium salt of g-hydroxybutyric acid used to treat narcolepsy, excessive sleepiness, and disturbed nighttime sleep. A study by Simonyan et al. [90] suggests that this medication has direct modulatory effects on abnormal neural activity of the dystonic network. This medication can raise blood pressure values due to the sodium content. However, research has shown a low frequency of cardiovascular adverse drug reactions and no association with cardiovascular risk [91]. Other than the cardiovascular risk in general, due to the symptoms of the disease, dystonia patients are prone to anxiety and depressive comorbidities, and the use of escitalopram could seem reasonable in patients with existing symptoms [92].

5.5. Future Neuromodulation Treatment Options and Vibrotactile Stimulation

The effectiveness of repetitive transcranial magnetic stimulation (rTMS), a non-invasive neuromodulation technique, in assessing cortical excitability and inhibition of laryngeal musculature might be one of the potential treatment options for LD. Previous neurophysiological findings demonstrated decreased intracortical inhibition in patients with adLD compared to healthy controls [8,11]. Application of low frequency (inhibitory) rTMS to the LMC might decrease the over-activation of the laryngeal muscles [93]. Given that adductor LD has been found to be associated with decreased cortical inhibition and that 1 Hz is known to increase intracortical inhibition, the purpose of the pilot study by Prudente et al. [93] was to examine the effects of 1200 pulses of 1 Hz rTMS delivered to LMC in people with adductor LD and healthy individuals. This is the first feasibility study testing effects of 1 Hz rTMS in LD. The authors tested only a single session of 1 Hz rTMS and observed acoustical measures changes pointing to beneficial effects on voice symptoms. Future studies would need to test the long-treatment duration of 1 Hz rTMS in LD. To test this hypothesis of the beneficial effects of five days of treatment of 1 Hz rTMS, a proof-of-concept, randomized study was recently registered on 27 October 2021 (ClinicalTrials.gov Identifier: NCT05095740, accessed day: 20 May 2022), and the estimated study completion date is 31 May 2025/2026.

Another non-invasive brain stimulation technique, transcranial direct current stimulation (tDCS), has not been reported in the assessment of LD according to the current state-of-the-art.

Further, a feasibility study was performed using vibrotactile stimulation (VTS) to treat LD [57]. The authors reported that 29 min of VTS in a one-day session improved the voice quality parameter (*smoot cepstral peak prominence*). Although a stimulation protocol by using VTS has been published, the optimal stimulation protocol for the treatment of LD is not yet known. After publishing a paper on a feasibility study of VTS, the authors started a clinical study, which is still ongoing, testing the effect of VTS for four weeks in patients with LD (ClinicalTrials.gov Identifier: NCT03746509, accessed day: 20 March 2022). The results have not yet been published, nor is their VTS stimulator commercially available. The same research group applied for a patent (the United States Patent Application Publication, Konczak et al., Pub. No. US 2019/0159953 A1, Pub. Date: 30 May 2019) where they protected the VTS solution of placing the vibrators on the laryngeal muscles over the skin in the form of a necklace placed around the neck.

6. Case Reports of LD Patients

6.1. Patient with adLD

6.1.1. Clinical Findings

A 55-year-old right-handed woman, a psychologist, started to present hoarseness in March 2015 (Video S1A,B, Supplementary Materials). The first endoscopic examination (Karl Storz) (April 2015) confirmed laryngitis, spindle-shaped thickening of the vocal cords, decreased stroboscopic amplitudes, and prolonged adduction of the vocal cords. Voice saving therapy, speech therapy, a light diet, and taking Iberogast® (Bayer AG, Kaiser-Wilhelm-Allee 1, 51373 Leverkusen, Germany) to improve digestion were recommended. The second examination (April 2016) confirmed dysphonia with thinner vocal cords, reduced Bernoulli effect, spasms during vocalization, extended closing phase, and reduced glottal wave. The vocal spasm was also detected during counting, muttering, and minor spasms in buzzing. Brain magnetic resonance imaging (MRI) was performed in October 2016 with normal finding. At the subsequent examination (January 2017), the dysphonia spastica was diagnosed. Spectral and multidimensional acoustic voice analysis showed that the spasm was partially reduced with prolonged phonation of vowel /i/ with high-frequency Fo (346 Hz). The vocal spasm was present in all verbal and vocal tasks except in whisper counting. Acoustic parameters of diadochokinesis (pa-pa) indicated a markedly long syllable duration and accelerated pronunciation change, as well as increased syllable variation. There were marked variations in frequency and amplitude in the analysis of vowel /a/ related to the quality of the voice and the frequency of tremors. Focal LD was diagnosed in February 2017. The first BoNT treatment with Dysport®, Galderma Laboratories, L.P., El Segundo, CA, USA (abobotulinumtoxinA) (15 units) was injected into the right vocal cord under electromyography (EMG) guidance. The second BoNT treatment was performed with Dysport® (abobotulinumtoxinA) (15 units) injected in both vocal cords under EMG. Therefore, the patient was treated with BoNT in 2017 with a short-term improvement of up to ten days with swallowing difficulties and refused further treatment. The brain MRI was again performed in March 2021 with a normal finding.

6.1.2. Evaluation of Corticobulbar and Corticospinal Excitability with Transcranial Magnetic Stimulation (TMS)

The corticospinal excitability measures (RMT, amplitude, and latency of motor evoked potentials for upper extremity muscles) and corticobulbar excitability measure (motor evoked potential latency from cricothyroid muscle) performed with single pulse transcranial magnetic stimulation (TMS) over the primary motor cortex (Nexstim NBS System 4 of the manufacturer Nexstim Plc., Helsinki, Finland) [4,94,95]. The MRI of the subject's head was performed with Siemens Magnetom Area having Tim (76 × 18) of strength 1.5 T. MRI images were used for the 3D reconstruction of individual brain anatomy. With the subject comfortably seated, the MRI is co-registered to the subject's head using the tracking system with Nexstim's unique forehead tracker. The eight-shaped magnetic coil was used, generating a biphasic pulse with a length of 289 µs. The coil with an inner winding diameter of 50 mm and an outer winding diameter of 70 mm was placed tangentially to the subject's skull over the primary motor cortex. The maximum electric field strength measured 25 mm below the coil in a spherical conductor model representing the human head was 172 V/m. The cSP was tested as an inhibitory cortical measure [94].

For recording the responses from the cricothyroid muscle, two hook wire electrodes (type 003-400160-6) (SGM d.o.o., Split, Croatia) were inserted into the cricothyroid muscle according to published methodology [4,96]. Surface electromyography electrodes (Ambu Blue Sensor BR, BR-50-K/12) were attached in a belly tendon fashion over the right APB muscle with the ground electrode over the dorsal surface of the APB muscle. Before insertion of the electrodes individually, the subject needs to slightly extend the neck and produce a high-pitch sound (i.e., /iiii . . . /). During this slight facilitation, it is helpful to palpate the contracted cricothyroid muscle belly between the thyroid and cricoid cartilages by marking this spot with the marker. Each hook wire electrode consists of Teflon-coated stainless steel wire 76 µm in diameter, passing through 27-gauge needles (0.4 mm), 13 mm in length. The recording wires have a stripped Teflon isolation of 2 mm at their tip and are curved to form the hook for anchoring them. The sampling rate was 3 kHz per channel, resolution 0.3 µV, scale −7.5–7.5 mV, CMRR > 90 dB, noise < 5 µV peak-to-peak, and frequency band 10–500 Hz. The RMT intensity for the upper extremity muscles (abductor pollicis brevis) was 49% of maximal stimulator output. Figure 1 (A)(B) presents positive cortical spots for primary motor cortical representation for upper extremity APB muscle and cricothyroid muscle with the recording of MEPs from APB and cricothyroid muscle. The single magnetic pulse intensity over the LMC was gradually increased from 51% to 80 % of maximal stimulator output that the subject could tolerate (reporting pain and discomfort due to activation of temporal musculature). Figure 2 shows application of a single magnetic pulse during vocalization, inducing motor evoked potential from the left cricothyroid muscle (latency of 11.3 ms) with no cSP induced in the cricothyroid muscle at 80 % of maximal stimulator output.

6.1.3. Electroneuronographic (ENG) Assessment of Motor and Sensory Nerves of Upper and Lower Extremity Muscles

There were no deviations in electroneurographic (ENG) measures for upper and lower extremity muscles. ENG assessment of lower and upper extremities included the following measures for motor nerves (n. peroneus and n. tibialis: distal motor latency, compound muscle action potential amplitude, compound muscle action potential duration, conduction velocity, and F-wave latency); and for sensory nerves (n. medianus and n. ulnaris: sensory nerve action potential amplitude, sensory nerve action potential latency, and conduction velocity). The electrophysiological examination was performed using the Medelec-Synergy EMG instrument (Oxford Instrument Co., Surrey, UK).

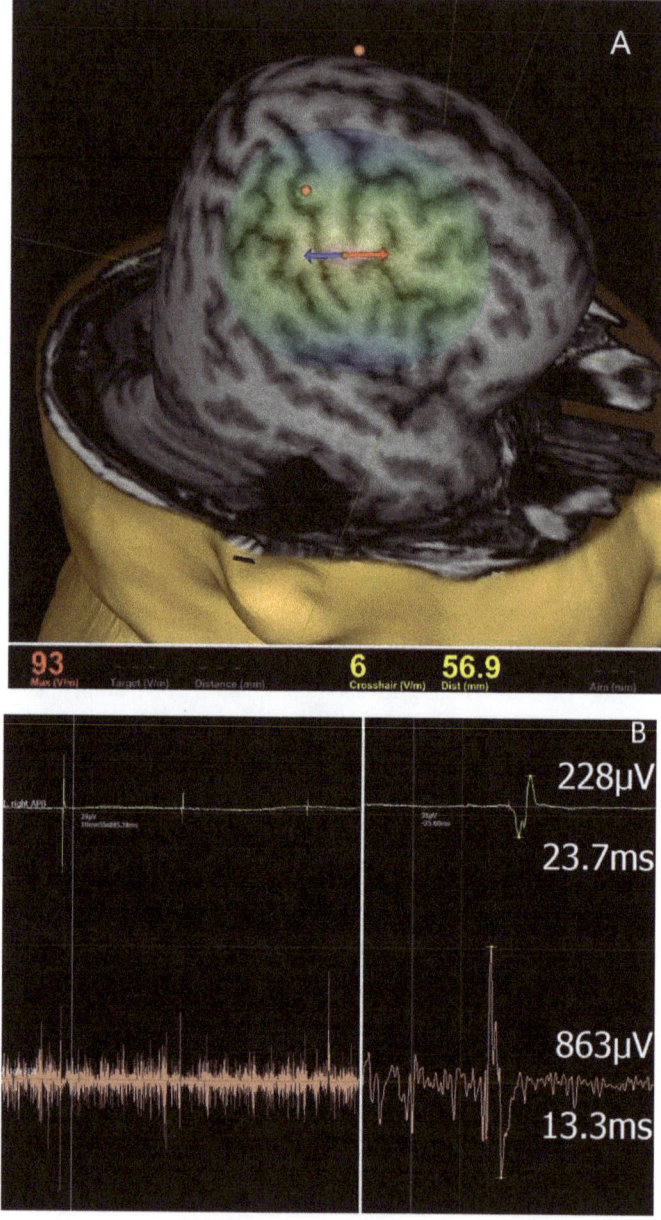

Figure 1. Primary motor cortical representation for the upper extremity left APB muscle and left cricothyroid muscle (**A**) with the recording of MEPs from APB and the cricothyroid muscle (**B**). Note: The orange spot on (**A**) depicts the cortical spot for APB muscle and MEP recording from APB muscle (**B**, upper channel, green color), and the orange spot with the position of the magnetic coil over the primary motor cortex (LMC) denotes the positive spot for inducing MEP in the cricothyroid muscle (lower channel on **B**, pink color). The latency of MEP in the cricothyroid muscle is 13.3 ms, and the amplitude of 863 µV, while the MEP latency of APB is 23.7 ms, and an amplitude of 228 µV. The stimulation intensity was 80% of maximal stimulator output with the subject engaged in phonation task (the left traces on **B** depict laryngeal muscle contractions in free-running electromyography).

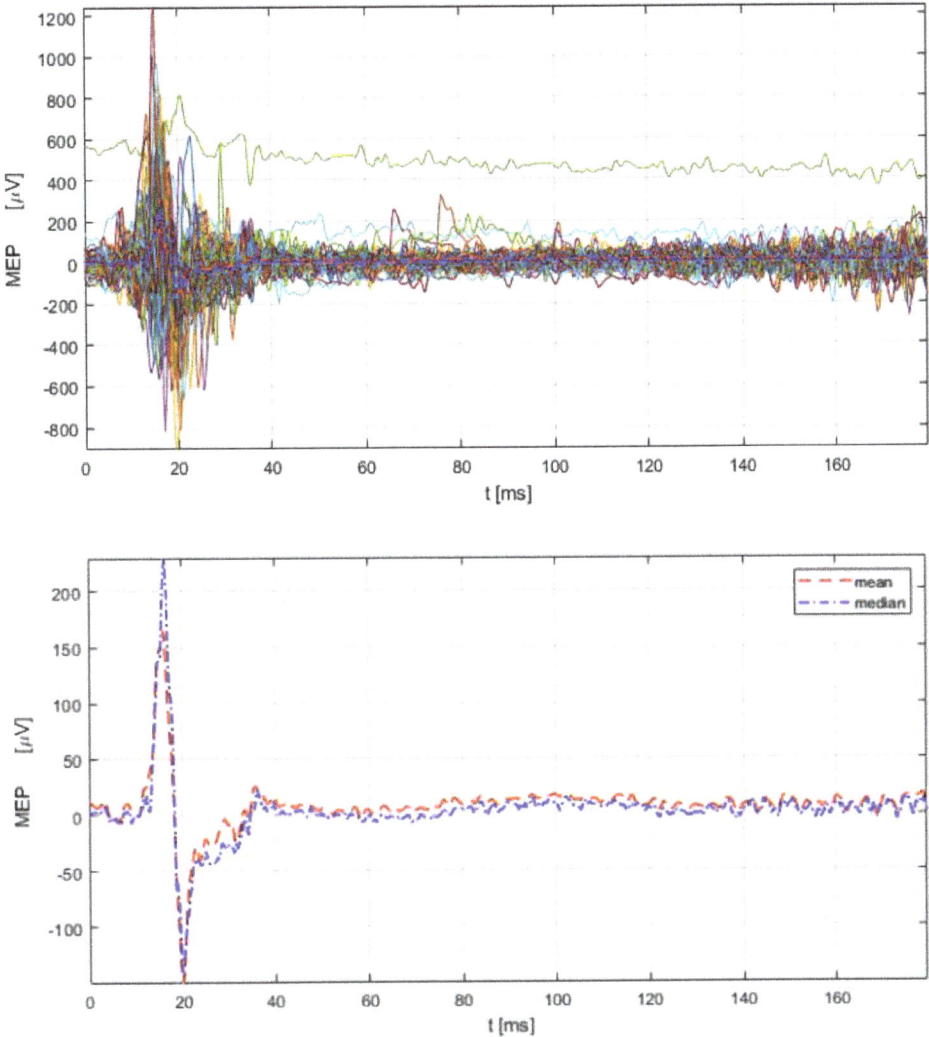

Figure 2. Mapping of the LMC (right hemisphere) and recording corticobulbar motor evoked (MEPs) from the cricothyroid muscle at intensities of 60–80% of the maximal stimulator output and with MEP latency of 11.3 ms. On the upper part of the figure are overlapped MEPs, and on the lower part are the mean and median of these responses. cSP could not be recorded.

6.1.4. Blood—DNA Analysis

Routine blood analysis, including white blood count, erythrocyte sedimentation rate, and C-reactive protein, were within the normal range. There were no abnormal findings in iron, manganese, parathyroid hormone, and serum homocysteine level. A blood sample was collected, and the DNA was extracted from dried blood spots on filter cards (CentoCard®) using standard, spin column-based methods, following the manufacturer's instructions. Targeted sequencing of the patient's DNA was performed using a next-generation sequencing (NGS) panel, including 88 dystonia-associated genes (Centogene, Rostock, Germany). Genomic DNA was enzymatically fragmented, and Illumina adapters were ligated to generate fragments for subsequent sequencing on the NovaSeq 6000 platform (Illumina), with the average coverage targeted to at least 100× or at least 99.5% of the target DNA covered 20×. All coding regions of the panel genes, 10 bp of flanking intronic sequences, and known pathogenic/likely pathogenic variants within these genes (coding and non-coding) were targeted for the analysis. Data analysis, including alignment to the hg19 human reference genome (Genome Reference Consortium GRCh37), variant calling, and annotation, were performed using validated in-house software. No clinically relevant variants, including copy number variations (CNVs), were identified in the panel genes.

6.1.5. Pharmacological Treatment Attempts

Medication treatment with trihexyphenidyl (Artane, anticholinergic drug) was introduced on 20 March 2021, with a dosage of 2 mg daily per six days and increasing by 2 mg every six days. The patient reached 8 mg and ended the treatment after two weeks due to severe side effects (red eyes, anxiety, distractibility, lethargy) and with no signs of voice symptoms improvement. Medication treatment with benzodiazepine (clonazepam) (Rivotril, Roche) was introduced on 24 June 2021, with a dosage of 0.5 mg daily per six days and increasing by 0.5 mg every six days. In four weeks of treatment, the patient reached 2 mg with side effects (drowsiness, fatigue, sadness, crying). The patient monocyte subsets (anti-inflammatory, inflammatory markers) were no different before and after treatment with a benzodiazepine. In the acoustic analysis of vowel /a/ there were still distinctive variations in the frequency of tremors after benzodiazepine medication.

6.1.6. Patient with adLD Conclusion

The patient had severe dysphagia, which necessitated discontinuation of BoNT treatment and beginning treatment with drugs recommended to treat dystonia [16,18,97]. The medication treatment with an anticholinergic drug (trihexyphenidyl) was classified as the first-line agent for symptomatic therapy in dystonia, however, no findings were reported for treatment of the LD. The adLD patient in our study could not reach the recommended daily therapeutic level of 15 mg of trihexyphenidyl due to severe side effects. Benzodiazepine (clonazepam) was introduced as the second-line agent, but still, no effect was noticed on acoustic voice measures (Figure 3A,B). The patient case also showed that there is no genetic basis for LD disease, and cSP could not be recorded in laryngeal muscle due to lack of inhibition or insufficient intensity (80% of maximal stimulator output was rather high over the lateral part of LMC providing discomfort to the subject). Previous studies reported inducing cSP ranging from 48% to 72% of the maximal stimulator output in adLD subjects and in healthy subjects from 50% to 67% of maximal stimulator output [11]. The case report also shows the problem in the length of time to make a final diagnosis. In this particular case, it took two years to make a valid diagnosis. The patient is under consideration for an experimental trial with rTMS and tDCS.

6.2. Patient with abLD

6.2.1. Clinical Findings

A 57-year-old male, by profession lawyer (judge) and singer of traditional Croatian a cappella singing, has had LD of the left vocal cord for three years. The patient noticed changes in his voice in January 2019 while singing in lower tones, and in June 2019, a breathless voice developed. LD was confirmed by endo-video-stroboscopy, acoustic voice analysis, and neurological evaluation for signs of regional dystonia, other movement disorders, or any other neurological deficit (lesion). Magnetic resonance imaging (MRI), and electroneuronography of upper and lower extremities revealed a normal finding, and electromyography confirmed possible spasms in the left cricothyroideus muscle. Although the treatment of choice for the patient's conditions was botulinum toxin treatment, the patient underwent a vocal cord augmentation procedure as a second opinion from a private practice otolaryngologist. Autologous fat vocal fold augmentation is a general surgical procedure used to repair glottal incompetence in patients with unilateral vocal fold paralysis. Autologous fat is harvested from the lower abdomen, and the small fat grafts are purified from other tissues. Under microscope control, the autologous fat is injected into the thyroarytenoid muscle using an applicator with a special gear mechanism. Spectral and multidimensional acoustic voice analysis showed voice breaks predominant in speech tasks (i.e., vocalization of sound /i/—number of voice breaks 5, Jitter (local) (%)—5.45, Shimmer (local, dB)—1.64), and partially reduced when coughing (number of voice breaks 2, Jitter (local) (%)—2.14, Shimmer (local, dB)—1.34) and singing (i.e., vocalization of high pitch sound /i/—number of voice breaks 3, Jitter (local) (%)—1.90, Shimmer (local, dB)—1.39).

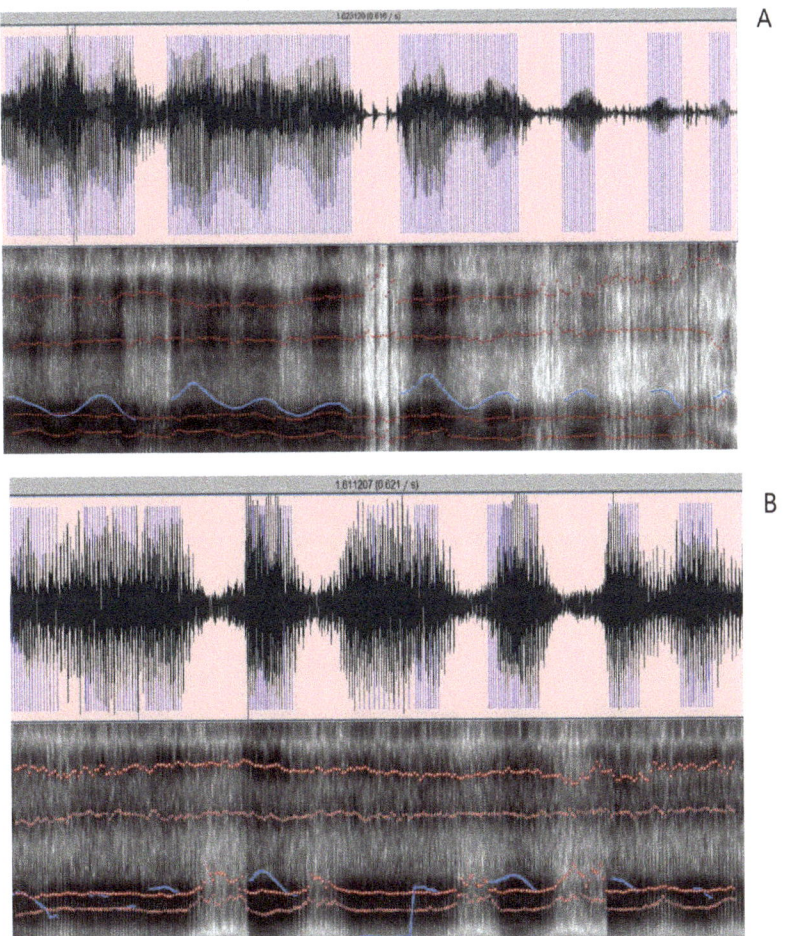

Figure 3. (**A**) The duration of the selection: 1.623120 s, Pitch: Median pitch: 199.863 Hz, Mean pitch: 200.121 Hz, Standard deviation: 17.163 Hz, Minimum pitch: 167.703 Hz, Maximum pitch: 247.906 Hz; Pulses: Number of pulses: 243, Number of periods: 237; Voicing: Fraction of locally unvoiced frames: 23.699% (41/173), Number of voice breaks (interrupted blue line): 5, Degree of voice breaks: 24.702% (0.426674 s/1.727257 s); Jitter: Jitter (local): 2.035%; Shimmer: Shimmer (local, dB): 0.714 dB; Mean harmonics-to-noise ratio: 8.846 dB. (**B**): The duration of the selection: 1.623120 s, Pitch: Median pitch: 179.098 Hz, Mean pitch: 169.509 Hz, Standard deviation: 35.773 Hz, Minimum pitch: 92.742 Hz, Maximum pitch: 218.821 Hz; Pulses: Number of pulses: 139, Number of periods: 129; Voicing: Fraction of locally unvoiced frames: 42.138% (67/159), Number of voice breaks (interrupted blue line): 8, Degree of voice breaks: 46.935% (0.756215 s/1.611207 s); Jitter: Jitter (local): 2.269%; Shimmer: Shimmer (local, dB): 0.915 dB; Mean harmonics-to-noise ratio: 4.313 dB.

Pneumo-phonic voice, calcification in the left cricoarytenoid joint, and lagging of the left vocal cord in adductor movements were indicators for conducting the phono-surgical intervention (November 2019). However, the autologous fat injection for medialization of the left vocal fold did not improve the voice symptoms. The recommended medication therapy included propranolol, coenzyme Q10, vitamin B1 disulfide, vitamin B6, vitamin B12, and magnesium. The patient refused medication treatment recommended for dystonia treatment [16,18,97].

6.2.2. Evaluation of Corticobulbar and Corticospinal Excitability with Transcranial Magnetic Stimulation (TMS)

The TMS technique was used for mapping the primary motor cortex for upper extremity hand and laryngeal muscle representation with a recording of RMT for upper extremity hand muscle (APB), motor evoked potentials from hand muscle (APB) at RMT, corticobulbar motor evoked potentials from laryngeal (cricothyroid muscle), and cSP from the cricothyroid muscle [4,8,11]. To facilitate the corticobulbar motor evoked potentials from the cricothyroid muscle to induce cSP, the subject vocalizes high pitch sound /i/ while slightly increasing the stimulation intensity starting from the referent RMT. RMT for the left hemisphere was 35% of maximal stimulator output, while the RMT intensity was 36% for the right hemisphere. Prolongations in cSP were detected in the right cricothyroid muscle (89.54 ± 21.9 ms) compared to cSP in the left cricothyroid muscle (44.78 ± 6.9 ms) [8] (Figure 4). The intensity of the left hemisphere primary motor cortex for cricothyroid muscle representation for cSP eliciting was of 63% of maximal stimulator output, while for the right hemisphere, it was 65% of maximal stimulator output.

6.2.3. Patient with adLD Conclusion

This case illustrates a rare case of abLD who did not benefit from the autologous fat injection. We have provided the first results of TMS application in evaluating the neurophysiological measure of cortical inhibition such as cSP in abLD. The patient is under consideration for BoNT treatment and an experimental trial with rTMS and tDCS.

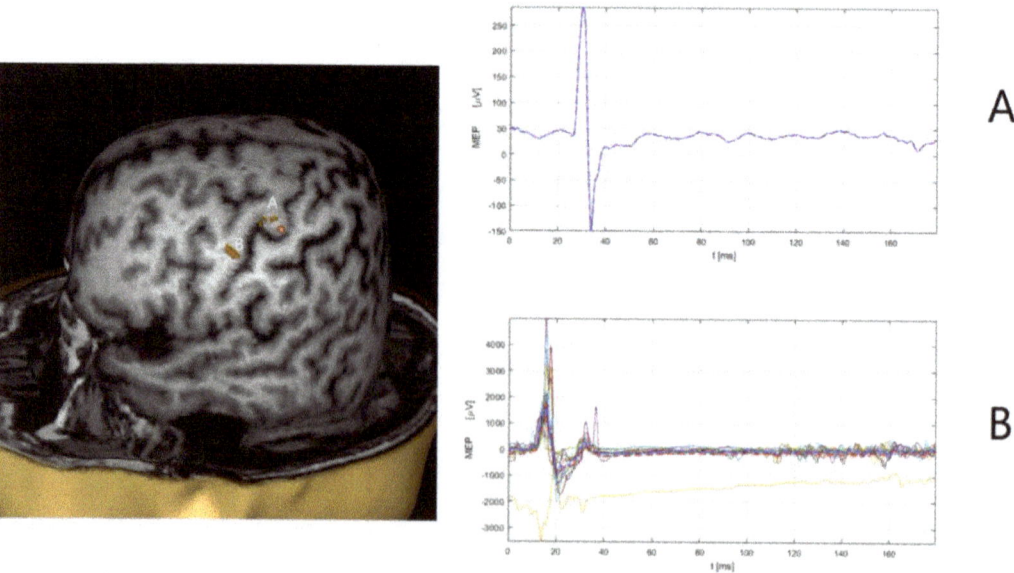

Figure 4. Cont.

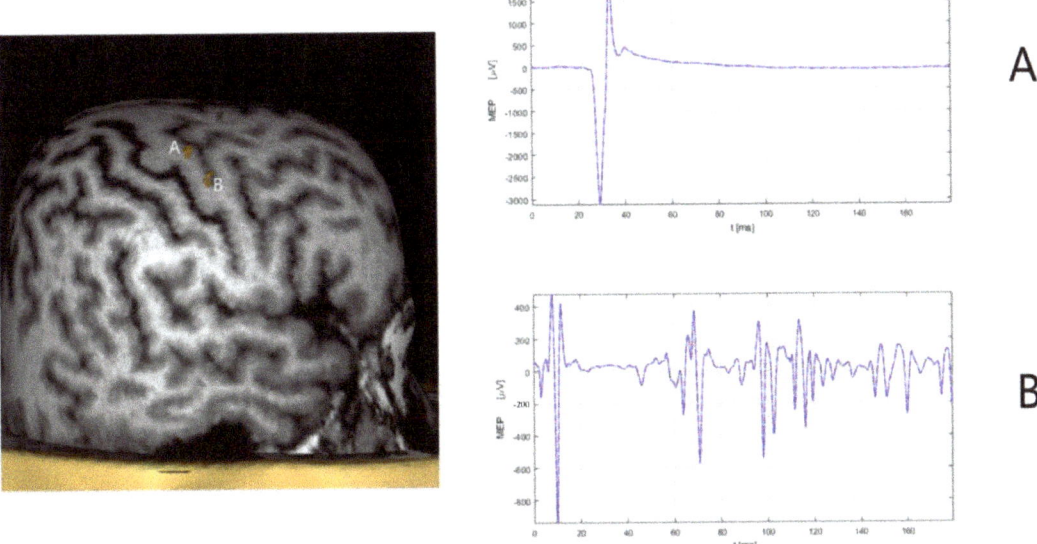

Figure 4. Transcranial magnetic stimulation (TMS) of the primary motor cortex for the upper extremity and laryngeal muscles. (**Upper**) TMS mapping of the left primary motor cortex for hand muscle representation (APB) and cricothyroid muscle representation with recording motor evoked potentials from the right-hand muscle (**A**), and corticobulbar motor evoked potentials from the right cricothyroid muscle (**B**). The latency of motor evoked potentials from the hand muscle is 23.61 ms with a peak-to-peak amplitude of 603.07 µV. The mean latency of corticobulbar motor evoked potentials is 11.67 ± 1.7 ms, and the cortical silent period (CST) duration of 89.54 ± 21.9 ms. (**Lower**) TMS mapping of the right primary motor cortex for hand muscle representation (APB) and cricothyroid muscle representation with recording motor evoked potentials from the left-hand muscle (**A**), and corticobulbar motor evoked potentials from the left cricothyroid muscle (**B**). The latency of motor evoked potentials from the hand muscle is 22.79 ms with a peak-to-peak amplitude of 106.07 µV. The mean latency of corticobulbar motor evoked potentials is 11.67 ± 1.7 ms, and the cortical silent period (CST) duration of 44.78 ± 6.9 ms.

7. Discussion

Diagnosis and treatment of LD remain challenging as underlying patho- and neurophysiology are unclear and require further studies. Currently, there is no cure for LD, and the disease is often treated with BoNT, speech and voice supportive therapy, and rarely by using medication due to side effects [16,17,19,97]. BoNTs are widely used for the treatment of LD [16,17,19]. Reliably good responses can be expected for the adLD with BoNT, reducing voice breaks and speaking effort and increasing quality of life [19]. However, BoNT therapy requires regular injections every three or several months to ensure continuity of benefits. Additionally, patients often experience bothersome side effects, including pain from injections, breathiness, dysphagia, and hypophonia. A less common side effect of BoNT is dysphagia which can be severe [17], as we reported in our case report of a patient with adLD. Through extensive research of the literature, it was found that LD is mostly treated with BoNT (56.6%), but rarely with other medications [97]. Pirio Richardson et al. [97] reported that benzodiazepines were used to treat 16 patients with LD, while muscle relaxants were used in 3 patients, dopaminergic drugs in 3 patients, and non–benzohypnotic drugs in 4 patients. According to a study by Pirio Richardson et al. [97] baclofen and anticholinergic drugs were not reported to be used in the treatment of LD.

Even though the medication treatment with an anticholinergic drug (trihexyphenidyl) was classified as the first-line agent for symptomatic therapy in dystonia [18], no findings were reported so far regarding the medication attempts for LD [18]. The adLD patient in our study could not reach the recommended daily therapeutic level of 15 mg of trihexyphenidyl due to severe side effects. Benzodiazepine (clonazepam) was introduced as the second-line agent [18], but no effect was noticed on acoustic voice measures. Both adLD and abLD patients in this report are currently with unchanged voice status, and further experimental trials are considered, such as rTMS or tDCS using inhibitory protocols such as 1 Hz [70].

Finally, the assessment of cSP with TMS in our two case reports of adLD and abLD patients points to altered intracortical inhibition mechanisms in LD, which is similar to the findings of Chen et al. [8,11]. The presented case of a male subject with abLD is an extremely rare type of LD, and according to our knowledge, it is the first case with a neurophysiological evaluation of cSP. Future studies with TMS are critical, involving a higher number of LD patients (both adLD and abLD types) investigating cSP from laryngeal muscle, as well as other neurophysiological measures such as SICI, LICI, and SAI [36–38,94]. A wider understanding of the neurophysiological basis of LD might lead to more efficient treatments, potentially involving noninvasive neuromodulation techniques such as rTMS or tDCS or vibrotactile stimulation of the laryngeal muscles.

The limitation of the present study relates to the neurophysiological assessment of the corticobulbar excitability by recording MEPs and assessment of cSP from non-targeted laryngeal muscles affected by LD disease. Future studies can adopt the procedures for the percutaneous introduction of recording electrodes into the target laryngeal muscles (i.e., thyroarytenoid muscle) affected by the LD [8,11].

8. Conclusions

Although LD diagnosis has improved, it remains unacceptably delayed [98,99], which is evident in our presented case of a female with adLD. Developed methodologies for mapping the corticobulbar pathway [4–8,11] provide a tool for assessing neurophysiological measures such as MEP responses from laryngeal muscles and cSP in LD patients. The recent neurophysiological studies with TMS point to the impaired intracortical inhibition measured with a non-invasive cSP measure. The current lack of full understanding of LD etiology and patho–neurophysiology contributes to limited therapeutic interventions, but hopefully, promising neuromodulatory techniques such as rTMS might bring new light to the treatment of LD disorder.

Supplementary Materials: The following supporting information can be downloaded at: https://www.mdpi.com/article/10.3390/jcm11123453/s1. Video S1: Patient speech before the diagnosis of focal adduction dystonia (year 2013) (A) and speech of the patient with focal adduction dystonia (year 2021) (B). (A) Original video caption in Croatian language: *Ja sam Maja Kandijaš Plejić, psiholog. Radim na poliklinici za djecu s teškoćama u razvoju Spektrum. Po svojoj bazičnoj edukaciji opremljena sam za dijagnostiku i pomaganje djeci koja su u problemu. Radeći ovaj posao osjećala sam da mi nešto nedostaje.* Video caption translation in the English language: *My name is Maja Kandijaš Plejić, I am a psychologist. I work at the Spektrum polyclinic for children with disabilities. According to my basic education, I provide diagnostic procedures and help children who are in trouble. Doing this job I felt like I was missing something.* (B) Original video caption in Croatian language: *Psiholog sam i radim na Poliklinici Meje za djecu s teškoćama u razvoju. Radim dijagnostiku i psihoterapiju. Dolaze djeca od vrlo male dobi, predškolska djeca, adolescent i dolaze obitelji koje su u problemima, rastave braka.* Video caption translation in the English language: *I am a psychologist and I work at the Meje Polyclinic for children with disabilities. I provide diagnostics and psychotherapy for children of young age, preschool children, adolescents, and families who are in trouble like divorces.* Table S1: Laryngeal Dystonia-Associated Genes.

Author Contributions: M.R.V.—conceptualization, methodology, investigation, data curation, writing—original draft preparation, visualization, resources; I.G.—methodology, investigation, resources, writing—original draft preparation, visualization; J.B.—methodology, writing—original draft preparation; V.K.—methodology, investigation, writing—review and editing; J.Š.—methodology, writing—review and editing, resources; I.K.—methodology, writing—review and editing; B.B.—methodology, writing—original draft preparation; I.B.—writing—review and editing, project administration; N.R.M.—conceptualization, methodology, investigation, data curation, writing—original draft preparation. All authors have read and agreed to the published version of the manuscript.

Funding: This research received no external funding.

Institutional Review Board Statement: The study was conducted in accordance with the Declaration of Helsinki and approved by the Institutional Review Board (or Ethics Committee) of the University of Split School of Medicine (protocol class code: 003-08/21-03/0003, No. 2181-198-03-04-21-0021, date of approval: 9 March 2021) for studies involving humans.

Informed Consent Statement: Informed consent was obtained from all subjects involved in the study. Written informed consent has been obtained from the patient(s) to publish this paper" if applicable. Written informed consent was obtained from the patient for publication of this Case report and any accompanying images and videos. A copy of the written consent is available for review by the corresponding author.

Data Availability Statement: Data is available on request from the corresponding author.

Conflicts of Interest: The authors declare no conflict of interest. The funders had no role in the design of the study; in the collection, analyses, or interpretation of data; in the writing of the manuscript, or in the decision to publish the results.

References

1. Amassian, V.E.; Anziska, B.J.; Cracco, J.B.; Cracco, R.Q.; Maccabee, P.J. Focal magnetic excitation of frontal cortex activates laryngeal muscles in man. *J. Physiol.* **1988**, *398*, 41.
2. Ertekin, C.; Turman, B.; Tarlacı, S.; Celik, M.; Aydogdu, I.; Secil, Y.; Kiyilioglu, N. Cricopharyngeal sphincter muscle responses to transcranial magnetic stimulation in normal subjects and in patients with dysphagia. *Clin. Neurophysiol.* **2000**, *112*, 86–94. [CrossRef]
3. Rödel, R.M.; Olthoff, A.; Tergau, F.; Simonyan, K.; Kraemer, D.; Markus, H.; Kruse, E. Human Cortical Motor Representation of the Larynx as Assessed by Transcranial Magnetic Stimulation (TMS). *Laryngoscope* **2004**, *114*, 918–922. [CrossRef]
4. Espadaler, J.; Rogić, M.; Deletis, V.; Leon, A.; Quijada, C.; Conesa, G. Representation of cricothyroid muscles at the primary motor cortex (M1) in healthy subjects, mapped by navigated transcranial magnetic stimulation (nTMS). *Clin. Neurophysiol.* **2012**, *123*, 2205–2211. [CrossRef]
5. Deletis, V.; Rogić, M.; Fernández-Conejero, I.; Gabarrós, A.; Jerončić, A. Neurophysiologic markers in laryngeal muscles indicate functional anatomy of laryngeal primary motor cortex and premotor cortex in the caudal opercular part of inferior frontal gyrus. *Clin. Neurophysiol.* **2014**, *125*, 1912–1922. [CrossRef]
6. Vidaković, M.R.; Schönwald, M.Z.; Rotim, K.; Jurić, T.; Vulević, Z.; Tafra, R.; Banožić, A.; Hamata, Ž.; Đogaš, Z. Excitability of contralateral and ipsilateral projections of corticobulbar pathways recorded as corticobulbar motor evoked potentials of the cricothyroid muscles. *Clin. Neurophysiol.* **2015**, *126*, 1570–1577. [CrossRef]
7. Deletis, V.; Fernandez-Conejero, I.; Ulkatan, S.; Costantino, P. Methodology for intraoperatively eliciting motor evoked potentials in the vocal muscles by electrical stimulation of the corticobulbar tract. *Clin. Neurophysiol.* **2009**, *120*, 336–341. [CrossRef]
8. Chen, M.; Summers, R.; Goding, G.S.; Samargia, S.; Ludlow, C.L.; Prudente, C.N.; Kimberley, T.J. Evaluation of the Cortical Silent Period of the Laryngeal Motor Cortex in Healthy Individuals. *Front. Neurosci.* **2017**, *11*, 88. [CrossRef]
9. Paulus, W.; Classen, J.; Cohen, L.G.; Large, C.H.; Di Lazzaro, V.; Nitsche, M.; Pascual-Leone, A.; Rosenow, F.; Rothwell, J.; Ziemann, U. State of the art: Pharmacologic effects on cortical excitability measures tested by transcranial magnetic stimulation. *Brain Stimul.* **2008**, *1*, 151–163. [CrossRef]
10. Wolters, A.; Ziemann, U.; Benecke, R. The cortical silent period. In *Oxford Handbook of Transcranial Stimulation*; Epstein, C.M., Wassermann, E.M., Ziemann, U., Eds.; Oxford University Press: New York, NY, USA, 2008; pp. 1–23.
11. Chen, M.; Summers, R.L.; Prudente, C.N.; Goding, G.S.; Samargia-Grivette, S.; Ludlow, C.L.; Kimberley, T.J. Transcranial magnetic stimulation and functional magnet resonance imaging evaluation of adductor spasmodic dysphonia during phonation. *Brain Stimul.* **2020**, *13*, 908–915. [CrossRef]
12. Whurr, R.; Lorch, M. Review of differential diagnosis and management of spasmodic dysphonia. *Curr. Opin. Otolaryngol. Head Neck Surg.* **2016**, *24*, 203–207. [CrossRef] [PubMed]
13. Simonyan, K.; Barkmeier-Kraemer, J.; Blitzer, A.; Hallett, M.; Houde, J.F.; Kimberley, T.J.; Ozelius, L.J.; Pitman, M.J.; Richardson, R.M.; Sharma, N.; et al. Laryngeal Dystonia. *Neurology* **2021**, *96*, 989–1001. [CrossRef] [PubMed]
14. Blitzer, A.; Brin, M.F.; Simonyan, K.; Ozelius, L.J.; Frucht, S. Phenomenology, genetics, and CNS network abnormalities in laryngeal dystonia: A 30-year experience. *Laryngoscope* **2017**, *128*, S1–S9. [CrossRef] [PubMed]
15. Guiry, S.; Worthley, A.; Simonyan, K. A separation of innate and learned vocal behaviors defines the symptomatology of spasmodic dysphonia. *Laryngoscope* **2018**, *129*, 1627–1633. [CrossRef] [PubMed]
16. Jankovic, J. Medical treatment of dystonia. *Mov. Disord.* **2013**, *28*, 1001–1012. [CrossRef] [PubMed]

17. Blitzer, A.; Brin, M.F.; Stewart, C.F. Botulinum toxin management of spasmodic dysphonia (laryngeal dystonia): A 12-year experience in more than 900 patients. *Laryngoscope* **2015**, *125*, 1751–1757. [CrossRef]
18. Termsarasab, P.; Thammongkolchai, T.; Frucht, S.J. Medical treatment of dystonia. *J. Clin. Mov. Disord.* **2016**, *3*, 1–18. [CrossRef]
19. Jinnah, H. Medical and Surgical Treatments for Dystonia. *Neurol. Clin.* **2020**, *38*, 325–348. [CrossRef]
20. Domingo, A.; Yadav, R.; Ozelius, L.J. Isolated dystonia: Clinical and genetic updates. *J. Neural Transm.* **2020**, *128*, 405–416. [CrossRef]
21. Lange, L.M.; Junker, J.; Loens, S.; Baumann, H.; Olschewski, L.; Schaake, S.; Madoev, H.; Petkovic, S.; Kuhnke, N.; Kasten, M.; et al. Genotype–Phenotype Relations for Isolated Dystonia Genes: MDSGene Systematic Review. *Mov. Disord.* **2021**, *36*, 1086–1103. [CrossRef]
22. Xiao, J.; Bastian, R.W.; Perlmutter, J.S.; Racette, B.A.; Tabbal, S.D.; Karimi, M.; Paniello, R.C.; Blitzer, A.; Batish, S.D.; Wszolek, Z.K.; et al. High-throughput mutational analysis of TOR1A in primary dystonia. *BMC Med. Genet.* **2009**, *10*, 24. [CrossRef] [PubMed]
23. Wilcox, R.A.; Winkler, S.; Lohmann, K.; Klein, C. Whispering dysphonia in an Australian family (DYT4): A clinical and genetic reappraisal. *Mov. Disord.* **2011**, *26*, 2404–2408. [CrossRef] [PubMed]
24. Lohmann, K.; Wilcox, R.A.; Winkler, S.; Ramirez, A.; Rakovic, A.; Park, J.S.; Arns, B.; Lohnau, T.; Groen, J.; Kasten, M.; et al. Whispering dysphonia (DYT4 dystonia) is caused by a mutation in the TUBB4 gene. *Ann. Neurol.* **2013**, *73*, 537–545.17. [CrossRef]
25. Djarmati, A.; Schneider, S.A.; Lohmann, K.; Winkler, S.; Pawlack, H.; Hagenah, J.; Brüggemann, N.; Zittel, S.; Fuchs, T.; Raković, A.; et al. Mutations in THAP1 (DYT6) and generalised dystonia with prominent spasmodic dysphonia: A genetic screening study. *Lancet. Neurol.* **2009**, *8*, 447–452. [CrossRef]
26. Xiao, J.; Zhao, Y.; Bastian, R.W.; Perlmutter, J.S.; Racette, B.A.; Tabbal, S.D.; Karimi, M.; Paniello, R.C.; Wszolek, Z.K.; Uitti, R.J.; et al. Novel THAP1 sequence variants in primary dystonia. *Neurology* **2010**, *74*, 229–238. [CrossRef]
27. Groen, J.L.; Yildirim, E.; Ritz, K.; Baas, F.; van Hilten, J.J.; van der Meulen, F.W.; Langeveld, T.P.; Tijssen, M.A. THAP1 mutations are infrequent in spasmodic dysphonia. *Mov. Disord.* **2011**, *26*, 1952–1954. [CrossRef]
28. Groen, J.L.; Kallen, M.C.; van de Warrenburg, B.P.; Speelman, J.D.; van Hilten, J.J.; Aramideh, M.; Boon, A.J.; Klein, C.; Koel-man, J.H.; Langeveld, T.P.; et al. Phenotypes and genetic architecture of focal primary torsion dystonia. *J. Neurol. Neurosurg. Psychiatry* **2012**, *83*, 1006–1011. [CrossRef]
29. LeDoux, M.S.; Xiao, J.; Rudzińska, M.; Bastian, R.W.; Wszolek, Z.K.; Van Gerpen, J.A.; Puschmann, A.; Momčilović, D.; Vemula, S.R.; Zhao, Y. Genotype-phenotype correlations in THAP1 dystonia: Molecular foundations and description of new cases. *Parkinsonism Relat. Disord.* **2012**, *18*, 414–425. [CrossRef]
30. de Gusmão, C.M.; Fuchs, T.; Moses, A.; Multhaupt-Buell, T.; Song, P.C.; Ozelius, L.J.; Franco, R.A.; Sharma, N. Dystonia-Causing Mutations as a Contribution to the Etiology of Spasmodic Dysphonia. *Otolaryngol. Head Neck Surg.* **2016**, *155*, 624–628. [CrossRef]
31. Kumar, K.R.; Davis, R.L.; Tchan, M.C.; Wali, G.M.; Mahant, N.; Ng, K.; Kotschet, K.; Siow, S.F.; Gu, J.; Walls, Z.; et al. Whole genome sequencing for the genetic diagnosis of heterogenous dystonia phenotypes. *Parkinsonism Relat. Disord.* **2019**, *69*, 111–118. [CrossRef]
32. Gultekin, M.; Prakash, N.; Ganos, C.; Mirza, M.; Bayramov, R.; Bhatia, K.P.; Mencacci, N.E. A Novel SGCE Nonsense Variant Associated With Marked Intrafamilial Variability in a Turkish Family With Myoclonus-Dystonia. *Mov. Disord. Clin. Pract.* **2019**, *6*, 479–482. [CrossRef] [PubMed]
33. Camargos, S.; Scholz, S.; Simón-Sánchez, J.; Paisán-Ruiz, C.; Lewis, P.; Hernandez, D.; Ding, J.; Gibbs, J.R.; Cookson, M.R.; Bras, J.; et al. DYT16, a novel young-onset dysto-nia-parkinsonism disorder: Identification of a segregating mutation in the stress-response protein PRKRA. *Lancet Neurol.* **2008**, *7*, 207–215. [CrossRef]
34. Camargos, S.; Lees, A.J.; Singleton, A.; Cardoso, F. DYT16: The original cases. *J. Neurol. Neurosurg. Psychiatry* **2012**, *83*, 1012–1014. [CrossRef] [PubMed]
35. Zech, M.; Castrop, F.; Schormair, B.; Jochim, A.; Wieland, T.; Gross, N.; Lichtner, P.; Peters, A.; Gieger, C.; Meitinger, T.; et al. DYT16 revisited: Exome sequencing identifies PRKRA mutations in a European dystonia family. *Mov. Disord.* **2014**, *29*, 1504–1510. [CrossRef]
36. Quadri, M.; Olgiati, S.; Sensi, M.; Gualandi, F.; Groppo, E.; Rispoli, V.; Graafland, J.; Breedveld, G.J.; Fabbrini, G.; Berardelli, A.; et al. PRKRA Mutation Causing Early-Onset Generalized Dystonia-Parkinsonism (DYT16) in an Italian Family. *Mov. Disord.* **2016**, *31*, 765–767. [CrossRef]
37. Charlesworth, G.; Plagnol, V.; Holmström, K.M.; Bras, J.; Sheerin, U.M.; Preza, E.; Rubio-Agusti, I.; Ryten, M.; Schneider, S.A.; Stamelou, M.; et al. Mutations in ANO3 cause dominant craniocervical dystonia: Ion channel implicated in pathogenesis. *Am. J. Hum. Genet.* **2012**, *91*, 1041–1050. [CrossRef]
38. Stamelou, M.; Charlesworth, G.; Cordivari, C.; Schneider, S.A.; Kägi, G.; Sheerin, U.M.; Rubio-Agusti, I.; Batla, A.; Houlden, H.; Wood, N.W.; et al. The phenotypic spectrum of DYT24 due to ANO3 mutations. *Mov. Disord.* **2014**, *29*, 928–934. [CrossRef]
39. Putzel, G.G.; Fuchs, T.; Battistella, G.; Rubien-Thomas, E.; Frucht, S.J.; Blitzer, A.; Ozelius, L.J.; Simonyan, K. GNAL mutation in isolated laryngeal dystonia. *Mov. Disord.* **2016**, *31*, 750–755. [CrossRef]
40. Zech, M.; Lam, D.D.; Francescatto, L.; Schormair, B.; Salminen, A.V.; Jochim, A.; Wieland, T.; Lichtner, P.; Peters, A.; Gieger, C.; et al. Recessive mutations in the α3 (VI) collagen gene COL6A3 cause early-onset isolated dystonia. *Am. J. Hum. Genet.* **2015**, *96*, 883–893. [CrossRef]

41. Meyer, E.; Carss, K.J.; Rankin, J.; Nichols, J.M.; Grozeva, D.; Joseph, A.P.; Mencacci, N.E.; Papandreou, A.; Ng, J.; Barral, S.; et al. Mutations in the histone methyltransferase gene KMT2B cause complex early-onset dystonia. *Nat. Genet.* **2017**, *49*, 223–237. [CrossRef]
42. Brás, A.; Ribeiro, J.A.; Sobral, F.; Moreira, F.; Morgadinho, A.; Januário, C. Early-onset oromandibular-laryngeal dys-tonia and Charlot gait: New phenotype of DYT-KMT2B. *Neurology* **2019**, *92*, 919. [CrossRef] [PubMed]
43. Carecchio, M.; Invernizzi, F.; Gonzàlez-Latapi, P.; Panteghini, C.; Zorzi, G.; Romito, L.; Leuzzi, V.; Galosi, S.; Reale, C.; Zibordi, F.; et al. Frequency and phenotypic spectrum of KMT2B dystonia in childhood: A single-center cohort study. *Mov. Disord.* **2019**, *34*, 1516–1527. [CrossRef] [PubMed]
44. Cif, L.; Demailly, D.; Lin, J.P.; Barwick, K.E.; Sa, M.; Abela, L.; Malhotra, S.; Chong, W.K.; Steel, D.; Sanchis-Juan, A.; et al. KMT2B-related disorders: Expansion of the phenotypic spectrum and long-term efficacy of deep brain stimulation. *Brain* **2020**, *143*, 3242–3261. [CrossRef] [PubMed]
45. Xavier, L.D.L.; Simonyan, K. The extrinsic risk and its association with neural alterations in spasmodic dysphonia. *Park. Relat. Disord.* **2019**, *65*, 117–123. [CrossRef]
46. Walter, U.; Blitzer, A.; Benecke, R.; Grossmann, A.; Dressler, D. Sonographic detection of basal ganglia abnormalities in spasmodic dysphonia. *Eur. J. Neurol.* **2013**, *21*, 349–352. [CrossRef]
47. Borujeni, M.J.S.; Esfandiary, E.; Almasi-Dooghaee, M. Childhood Laryngeal Dystonia Following Bilateral Globus Pallidus Abnormality: A Case Study and Review of Literature. *Iran. J. Otorhinolaryngol.* **2017**, *29*, 47–52.
48. Kiyuna, A.; Kise, N.; Hiratsuka, M.; Kondo, S.; Uehara, T.; Maeda, H.; Ganaha, A.; Suzuki, M. Brain Activity in Patients With Adductor Spasmodic Dysphonia Detected by Functional Magnetic Resonance Imaging. *J. Voice* **2017**, *31*, 379. [CrossRef]
49. Simonyan, K.; Berman, B.; Herscovitch, P.; Hallett, M. Abnormal Striatal Dopaminergic Neurotransmission during Rest and Task Production in Spasmodic Dysphonia. *J. Neurosci.* **2013**, *33*, 14705–14714. [CrossRef]
50. Simonyan, K.; Ludlow, C.L. Abnormal Activation of the Primary Somatosensory Cortex in Spasmodic Dysphonia: An fMRI Study. *Cereb. Cortex* **2010**, *20*, 2749–2759. [CrossRef]
51. Simonyan, K.; Tovar-Moll, F.; Ostuni, J.; Hallett, M.; Kalasinsky, V.F.; Lewin-Smith, M.R.; Rushing, E.J.; Vortmeyer, A.O.; Ludlow, C.L. Focal white matter changes in spasmodic dysphonia: A combined diffusion tensor imaging and neuropathological study. *Brain* **2007**, *131*, 447–459. [CrossRef]
52. Kanazawa, Y.; Kishimoto, Y.; Tateya, I.; Ishii, T.; Sanuki, T.; Hiroshiba, S.; Aso, T.; Omori, K.; Nakamura, K. Hyperactive sensorimotor cortex during voice perception in spasmodic dysphonia. *Sci. Rep.* **2020**, *10*, 1–11. [CrossRef] [PubMed]
53. Haslinger, B.; Erhard, P.; Dresel, C.; Castrop, F.; Roettinger, M.; Ceballos-Baumann, A.O. "Silent event-related" fMRI reveals reduced sensorimotor activation in laryngeal dystonia. *Neurology* **2005**, *65*, 1562–1569. [CrossRef] [PubMed]
54. Ali, S.O.; Thomassen, M.; Schulz, G.M.; Hosey, L.A.; Varga, M.; Ludlow, C.L.; Braun, A.R. Alterations in CNS Activity Induced by Botulinum Toxin Treatment in Spasmodic Dysphonia: An H 2 15 O PET Study. *J. Speech Lang. Hear. Res.* **2006**, *49*, 1127–1146. [CrossRef]
55. Kostic, V.S.; Agosta, F.; Sarro, L.; Tomić, A.; Kresojević, N.; Galantucci, S.; Svetel, M.; Valsasina, P.; Filippi, M. Brain structural changes in spasmodic dysphonia: A multimodal magnetic resonance imaging study. *Park. Relat. Disord.* **2016**, *25*, 78–84. [CrossRef]
56. Kirke, D.N.; Battistella, G.; Kumar, V.; Rubien-Thomas, E.; Choy, M.; Rumbach, A.; Simonyan, K. Neural correlates of dystonic tremor: A multimodal study of voice tremor in spasmodic dysphonia. *Brain Imaging Behav.* **2016**, *11*, 166–175. [CrossRef]
57. Khosravani, S.; Mahnan, A.; Yeh, I.-L.; Aman, J.E.; Watson, P.J.; Zhang, Y.; Goding, G.; Konczak, J. Laryngeal vibration as a non-invasive neuromodulation therapy for spasmodic dysphonia. *Sci. Rep.* **2019**, *9*, 1–11. [CrossRef]
58. Bianchi, S.; Fuertinger, S.; Ba, H.H.; Frucht, S.J.; Simonyan, K. Functional and structural neural bases of task specificity in isolated focal dystonia. *Mov. Disord.* **2019**, *34*, 555–563. [CrossRef]
59. Di Lazzaro, V.; Pilato, F.; Dileone, M.; Profice, P.; Ranieri, F.; Ricci, V.; Bria, P.; Tonali, P.; Ziemann, U. Segregating two inhibitory circuits in human motor cortex at the level of GABAA receptor subtypes: A TMS study. *Clin. Neurophysiol.* **2007**, *118*, 2207–2214. [CrossRef]
60. Turco, C.V.; El-Sayes, J.; Locke, M.B.; Chen, R.; Baker, S.; Nelson, A.J. Effects of lorazepam and baclofen on short- and long-latency afferent inhibition. *J. Physiol.* **2018**, *596*, 5267–5280. [CrossRef]
61. Turco, C.V.; El-Sayes, J.; Savoie, M.J.; Fassett, H.J.; Locke, M.B.; Nelson, A.J. Short- and long-latency afferent inhibition; uses, mechanisms and influencing factors. *Brain Stimul.* **2018**, *11*, 59–74. [CrossRef]
62. Richardson, S.P.; Bliem, B.; Lomarev, M.; Shamim, E.; Dang, N.; Hallett, M. Changes in short afferent inhibition during phasic movement in focal dystonia. *Muscle Nerve* **2007**, *37*, 358–363. [CrossRef] [PubMed]
63. Simonetta-Moreau, M.; Lourenço, G.; Sangla, S.; Mazières, L.; Vidailhet, M.; Meunier, S. Lack of inhibitory interaction between somatosensory afferent inputs and intracortical inhibitory interneurons in focal hand dystonia. *Mov. Disord.* **2006**, *21*, 824–834. [CrossRef] [PubMed]
64. Zittel, S.; Helmich, R.C.; Demiralay, C.; Münchau, A.; Bäumer, T. Normalization of sensorimotor integration by repetitive transcranial magnetic stimulation in cervical dystonia. *J. Neurol.* **2015**, *262*, 1883–1889. [CrossRef] [PubMed]
65. McCambridge, A.B.; Bradnam, L.V. Cortical neurophysiology of primary isolated dystonia and non-dystonic adults: A meta-analysis. *Eur. J. Neurosci.* **2020**, *53*, 1300–1323. [CrossRef]
66. Aoki, K.R. Pharmacology and Immunology of Botulinum Neurotoxins. *Int. Ophthalmol. Clin.* **2005**, *45*, 25–37. [CrossRef]

67. Blitzer, A.; Brin, M.F.; Stewart, C.F. Botulinum toxin management of spasmodic dysphonia (laryngeal dystonia): A 12-year experience in more than 900 patients. *Laryngoscope* **1998**, *108*, 1435–1441. [CrossRef]
68. Meyer, T.K.; Blitzer, A.B. Spasmodic Dysphonia. In *Handbook of Dystonia*; Stacy, M.A., Ed.; Informa Healthcare USA Inc.: New York, NY, USA, 2007; pp. 179–188.
69. Meyer, T.K. The treatment of laryngeal dystonia (spasmodic dysphonia) with botulinum toxin injections. *Oper. Tech. Otolaryngol. Neck Surg.* **2012**, *23*, 96–101. [CrossRef]
70. Sulica, L.; Blitzer, A. Botulinum toxin treatment of upper esophageal sphincter hyperfunction. *Oper. Tech. Otolaryngol. Neck Surg.* **2004**, *15*, 107–109. [CrossRef]
71. Naumann, M.; Jankovic, J. Safety of botulinum toxin type A: A systematic review and meta-analysis. *Curr. Med. Res. Opin.* **2004**, *20*, 981–990. [CrossRef]
72. Mejia, N.I.; Vuong, K.D.; Jankovic, J. Long-term botulinum toxin efficacy, safety, and immunogenicity. *Mov. Disord.* **2005**, *20*, 592–597. [CrossRef]
73. Currà, A.; Berardelli, A. Do the unintended actions of botulinum toxin at distant sites have clinical implications? *Neurology* **2009**, *72*, 1095–1099. [CrossRef] [PubMed]
74. Bomba-Warczak, E.; Vevea, J.D.; Brittain, J.M.; Figueroa-Bernier, A.; Tepp, W.H.; Johnson, E.A.; Yeh, F.L.; Chapman, E.R. Interneuronal Transfer and Distal Action of Tetanus Toxin and Botulinum Neurotoxins A and D in Central Neurons. *Cell Rep.* **2016**, *16*, 1974–1987. [CrossRef] [PubMed]
75. Davidson, B.J.; Ludlow, C.L. Long-Term Effects of Botulinum Toxin Injections in Spasmodic Dysphonia. *Ann. Otol. Rhinol. Laryngol.* **1996**, *105*, 33–42. [CrossRef] [PubMed]
76. Witmanowski, H.; Błochowiak, K. The whole truth about botulinum toxin—A review. *Adv. Dermatol. Allergol.* **2020**, *37*, 853–861. [CrossRef]
77. Santos, V.J.B.; Mattioli, F.M.; Mattioli, W.M.; Daniel, R.J.; Cruz, V.P.M. Laryngeal dystonia: Case report and treatment with botulinum toxin. *Braz. J. Otorhinolaryngol.* **2006**, *72*, 425–427. [CrossRef]
78. Evidente, V.G.H.; Ponce, F.A.; Evidente, M.H.; Lambert, M.; Garrett, R.; Sugumaran, M.; Lott, D.G. Adductor Spasmodic Dysphonia Improves with Bilateral Thalamic Deep Brain Stimulation: Report of 3 Cases Done Asleep and Review of Literature. *Tremor Other Hyperkinetic Mov.* **2020**, *10*. [CrossRef]
79. Krüger, M.T.; Hu, A.; Honey, C.R. Deep Brain Stimulation for Spasmodic Dysphonia: A Blinded Comparison of Unilateral and Bilateral Stimulation in Two Patients. *Ster. Funct. Neurosurg.* **2020**, *98*, 200–205. [CrossRef]
80. Poologaindran, A.; Ivanishvili, Z.; Morrison, M.D.; Rammage, L.A.; Sandhu, M.K.; Polyhronopoulos, N.E.; Honey, C.R. The effect of unilateral thalamic deep brain stimulation on the vocal dysfunction in a patient with spasmodic dysphonia: Interrogating cerebellar and pallidal neural circuits. *J. Neurosurg.* **2018**, *128*, 575–582. [CrossRef]
81. Stewart, C.F.; Sinclair, C.F.; Kling, I.F.; Diamond, B.E.; Blitzer, A. Adductor focal laryngeal Dystonia: Correlation between clinicians' ratings and subjects' perception of Dysphonia. *J. Clin. Mov. Disord.* **2017**, *4*, 20. [CrossRef]
82. Fulmer, S.L.; Merati, A.L.; Blumin, J.H. Efficacy of laryngeal botulinum toxin injection: Comparison of two techniques. *Laryngoscope* **2011**, *121*, 1924–1928. [CrossRef]
83. Risch, V.; Staiger, A.; Ziegler, W.; Ott, K.; Schölderle, T.; Pelykh, O.; Bötzel, K. How Does GPi-DBS Affect Speech in Primary Dystonia? *Brain Stimul.* **2015**, *8*, 875–880. [CrossRef] [PubMed]
84. Reese, R.; Gruber, D.; Schoenecker, T.; Bäzner, H.; Blahak, C.; Capelle, H.H.; Falk, D.; Herzog, J.; Pinsker, M.O.; Schneider, G.H.; et al. Long-term clinical outcome in meige syndrome treated with internal pallidum deep brain stimulation. *Mov. Disord.* **2011**, *26*, 691–698. [CrossRef] [PubMed]
85. Limotai, N.; Go, C.; Oyama, G.; Hwynn, N.; Zesiewicz, T.; Foote, K.; Bhidayasiri, R.; Malaty, I.; Zeilman, P.; Rodríguez, R.; et al. Mixed results for GPi-DBS in the treatment of cranio-facial and cranio-cervical dystonia symptoms. *J. Neurol.* **2011**, *258*, 2069–2074. [CrossRef] [PubMed]
86. Tisch, S.; Kumar, K.R. Pallidal Deep Brain Stimulation for Monogenic Dystonia: The Effect of Gene on Outcome. *Front. Neurol.* **2021**, *11*, 630391. [CrossRef]
87. Barrett, M.J.; Bressman, S. Genetics and Pharmacological Treatment of Dystonia. *Int. Rev. Neurobiol.* **2011**, *98*, 525–549. [CrossRef]
88. Sy, M.A.C.; Fernandez, H.H. Dystonia and leveraging oral pharmacotherapy. *J. Neural Transm.* **2021**, *128*, 521–529. [CrossRef]
89. Lizarraga, K.J.; Al-Shorafat, D.; Fox, S. Update on current and emerging therapies for dystonia. *Neurodegener. Dis. Manag.* **2019**, *9*, 135–147. [CrossRef]
90. Simonyan, K.; Frucht, S.; Blitzer, A.; Sichani, A.H.; Rumbach, A.F. A novel therapeutic agent, sodium oxybate, improves dystonic symptoms via reduced network-wide activity. *Sci. Rep.* **2018**, *8*, 1–8. [CrossRef]
91. Avidan, A.Y.; Kushida, C.A. The sodium in sodium oxybate: Is there cause for concern? *Sleep Med.* **2020**, *75*, 497–501. [CrossRef]
92. Escobar, A.M.; Martino, D.; Goodarzi, Z. The prevalence of anxiety in adult-onset isolated dystonia: A systematic review and meta-analysis. *Eur. J. Neurol.* **2021**, *28*, 4238–4250. [CrossRef]
93. Prudente, C.N.; Chen, M.; Stipancic, K.L.; Marks, K.L.; Samargia-Grivette, S.; Goding, G.S.; Green, J.R.; Kimberley, T.J. Effects of low-frequency repetitive transcranial magnetic stimulation in adductor laryngeal dystonia: A safety, feasibility, and pilot study. *Exp. Brain Res.* **2021**, *240*, 561–574. [CrossRef] [PubMed]

14. Rossini, P.M.; Burke, D.; Chen, R.; Cohen, L.G.; Daskalakis, Z.; Di Iorio, R.; Di Lazzaro, V.; Ferreri, F.; Fitzgerald, P.B.; George, M.S.; et al. Non-invasive electrical and magnetic stimulation of the brain, spinal cord, roots and peripheral nerves: Basic principles and procedures for routine clinical and research application. *An updated report from an IFCN Committee. Clin. Neurophysiol.* **2015**, *126*, 1071–1107. [CrossRef] [PubMed]
15. Soda, J.; Vidakovic, M.R.; Lorincz, J.; Jerkovic, A.; Vujovic, I. A Novel Latency Estimation Algorithm of Motor Evoked Potential Signals. *IEEE Access* **2020**, *8*, 193356–193374. [CrossRef]
16. Deletis, V.; Fernández-Conejero, I.; Ulkatan, S.; Rogić, M.; Carbó, E.L.; Hiltzik, D. Methodology for intra-operative recording of the corticobulbar motor evoked potentials from cricothyroid muscles. *Clin. Neurophysiol.* **2011**, *122*, 1883–1889. [CrossRef] [PubMed]
17. Richardson, S.P.; Wegele, A.R.; Skipper, B.; Deligtisch, A.; Jinnah, H.; Dystonia Coalition Investigators. Dystonia treatment: Patterns of medication use in an international cohort. *Neurology* **2017**, *88*, 543–550. [CrossRef]
18. Creighton, F.X.; Hapner, E.; Klein, A.; Rosen, A.; Jinnah, H.A.; Johns, M.M. Diagnostic Delays in Spasmodic Dysphonia: A Call for Clinician Education. *J. Voice* **2015**, *29*, 592–594. [CrossRef]
19. Macerollo, A.; Superbo, M.; Gigante, A.; Livrea, P.; Defazio, G. Diagnostic delay in adult-onset dystonia: Data from an Italian movement disorder center. *J. Clin. Neurosci.* **2015**, *22*, 608–610. [CrossRef]

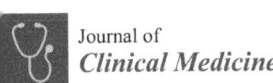

Review

Motor Skills and Visual Deficits in Developmental Coordination Disorder: A Narrative Review

Elena Pinero-Pinto [1], Rita Pilar Romero-Galisteo [2,*], María Carmen Sánchez-González [3], Isabel Escobio-Prieto [1,4], Carlos Luque-Moreno [1,4] and Rocío Palomo-Carrión [5]

1. Department of Physical Therapy. Faculty of Nursing, Physiotherapy and Podiatry, University of Seville, 41009 Seville, Spain
2. Department of Physiotherapy, Faculty of Science Health, University of Málaga, 29016 Málaga, Spain
3. Department of Physics of Condensed Matter, Optics Area, University of Seville, 41012 Seville, Spain
4. Instituto de Biomedicina de Sevilla (IBIS), 41013 Seville, Spain
5. Department of Nursing, Physiotherapy and Occupational Therapy, Faculty of Physiotherapy and Nursing, University of Castilla-La Mancha, 45071 Toledo, Spain
* Correspondence: rpromero@uma.es

Abstract: Background: Developmental coordination disorder (DCD) is a developmental disorder in which numerous comorbidities seem to coexist, such as motor and visual impairment and some executive functions; Methods: A narrative review on motor and visual deficits in children with DCD was carried out; Results and Discussion: Fine and gross motor skills are affected in children with DCD. In addition, they seem to be related to visual deficits, such as difficulty in visual perception, sensory processing and visual memory. Limitations have also been found in accommodation. Interventions in children with DCD should be aimed at improving both aspects, since vision affects motor skills and vice versa; Conclusions: In children with DCD, who present a marked deficit in global shape processing, it causes an association between deficiencies in visual perception and motor skills.

Keywords: developmental coordination disorder; visual deficits; motor skills; review; motor skills deficits; vision impairments; motor performance

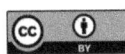

1. Introduction

Developmental coordination disorder (DCD) is a heterogeneous condition occurring in nearly 6% of the general population [1]. It appears that performance deficits may be related to functional and structural problems in a distributed neural network that supports motor control and learning [2].

The onset of symptoms is determined at an early age [3]. The main motor deficits described in the DSM-V are voluntary gaze control during movement, dependent motor training/learning, cognitive/motor integration and atypical motor network functioning [3]. Motor control deficits in DCD depend on the nature of the task to be performed. Deficits are evident for dual tasks and tasks that require greater temporal or spatial precision, or a more complex planning that requires some adaptation/adjustment at the perceptual-motor level to maintain stability [2]. In addition to motor impairments, which may affect all motor skills or only some motor skills [4–6], the literature reports other frequent impairments, such as visual [1,7,8], cognitive [9–11] and reduced executive functions [1,12].

In order to acquire proper motor skills, adequate visual feedback is necessary [13]. Children with DCD present some difficulties in sensory processing and integration [14,15], especially in visual perception [16,17]. These deficits in visual perception, as well as other visual disturbances present in children with DCD, appear to affect motor skills [15,16,18].

Children with visual deficits and a condition that affects their neurodevelopment may require extensive and specialized help, although there is no evidence on the most effective strategies for visual improvement in children with DCD [19]. The objective of this narrative review is to characterize the state of the art on visual deficiencies in individuals with DCD and their influence on motor deficits.

2. Materials and Methods

This narrative review presents an overview of the currently available literature regarding the epidemiology of visual and motor deficits in DCD and the intervention on these deficits. The study was based on reviews, original articles, meta-analyses and intervention guides published in English.

2.1. Information Sources

A literature search was performed from 1 August 2022 to 30 September 2022 using Web of Science, PubMed, Scopus, and Cinahl. The search was performed by two reviewers separately. The searches were carried out in the time period from 2002 to 2022. Any disagreements between the two reviewers were resolved by a third unblinded reviewer. Articles were screened by title and abstract, and subsequently, the full texts of the selected articles were examined.

2.2. Search Strategy

The literature search used various combinations of the keywords "developmental coordination disorder" AND "motor skills" OR "motor disorder" OR "motor skills disorders" OR "Motor Performance" in combination with one or more of the following: "vision", "visual", "vergence", "strabismus", "eye movements", "phoria", "stereovision", "stereoacuity", "refractive errors", "vision impairments" and "visual acuity". Those studies relevant to visual disturbances, motor disturbances and both deficits in combination with each other were selected, with the aim of identifying the relationship between them. Articles that were irrelevant to the scope of this review were excluded. Additional literature was identified from the reference lists cited in the initially identified articles.

2.3. Eligibility Criteria

The selection criteria included publications that described the visual characteristics of children with DCD, as well as those that described motor deficits in the same population, and those that included visual and motor variables in their intervention in these children. They had to be available in full text and written in English. Articles were excluded if: (1) they did not report data on motor and/or visual deficits in DCD; (2) the patients included were adults; (3) the article was a letter, conference abstract or study protocol. After applying electronic filters, duplicates and unintelligible articles were removed by including them in Mendeley (Mendeley Software, London, UK), which is a bibliographic software used to acquire and organize all references. Manual selection of titles and abstracts was performed immediately by two different reviewers. The selected eligible articles underwent a full-text review by two independent investigators.

2.4. Data Collection Process

Data were extracted using a standardized form, which included the following information: (1) names of the authors and year of publication, (2) type of study, (3) variable analyzed (visual/motor/both/intervention), and (4) relevant data.

2.5. Quality Assessment of Narrative Review Articles

To carry out the evaluation of this narrative review, we used the SANRA tool, which is a brief scale for the quality assessment of narrative review articles. SANRA's internal consistency and item-total correlation are sufficient, with satisfactory inter-rater reliability. This tool consists of 6 items: explanation of the review's importance (item 1) and statement of the aims (item 2) of the review, description of the literature search (item 3), referencing (item 4), scientific reasoning (item 5), and presentation of relevant and appropriate endpoint data (item 6). Two reviewers external to this study administered the SANRA tool to determine the quality of the study.

3. Results

3.1. Selection of Sources of Evidence

The search in the database, using the keywords mentioned above without any filter, resulted in 830 documents. After removing duplicates and articles that could not be read by Mendeley, a total of 394 articles remained in the sample. The manual selection of titles and abstracts resulted in the exclusion of 350 studies, leading to 44 eligible studies. A total of 4 papers were excluded from the study, since the data they provided were not relevant in relation to visual and motor skills in children with DCD. The selected studies are shown in Figure 1. Most of the selected studies were descriptive and experimental studies.

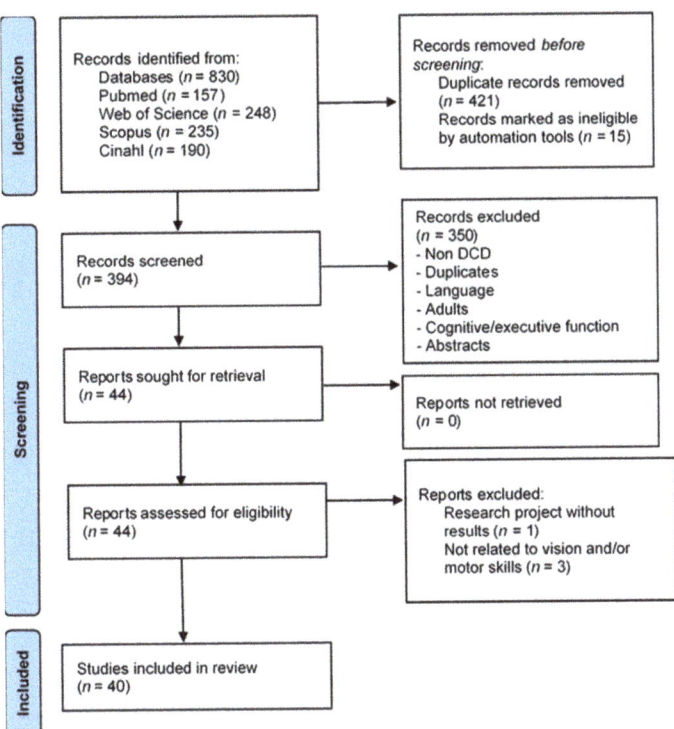

Figure 1. Schematic representation of the strategy for the selection of final articles.

3.2. Study Characteristics

A total of 7 articles addressed the motor skills of children with DCD with some involvement of the visual system [9,10,20–24]. Another 8 articles addressed the visual characteristics of children with DCD [25–32]. Of the 40 articles, 17 addressed the relationship between motor skills and vision in children with DCD, of which 10 investigated fine motor skills [4,8,33–40] and another 7 investigated gross motor skills [5,7,41–45]. The remaining 8 articles deal with visual intervention that influences the motor development of children with DCD [46–53]. Table 1 shows the specific characteristics of the selected studies, such as the type of study, the variable studied, and other relevant data.

Table 1. Characteristics of the selected studies.

Author (Date)	Design	n (Mean Age, Years)	Motor Skills	Visual Deficit	Fine Motor Skills	Gross Motor Skills	Visual/Motor Intervention
Van Dyck et al. (2022) [9]	D	50 (9)	•				
Adams et al. (2014) [20]	SR	-	•				
Opitz et al. (2020) [10]	D	24 (8.5)	•				
Tsai et al. (2008) [21]	D	64 (9.5)	•				
Geuze (2003) [22]	RCT	24 (9)	•				
Reynolds et al. (2017) [23]	D	29 (9.5)	•				
Grohs et al. (2021) [24]	CH	26 (10.6)	•				
Creavin et al. (2014) [25]	CS	7154 (7.5)		•			
Bilbao and Piñero (2021) [26]	ES	7 (9.5)		•			
Sumner et al. (2018) [27]	D	23 (8.9)		•			
Robert et al. (2014) [28]	D	27 (9)		•			
Gómez et al. (2017) [30]	D	20 (8.5)		•			
González et al. (2016) [29]	D	10 (10)		•			
Kagerer et al. (2004) [31]	ES	7 (8)		•			
Crawford and Dewey (2008) [32]	D	27 (8.8)		•			
Rafique and Northway (2015) [33]	D	9 (10.3)			•		
Rafique and Northway (2021) [34]	D	24 (10.4)			•	•	
Licari et al. (2018) [35]	D	11 (9.4)			•		
Braddick and Atkinson (2013) [36]	NR	-			•		
Arthur et al. (2021) [37]	D	19 (10)			•		
Wilmut et al. (2006) [38]	D	7 (7.5)			•		
Zoia et al. (2005) [4]	D	19 (9)			•		
Prunty et al. (2016) [8]	D	28 (11)			•		
Nobusako et al. (2018) [39]	ES	29 (9.8)			•		
Nobusako et al. (2021) [40]	ES	19 (9.3)			•		
Bair et al. (2012) [41]	ES	20 (9.1)				•	
Cherng et al. (2007) [5]	ES	20 (5)				•	
Fong et al. (2012) [42]	ES	22 (7.6)				•	
Bair et al. (2011) [43]	ES	11 (7.2)				•	
Deconinck et al. (2006) [44]	D	12 (7.8)				•	
Deconinck et al. (2008) [45]	ES	10 (7)				•	
Tsai et al. (2008) [21]	D	60 (10)				•	
Norouzi et al. (2021) [46]	ES	20 (8.5)					•
Miles et al. (2015) [47]	RCT	30 (9)					•
Wood et al. (2017) [48]	RCT	21 (8.6)					•
Coetzee and Pienaar (2013) [49]	CO	32 (7.9)					•
Fong et al. (2016) [50]	RCT	88 (7.7)					•
Wilson et al. (2016) [51]	RCT	54 (8)					•
Deconinck et al. (2009) [52]	ES	13 (9)					•
Slowinski et al. (2019) [53]	RTC *	21 (8.5)					•

n: sample size of children with DCD; D: Descriptive (not specified); SR: Systematic Review; RCT: Randomized Clinical Trial; CH: Cohort Study; CS: Cross sectional Study; ES: Experimental Study; NR: Narrative Review; CO: Cross-Over study; *: Pseudo-Randomized.

A total of 17 selected articles were descriptive studies, although some did not specify it [4,7–10,21,23,27–30,32–35,37,38,44]. Another 18 were experimental, including the RTCs [5,22,26,31,39–43,45–53]. The rest were other types of studies [20,24,25,36].

3.3. Quality Assessment of This Narrative Review Article

Two reviewers external to the research (MPS and JMSG) administered the SANRA tool to this narrative review to determine its quality level. The minimum score in each item is 0 and the maximum is 2, from lowest to highest quality in each item. The sum score of both reviewers is 11, with some difference that can be observed in Table 2.

Table 2. Scores obtained by the two reviewers in the SANRA narrative review quality tool.

Reviewer	Item 1	Item 2	Item 3	Item 4	Item 5	Item 6	Sum Score
1	2	1	2	2	2	2	11
2	2	2	2	2	2	1	11

4. Discussion

4.1. DCD Motor Skills

Seven studies examine the motor characteristics of children with DCD [9,10,20–24]. Children with DCD have fine and/or gross motor skills below the level expected for their age and learning opportunities [9]. According to the diagnostic criteria of the DSM-V [3], people with DCD acquire motor coordination below expectations for their chronological age and present clumsiness, inaccuracy in the performance of motor skills or slowness. The motor deficit described seems to interfere with activities of daily living, academic activities, or age-related leisure activities, although it has not been related to a medical condition or disease.

Research shows that children with DCD exhibit slower, more variable reaction times compared to typically developing children as a result of either slower processing speed, inefficient preparation of movement or both [15]. Motor planning appears to be impaired in DCD on most but not all tasks. Tests of visuomotor adaptation have shown that children with DCD present a lower capacity to adapt their movement to different task constraints. This has been shown by a higher movement variability, lower movement accuracy and/or longer movement durations [15]. Movement times or durations are frequently reported to be longer in children with DCD than in typically developing children, probably as a result of a stronger reliance on visual information for movement control [20].

Children with DCD also show delayed postural adjustment time [20]. Acquiring postural control requires the ability to integrate inputs from the somatosensory, visual, and vestibular systems and to use the integrated sensory signals to generate coordinated motor actions [42]. Opitz et al. [10] reported that children with DCD improved their reaction times when they were learning motor sequences, but showed less accuracy in distinguishing between different sequences. This impaired explicit discrimination was observed in different domains, including the visuospatial and temporal domain.

Motor control strategies to regulate muscle activity are less uniform and consistent than in typically developing children [42]. Different studies analyze postural patterns in children with DCD [5,21,22,42,50]. Alterations are found in the timing and pattern of activation of the postural muscles used to maintain posture during goal-directed reaching. The normal sequence of muscle activation from distal to proximal in disturbed standing was replaced by a pattern of activation from proximal to distal. Balance problems have also been found, with greater coactivation of leg muscles when standing on their non-preferred leg [21]. All of these neuromuscular deficits can affect the motor strategies used by these children for postural control.

Imitation and visual learning are essential for motor development; therefore, it is possible that imitation difficulties have an impact on the acquisition of movement in children with DCD [23]. To achieve a correct imitation, the integration of multiple sensory systems is required. That is why deficits in imitation could also be a consequence of dysfunction of processes that have also been associated with DCD, such as visual attention or processing, memory and executive function, sensory-perception function, or motor learning and adaptation. Furthermore, they are unlikely to be limited to a single area.

The difficulty in acquiring movement skills in children with DCD may be due, among other things, to a deficit in imitation and observational learning. Motor control is the ability to initiate and produce intentional, coordinated and precise movements [24], which are aspects that can be affected by coordination deficits and imitation deficits.

There are few studies looking at limb function in children with DCD [36–38]. Deficits found in manual skills in children with DCD include slower reaction time, reduced accuracy, and more variable speed of movement when reaching [4,24,36]. In relation to bimanual coordination in children with DCD, the scientific literature suggests that the deficits may be more evident in the non-dominant limb, in addition to the fact that children with DCD may also show difficulty with coupling between limbs [24]. In the most difficult bimanual tasks, bilateral deficits in spatiotemporal metrics are observed in children with DCD [46].

4.2. DCD Visual Deficits

A total of 8 studies have analyzed the visual disturbances that occur in children with DCD [25–32]. Children with severe DCD have abnormalities in binocular vision, refractive errors, and ocular alignment [25]. Accommodation abnormalities, which contribute to impaired motor skills in children with DCD, have also been found [33,34]. The study developed by Bilbao and Piñero [26], resolves that children with DCD have a significantly lower amplitude of accommodation and a trend of greater exophoria compared to those with other developmental disorders.

Sumner et al. [27] found deficits in maintaining participation in fixation and following tasks with more antisaccade errors in a group of children with DCD compared to a control group. Some studies [25,28] that analyzed eye-tracking records showed abnormal eye movements in children with DCD (on screen, the number of fixations was higher and the duration of each fixation was shorter in children with DCD than in control children). These children also made more saccadic eye movements. However, other authors [30] found no relationship between the imprecision of eye movements and the imprecision of numerical estimation in children with DCD. Gonzalez et al. [29] explain how cognitive control influences saccadic eye movements in children with DCD. It appears that these children are competent in executing saccades during reflexive conditions (without cues), but show deficiencies in more complex control processes involving prediction and inhibition.

In typically developing children, soft horizontal seeking is mature by the age of 7 years, whereas soft vertical seeking is not mature until late adolescence. Robert et al. [28] hypothesize that children with DCD have a late maturation of both search systems. In their study, horizontal pursuit gain was similar in both populations, but vertical pursuit gain was significantly impaired, that is, it was more saccadic in children with DCD than in typically developing children. Some atypical ocular motility has been identified in patients with DCD [27], especially with regard to poor sustained engagement in fixation in DCD subjects. There also appear to be differences in gaze behavior compared to control groups [37]. Gaze training was investigated to verify whether it retrospectively generated benefits in movement organization [53].

Children with DCD often have deficits in sensory processing and visual perception [9,14,18,31,50,54]. Children with DCD perform significantly worse on the visual perception test compared to typically developing children, although the deficits are not common to all children with DCD. This means that there is great variability in the visuoperceptive clinic of children with DCD [17]. Nevertheless, Crawford and Dewey [32] suggest that DCD alone is not associated with visual perception problems. According to these authors, the presence of concurrent disorders could be the key to visual perception deficits in children with DCD. However, the number of concurrent deficits present in DCD is associated with the severity of visual perception dysfunction. For example, deficits in visual memory skills appear to be a specific area of difficulty for children with DCD and concurrent reading disability and/or attention deficit hyperactivity disorder.

4.3. Relationship between Vision and Motor Skills

Of the selected studies, we found 17 that relate vision and motor skills, 10 of them in relation to fine motor skills [4,8,33–40] and the other 7 on gross motor skills [5,7,41–45].

In order to acquire proper motor skills, adequate visual feedback is necessary [13]. It is quite possible that impaired visuomotor integration could be a phenomenon that affects the results in all tasks. The most frequently observed deficit in DCD involves the processing of visual information, which is an aspect that determines motor behavior [20]. Children with DCD use somatosensory information for postural control as effectively as children with normal development. Somatosensory function normally matures at the age of 3–4 years and is not affected by DCD, as the results of Fong et al. [42] demonstrate. Thus, children with DCD partially compensate their balance problem by relying on somatosensory input. Visual-spatial processing and visual-kinesthetic integration are prerequisites for the successful maintenance of stability, and they are usually impaired in children with DCD [5,42,45].

In this line, the study carried out by Cheng et al. [6] examined the extent to which the motor deficits of children with DCD, evaluated with the Movement Assessment Battery for Children-2 (MABC-2), are linked to their visual perception abilities. Results indicated that poor performance within DCD on tasks such as static visual discrimination, visual sequential memory and eye-hand sequential coupling will negatively affect performance in MABC-2 or in tasks of daily living. For typically developing children, visual perceptual skills did not correlate with their motor skills. Based on these results, children with DCD may have trouble coordinating visual cues to perform motor tasks. A similar study was carried out by Van Waelvelde et al. [16]. In this case, children with DCD also performed significantly worse than the control group on all measures. The visual discrimination task was not significantly correlated with any of the motor tasks. In this case, the association between visual perceptual deficits and motor tasks was shown to be task-specific.

On the other hand, the relationship between accommodation and motor tasks in children with DCD has also been studied [33,34]. These children had significantly poorer accommodation facility and amplitude dynamics compared to the control group. Therefore, the results indicate a relationship between the alteration of accommodation and motor skills; more specifically, accommodation abnormalities were correlated with the performance of visuomotor, upper extremity and fine dexterity tasks [33]. Children with DCD exhibit reliance on accommodative feedback only on visuomotor and upper extremity tasks. Thus, children with DCD may be less dependent on visual feedback obtained from accommodation, as they have adaptive mechanisms to overcome faulty information when there are oculomotor abnormalities [34].

Micheletti et al. [54] suggest that two distinct visually related components, associated with global shape and global motion sensitivity, contribute to DCD differently across the range of severity of the disorder. In their study, the results within the DCD group indicate that the relationship between motor skill deficits and global visual perception is more complex than the comparison with typically developing controls indicates. When a marked deficit in global shape processing is present, as occurs in children with DCD, this dominates the association between deficits in visual perception and motor skills.

4.3.1. Vision Deficits and Fine Motor Skills

A total of 10 articles were selected based on the theme of fine motor skills and vision [4,8,33–40]. The scientific literature shows that manual functions are more affected by vision and its effects in children with DCD [34]. Manual motor tasks, with visual support, which requires predictive control, are affected in children with DCD [18]. Catching performance in children with DCD probably reflects a combination of errors in paying attention to visual information and organization of movement [35]. Children with DCD are less able to use a predictive strategy during visuo-manual follow-up with intermittent occlusion. They are also less proficient at tracking a moving target than typically developing children. Ferguson et al. [18] showed that children in the DCD group made more changes to their trajectory and more recovery movements. Moreover, tracking performance deteriorates when visual feedback is reduced. Other authors [36] also defend that certain deficits, such as DCD, present abnormal visuomanual actions, which are observed in bimanual coordination and in the visual guidance of the action in the task and failures in motor planning. Initially, the study of Arthur et al. [37] does not agree with this fact, since they did not find evidence to support the proposition that children with DCD coordinate their hands and eyes in a non-predictive way. However, in a later exploratory follow-up analysis, they did find differences in fundamental eye movement patterns between groups, and children in the DCD group showed some evidence of atypical visual sampling strategies and gaze-anchoring behaviors during the task.

Regarding eye-hand coordination in children with DCD, the study by Wilmut et al. [38] concludes that there is no evidence of a problem in the speed or precision of simple movements, although they observed difficulty in linking sequential changes of gaze and hand required to complete everyday tasks or typical assessment items. Along the same lines, Grohs et al. [24] reported that children with DCD presented greater variability in the speed of the dominant limb, as well as greater deviations from the ideal trajectory of the non-dominant limb. Similarly, when reaching for a target, the trajectories followed by the DCD group were longer and more curved than those of the control group in the study of Zoia et al. [4]. Moreover, deceleration times were longer for the DCD group. This study concludes that the use of visual feedback by children with DCD may be different from that of typically developing children. However, it seems that there is no consensus on the relationship between the deficit in visual perception and handwriting skills. Prunty et al. [8] examined the role of visual perception and visuomotor integration in the identification and explanation of writing difficulties (speed, legibility, and excessive pauses) in children with DCD; these authors found that, although the DCD group scored poorly on measures of visual perception, these were not predictive of their handwriting performance.

Overall, increased visual bias has been found to correlate with poor manual dexterity in children with DCD [40]. The study of Nobusako et al. [39] demonstrated that DCD children with clumsy manual dexterity have deficits in visuomotor temporal integration and automatic imitation function. In addition, they revealed a significant correlation between manual dexterity and visuomotor temporal integration measures. The results indicated that visuomotor temporal integration is the strongest predictor of poor manual dexterity.

4.3.2. Vision Deficits and Gross Motor Skills

Seven articles were found that related gross motor skills and vision [5,7,41–45]. According to Bair et al. [41], the postural body schema and the development of the dorsal stream are useful in explaining the reweighting of low vision. The lack of multisensory fusion supports the notion that optimal multisensory integration is a slow developmental process and is vulnerable in children with DCD.

Among the gross motor skills, balance or stability in standing posture stands out. Several studies have explored the influence of vision on standing balance in children with DCD [5,21,22,41–43]. For example, Cherng et al. [5] showed that the standing stability of children with DCD was significantly poorer than that of control children subjected to different sensory conditions (visual and somatosensory inputs). The results suggest that children with DCD experience more difficulty in coping with altered sensory input, which has also been reported by Deconinck et al. [45]. In all conditions that the children were subjected to, the mean postural sway velocity was greater for children with DCD. It also revealed a greater reliance on vision in children with DCD when standing on a firm surface. These results suggest that postural control problems may still be associated with difficulties reappraising sensory information in response to environmental demands. Tsai et al. [21] were more precise in their study, since they discriminated between the dominant and non-dominant leg and between sexes. DCD children showed more difficulty standing on the non-dominant leg with their eyes open and closed. In addition, while the boys showed results similar to those of the total group, the girls with DCD only obtained significant differences in three conditions with eyes closed, but not with eyes open. Geuze [22] corroborates these results. In their study, DCD children had more difficulty standing on one leg with their eyes closed. While standing on the non-preferred leg, the DCD children's electromyograms showed slightly greater coactivation of lower and upper leg muscles. If standing was disturbed, children with DCD took longer to regain their posture. However, children with DCD learned to compensate for the disturbance in a few attempts. In difficult or novel situations, children with DCD appear to suffer from increased postural sway as a result of suboptimal balance control. To facilitate standing postural control, Bair et al. [43] suggest that children with DCD benefit from the use of vision in combination with tactile information, possibly due to their less developed internal models of body orientation and self-motion. Internal model deficits, among other postural deficits, may increase balance impairment in children with DCD.

According to Tsai [7], DCD children performed significantly worse than the control group, although only visual perception and motor skills with timed responses were significantly correlated. Therefore, visual perception related to motor performance has a speed component in these children. This is also related to the results of Deconinck et al. [44] regarding the relationship of vision and gait in children with DCD. These authors suggest that children with DCD are more dependent on global visual flow information than typically developing children for maintenance of balance and speed control during gait. This increased reliance on visual control could be associated with an underdeveloped internal sensorimotor model.

4.4. Interventions for Vision and Motor Deficits in DCD

Of the selected studies, 8 refer to visual intervention as a therapy that directly influences the motor skills of children with DCD [46–48,50–53]. Children with DCD who meet diagnostic criteria generally need treatment. The indications for intervention essentially depend on the influence of the diagnosis on activities of daily living. However, in some cases, the diagnosis does not indicate treatment [2].

If DCD requirements are met but there are motor problems in performing tasks of daily living and in educational and social support, then strategies for participation in all environmental contexts should be implemented. This is common in children under 5 years of age who have significant motor problems but do not meet all the diagnostic criteria for DCD. Recommendation 17 of the International clinical practice recommendations on intervention in children with DCD is that evidence of effectiveness, including regimen and dose, should be considered when planning intervention. In the case of co-occurring disorders, they recommend that intervention priorities be established according to the type and severity of each disorder, and in consultation with the child and family [2].

There are different studies that analyze the effect of visual training to improve motor skills in children with DCD [46–48]. Quiet-Eye Training (QET) has been shown to be more effective than traditional training methods in teaching a throw and catch task. In the study of Miles et al. [47], QET improved DCD children's ability to focus on a target on the wall before throwing, as well as better anticipation and tracking of the ball, which translates into better catching technique. QET could be an effective adjunct for therapists teaching visual-motor skills to children with DCD. Along the same lines, Norouzi Seyed Hosseini et al. [46] analyzed the effect of TQT on the bimanual coordination of children with DCD. The results indicated that the coordination mode performance was strongly influenced by the QET. Therefore, they conclude that the successful performance of a bimanual linear task depends mainly on the availability of visual feedback. Similarly, Wood et al. [48] have been shown to improve the ability to throw and catch a ball in children with DCD through TCE, which in turn also alleviates the negative psychosocial impact of these motor skill deficits. All parents of children with DCD in this study reported improvements in their children's confidence, social skills, and predilection for physical activity after testing.

Coetzee and Pienaar [49] carried out a vision therapy program in children with DCD to verify whether visual motor problems improved. The vision therapy program lasted 18 weeks and was carried out once a week, with 40 min per session. A 75–100% improvement in visual tracking, fixation, ocular alignment, and convergence was reported in children with DCD, who underwent an 18-week vision therapy program [49].

The study of Nobusako et al. [39] suggested that improving visuomotor ability temporal integration can be an effective rehabilitation strategy for DCD. Therefore, it is necessary to develop new neurorehabilitation techniques that favor visuomotor temporal integration. In the same line, Fong et al. [50] showed that task-specific balance training marginally improves somatosensory function and somewhat improves balance performance in children with DCD. It appears that, by improving motor function, it is also possible to improve deficits in visual function.

In another sense, results suggest that motor imagery is accessible to children with DCD, but less refined/developed compared with healthy controls [20,51]. Different studies found that children with DCD were able to perform motor imagery, although with a slower and less accurate rate of mental transformation than controls [20,52,55,56]. The motor imaging deficit observed in children with DCD is associated with motor imaging accuracy, rather than vividness [56]. Generally, it seems that children with DCD may incorporate motor imagery adequately for simple tasks, but may use it less consistently than typically developing children. In motor planning tasks, it is important to systematically vary the complexity of motor imagery tasks to identify the specific capacities of the child with DCD [20]. As such, motor imagery can be voluntarily incorporated to reinforce the relationship between the (simulated) motor output signal and the resulting behavior of the physical system. The results of motor imagery training in improved skill and function are pervasive in motor learning. In a motor imagery training study, Wilson et al. [51] showed training effects comparable to conventional physical therapy. The mechanism of change could be related to the training of predictive models of action with repeated mental simulation.

4.5. Limitations and Strengths

Despite its narrative nature, the present study provides a comprehensive and systematic overview on visual disturbances in children with DCD and their possible influence on motor deficits.

However, we are aware that some documents may have been lost. A lack of consistent data in the reports, which are not always supported by numbers and statistics, suggests the need for more transparent and objective studies based on standardized reports. However, to our knowledge, this is the first study to describe related visual and motor impairments in children with DCD.

5. Conclusions and Clinical Implications

In children with DCD, the literature seems to indicate that there is a clear association between visual deficits and motor skills, both fine and gross. Future research should delve into this last relationship at the functional level to enable effective interventions. Due to the lack of homogeneity in the current studies on the relationship between vision and motor skills in children with DCD, more randomized clinical trials, as well as descriptive studies that analyze this relationship in depth, are necessary to establish a correct intervention for these children. It would be interesting for future research to use a fuller overview of methods, intervention and findings so that comparisons can be made between different studies.

Author Contributions: Conceptualization, E.P.-P. and R.P.-C.; methodology, R.P.R.-G.; investigation, E.P.-P.; writing—original draft preparation, E.P.-P. and M.C.S.-G.; writing—review and editing, E.P.-P. and I.E.-P.; visualization, C.L.-M.; supervision, C.L.-M.; project administration, R.P.R.-G. and R.P.-C. All authors have read and agreed to the published version of the manuscript.

Funding: This research received no external funding.

Institutional Review Board Statement: Not applicable.

Informed Consent Statement: Not applicable.

Data Availability Statement: Not applicable.

Conflicts of Interest: The authors declare no conflict of interest.

References

1. Farmer, M.; Echenne, B.; Drouin, R.; Bentourkia, M. Insights in Developmental Coordination Disorder. *Curr. Pediatr. Rev.* **2017**, *13*, 111–119. [CrossRef] [PubMed]
2. Blank, R.; Barnett, A.L.; Cairney, J.; Green, D.; Kirby, A.; Polatajko, H.; Rosenblum, S.; Smits-Engelsman, B.; Sugden, D.; Wilson, P.; et al. International clinical practice recommendations on the definition, diagnosis, assessment, intervention, and psychosocial aspects of developmental coordination disorder. *Dev. Med. Child Neurol.* **2019**, *61*, 242–286. [CrossRef] [PubMed]
3. American Psychiatric Association. *Diagnostic and Statistical Manual of Mental Disorders*, 5th ed.; American Psychiatric Association: Arlington, VA, USA, 2013; ISBN 0-89042-555-8.
4. Zoia, S.; Castiello, U.; Blason, L.; Scabar, A. Reaching in children with and without developmental coordination disorder under normal and perturbed vision. *Dev. Neuropsychol.* **2005**, *27*, 257–273. [CrossRef] [PubMed]
5. Cherng, R.J.; Hsu, Y.W.; Chen, Y.J.; Chen, J.Y. Standing balance of children with developmental coordination disorder under altered sensory conditions. *Hum. Mov. Sci.* **2007**, *26*, 913–926. [CrossRef]
6. Cheng, C.H.; Ju, Y.Y.; Chang, H.W.; Chen, C.L.; Pei, Y.C.; Tseng, K.C.; Cheng, H.Y.K. Motor impairments screened by the movement assessment battery for children-2 are related to the visual-perceptual deficits in children with developmental coordination disorder. *Res. Dev. Disabil.* **2014**, *35*, 2172–2179. [CrossRef]
7. Tsai, C.L.; Wu, S.K. Relationship of visual perceptual deficit and motor impairment in children with developmental coordination disorder. *Percept. Mot. Skills* **2008**, *107*, 457–472. [CrossRef]
8. Prunty, M.; Barnett, A.L.; Wilmut, K.; Plumb, M. Visual perceptual and handwriting skills in children with Developmental Coordination Disorder. *Hum. Mov. Sci.* **2016**, *49*, 54–65. [CrossRef]
9. Van Dyck, D.; Baijot, S.; Aeby, A.; De Tiège, X.; Deconinck, N. Cognitive, perceptual, and motor profiles of school-aged children with developmental coordination disorder. *Front. Psychol.* **2022**, *13*, 1–22. [CrossRef]
10. Opitz, B.; Brady, D.; Leonard, H.C. Motor and non-motor sequence prediction is equally affected in children with developmental coordination disorder. *PLoS ONE* **2020**, *15*, e0232562. [CrossRef]
11. Wilson, P.; Ruddock, S.; Rahimi-Golkhandan, S.; Piek, J.; Sugden, D.; Green, D.; Steenbergen, B. Cognitive and motor function in developmental coordination disorder. *Dev. Med. Child Neurol.* **2020**, *62*, 1317–1323. [CrossRef]
12. Vaivre-Douret, L. Executive function in persisting versus remitting developmental coordination disorder. *Dev. Med. Child Neurol.* **2020**, *62*, 1235. [CrossRef] [PubMed]
13. Lino, F.; Chieffo, D.P.R. Developmental Coordination Disorder and Most Prevalent Comorbidities: A Narrative Review. *Children* **2022**, *9*, 1095. [CrossRef] [PubMed]
14. Allen, S.; Casey, J. Developmental coordination disorders and sensory processing and integration: Incidence, associations and co-morbidities. *Br. J. Occup. Ther.* **2017**, *80*, 549–557. [CrossRef] [PubMed]
15. Coats, R.O.A.; Britten, L.; Utley, A.; Astill, S.L. Multisensory integration in children with Developmental Coordination Disorder. *Hum. Mov. Sci.* **2015**, *43*, 15–22. [CrossRef]
16. Van Waelvelde, H.; De Weerdt, W.; De Cock, P.; Smits-Engelsman, B.C.M. Association between visual perceptual deficits and motor deficits in children with developmental coordination disorder. *Dev. Med. Child Neurol.* **2004**, *46*, 661–666. [CrossRef]
17. Tsai, C.L.; Wilson, P.H.; Wu, S.K. Role of visual-perceptual skills (non-motor) in children with developmental coordination disorder. *Hum. Mov. Sci.* **2008**, *27*, 649–664. [CrossRef]
18. Ferguson, G.D.; Duysens, J.; Smits-Engelsman, B.C.M. Children with Developmental Coordination Disorder are deficient in a visuo-manual tracking task requiring predictive control. *Neuroscience* **2015**, *286*, 13–26. [CrossRef]
19. Williams, C.; Northstone, K.; Borwick, C.; Gainsborough, M.; Roe, J.; Howard, S.; Rogers, S.; Amos, J.; Woodhouse, J.M. How to help children with neurodevelopmental and visual problems: A scoping review. *Br. J. Ophthalmol.* **2014**, *98*, 6. [CrossRef]
20. Adams, I.L.J.; Lust, J.M.; Wilson, P.H.; Steenbergen, B. Compromised motor control in children with DCD: A deficit in the internal model?-A systematic review. *Neurosci. Biobehav. Rev.* **2014**, *47*, 225–244. [CrossRef]
21. Tsai, C.L.; Wu, S.K.; Huang, C.H. Static balance in children with developmental coordination disorder. *Hum. Mov. Sci.* **2008**, *27*, 142–153. [CrossRef]
22. Geuze, R.H. Static balance and developmental coordination disorder. *Hum. Mov. Sci.* **2003**, *22*, 527–548. [CrossRef] [PubMed]
23. Reynolds, J.E.; Kerrigan, S.; Elliott, C.; Lay, B.S.; Licari, M.K. Poor Imitative Performance of Unlearned Gestures in Children with Probable Developmental Coordination Disorder. *J. Mot. Behav.* **2017**, *49*, 378–387. [CrossRef] [PubMed]
24. Grohs, M.N.; Hawe, R.L.; Dukelow, S.P.; Dewey, D. Unimanual and bimanual motor performance in children with developmental coordination disorder (DCD) provide evidence for underlying motor control deficits. *Sci. Rep.* **2021**, *11*, 1–13. [CrossRef] [PubMed]
25. Creavin, A.L.; Lingam, R.; Northstone, K.; Williams, C. Ophthalmic abnormalities in children with developmental coordination disorder. *Dev. Med. Child Neurol.* **2014**, *56*, 164–170. [CrossRef] [PubMed]
26. Bilbao, C.; Piñero, D.P. Distribution of Visual and Oculomotor Alterations in a Clinical Population of Children with and without Neurodevelopmental Disorders. *Brain Sci.* **2021**, *11*, 351. [CrossRef]
27. Sumner, E.; Hutton, S.B.; Kuhn, G.; Hill, E.L. Oculomotor atypicalities in Developmental Coordination Disorder. *Dev. Sci.* **2018**, *21*, 1–12. [CrossRef]

28. Robert, M.P.; Ingster-Moati, I.; Albuisson, E.; Cabrol, D.; Golse, B.; Vaivre-Douret, L. Vertical and horizontal smooth pursuit eye movements in children with developmental coordination disorder. *Dev. Med. Child Neurol.* **2014**, *56*, 595–600. [CrossRef]
29. Gonzalez, C.C.; Mon-Williams, M.; Burke, S.; Burke, M.R. Cognitive Control of Saccadic Eye Movements in Children with Developmental Coordination Disorder. *PLoS ONE* **2016**, *11*, e0165380. [CrossRef]
30. Gomez, A.; Piazza, M.; Jobert, A.; Dehaene-Lambertz, G.; Huron, C. Numerical abilities of school-age children with Developmental Coordination Disorder (DCD): A behavioral and eye-tracking study. *Hum. Mov. Sci.* **2017**, *55*, 315–326. [CrossRef]
31. Kagerer, F.A.; Bo, J.; Contreras-Vidal, J.L.; Clark, J.E. Visuomotor adaptation in children with developmental coordination disorder. *Motor Control* **2004**, *8*, 450–460. [CrossRef]
32. Crawford, S.G.; Dewey, D. Co-occurring disorders: A possible key to visual perceptual deficits in children with developmental coordination disorder? *Hum. Mov. Sci.* **2008**, *27*, 154–169. [CrossRef] [PubMed]
33. Rafique, S.A.; Northway, N. Relationship of ocular accommodation and motor skills performance in developmental coordination disorder. *Hum. Mov. Sci.* **2015**, *42*, 1–14. [CrossRef] [PubMed]
34. Rafique, S.A.; Northway, N. Reliance on visual feedback from ocular accommodation on motor skills in children with developmental coordination disorder and typically developing controls. *Hum. Mov. Sci.* **2021**, *76*, 1–10. [CrossRef]
35. Licari, M.K.; Reynolds, J.E.; Tidman, S.; Ndiaye, S.; Sekaran, S.N.; Reid, S.L.; Lay, B.S. Visual tracking behaviour of two-handed catching in boys with developmental coordination disorder. *Res. Dev. Disabil.* **2018**, *83*, 280–286. [CrossRef] [PubMed]
36. Braddick, O.; Atkinson, J. Visual control of manual actions: Brain mechanisms in typical development and developmental disorders. *Dev. Med. Child Neurol.* **2013**, *55* (Suppl. 4), 13–18. [CrossRef]
37. Arthur, T.; Harris, D.J.; Allen, K.; Naylor, C.E.; Wood, G.; Vine, S.; Wilson, M.R.; Tsaneva-Atanasova, K.; Buckingham, G. Visuo-motor attention during object interaction in children with developmental coordination disorder. *Cortex* **2021**, *138*, 318–328. [CrossRef]
38. Wilmut, K.; Wann, J.P.; Brown, J.H. Problems in the coupling of eye and hand in the sequential movements of children with Developmental Coordination Disorder. *Child. Care. Health Dev.* **2006**, *32*, 665–678. [CrossRef]
39. Nobusako, S.; Sakai, A.; Tsujimoto, T.; Shuto, T.; Nishi, Y.; Asano, D.; Furukawa, E.; Zama, T.; Osumi, M.; Shimada, S.; et al. Deficits in Visuo-Motor Temporal Integration Impacts Manual Dexterity in Probable Developmental Coordination Disorder. *Front. Neurol.* **2018**, *9*, 1–15. [CrossRef]
40. Nobusako, S.; Osumi, M.; Furukawa, E.; Nakai, A.; Maeda, T.; Morioka, S. Increased visual bias in children with developmental coordination disorder: Evidence from a visual-tactile temporal order judgment task. *Hum. Mov. Sci.* **2021**, *75*, 1–12. [CrossRef]
41. Bair, W.N.; Kiemel, T.; Jeka, J.J.; Clark, J.E. Development of multisensory reweighting is impaired for quiet stance control in children with developmental coordination disorder (DCD). *PLoS ONE* **2012**, *7*, e40932. [CrossRef]
42. Fong, S.S.M.; Tsang, W.W.N.; Ng, G.Y.F. Altered postural control strategies and sensory organization in children with developmental coordination disorder. *Hum. Mov. Sci.* **2012**, *31*, 1317–1327. [CrossRef]
43. Bair, W.N.; Barela, J.A.; Whitall, J.; Jeka, J.J.; Clark, J.E. Children with Developmental Coordination Disorder benefit from using vision in combination with touch information for quiet standing. *Gait Posture* **2011**, *34*, 183–190. [CrossRef] [PubMed]
44. Deconinck, F.J.A.; De Clercq, D.; Savelsbergh, G.J.P.; Van Coster, R.; Oostra, A.; Dewitte, G.; Lenoir, M. Visual contribution to walking in children with Developmental Coordination Disorder. *Child. Care. Health Dev.* **2006**, *32*, 711–722. [CrossRef] [PubMed]
45. Deconinck, F.J.A.; De Clercq, D.; Van Coster, R.; Oostra, A.; Dewitte, G.; Savelsbergh, G.J.P.; Cambier, D.; Lenoir, M. Sensory contributions to balance in boys with developmental coordination disorder. *Adapt. Phys. Activ. Q.* **2008**, *25*, 17–35. [CrossRef] [PubMed]
46. Norouzi Seyed Hosseini, R.; Norouzi, E.; Soleymani, M. Effects of Quiet Eye Training on Performance of Bimanual Coordination in Children with DCD. *Iran. J. Child Neurol.* **2021**, *15*, 43–54. [CrossRef]
47. Miles, C.A.L.; Wood, G.; Vine, S.J.; Vickers, J.N.; Wilson, M.R. Quiet eye training facilitates visuomotor coordination in children with developmental coordination disorder. *Res. Dev. Disabil.* **2015**, *40*, 31–41. [CrossRef]
48. Wood, G.; Miles, C.A.L.; Coyles, G.; Alizadehkhaiyat, O.; Vine, S.J.; Vickers, J.N.; Wilson, M.R. A randomized controlled trial of a group-based gaze training intervention for children with Developmental Coordination Disorder. *PLoS ONE* **2017**, *12*, e0171782. [CrossRef]
49. Coetzee, D.; Pienaar, A.E. The effect of visual therapy on the ocular motor control of seven- to eight-year-old children with developmental coordination disorder (DCD). *Res. Dev. Disabil.* **2013**, *34*, 4073–4084. [CrossRef]
50. Fong, S.S.M.; Guo, X.; Liu, K.P.Y.; Ki, W.Y.; Louie, L.H.T.; Chung, R.C.K.; Macfarlane, D.J. Task-Specific Balance Training Improves the Sensory Organisation of Balance Control in Children with Developmental Coordination Disorder: A Randomised Controlled Trial. *Sci. Rep.* **2016**, *6*, 1–8. [CrossRef]
51. Wilson, P.H.; Thomas, P.R.; Maruff, P. Motor Imagery Training Ameliorates Motor Clumsiness in Children. *J. Child Neurol.* **2016**, *17*, 491–498. [CrossRef]
52. Deconinck, F.J.A.; Spitaels, L.; Fias, W.; Lenoir, M. Is developmental coordination disorder a motor imagery deficit? *J. Clin. Exp. Neuropsychol.* **2009**, *31*, 720–730. [CrossRef] [PubMed]
53. Słowiński, P.; Baldemir, H.; Wood, G.; Alizadehkhaiyat, O.; Coyles, G.; Vine, S.; Williams, G.; Tsaneva-Atanasova, K.; Wilson, M. Gaze training supports self-organization of movement coordination in children with developmental coordination disorder. *Sci. Rep.* **2019**, *9*, 1–11. [CrossRef] [PubMed]

54. Micheletti, S.; Corbett, F.; Atkinson, J.; Braddick, O.; Mattei, P.; Galli, J.; Calza, S.; Fazzi, E. Dorsal and Ventral Stream Function in Children With Developmental Coordination Disorder. *Front. Hum. Neurosci.* **2021**, *15*, 703217. [CrossRef] [PubMed]
55. Williams, J.; Thomas, P.R.; Maruff, P.; Butson, M.; Wilson, P.H. Motor, visual and egocentric transformations in children with Developmental Coordination Disorder. *Child. Care. Health Dev.* **2006**, *32*, 633–647. [CrossRef]
56. Fuchs, C.T.; Caçola, P. Differences in accuracy and vividness of motor imagery in children with and without Developmental Coordination Disorder. *Hum. Mov. Sci.* **2018**, *60*, 234–241. [CrossRef]

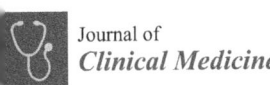

The Impact of Nonmotor Symptoms on Health-Related Quality of Life in Parkinson's Disease: A Network Analysis Approach

Konstantin G. Heimrich [1,*], Aline Schönenberg [2], Diego Santos-García [3], Pablo Mir [4,5], COPPADIS Study Group [6,†] and Tino Prell [2]

1. Department of Neurology, Jena University Hospital, Am Klinikum 1, 07747 Jena, Germany
2. Department of Geriatrics, Halle University Hospital, Ernst-Grube-Straße 40, 06120 Halle, Germany
3. Department of Neurology, CHUAC (Complejo Hospitalario Universitario de A Coruña), c/As Xubias 84, 15006 A Coruña, Spain
4. Unidad de Trastornos del Movimiento, Servicio de Neurología y Neurofisiología Clínica, Instituto de Biomedicina de Sevilla, Hospital Universitario Virgen del Rocío/CSIC/Universidad de Sevilla, 41013 Seville, Spain
5. Centro de Investigación Biomédica en Red Sobre Enfermedades Neurodegenerativas (CIBERNED), 28031 Madrid, Spain
6. Fundación Española de Ayuda a la Investigación en Enfermedades Neurodegenerativas y/o de Origen Genético, Calle Antonio J de Sucre 1A, 15179 Oleiros, Spain
* Correspondence: konstantin.heimrich@med.uni-jena.de
† Membership of the COPPADIS Study Group is provided in the Appendix A.

Abstract: Nonmotor symptoms negatively affect health-related quality of life (HRQoL) in patients with Parkinson's disease (PD). However, it is unknown which nonmotor symptoms are most commonly associated with HRQoL. Considering the complex interacting network of various nonmotor symptoms and HRQoL, this study aimed to reveal the network structure, explained HRQoL variance, and identify the nonmotor symptoms that primarily affect HRQoL. We included 689 patients with PD from the Cohort of Patients with Parkinson's Disease in Spain (COPPADIS) study who were rated on the Nonmotor Symptoms Scale in Parkinson's disease (NMSS) and the Parkinson´s Disease Questionnaire 39 (PDQ-39) at baseline. Network analyses were performed for the 30 items of the NMSS and both the PDQ-39 summary index and eight subscales. The nodewise predictability, edge weights, strength centrality, and bridge strength were determined. In PD, nonmotor symptoms are closely associated with the mobility, emotional well-being, cognition, and bodily discomfort subscales of the PDQ-39. The most influential nonmotor symptoms were found to be fatigue, feeling sad, hyperhidrosis, impaired concentration, and daytime sleepiness. Further research is needed to confirm whether influencing these non-motor symptoms can improve HRQoL.

Keywords: Parkinson disease; nonmotor symptoms; quality of life; cognition; depression; fatigue; hyperhidrosis; disorders of excessive somnolence; network analysis; NMSS; PDQ-39

1. Introduction

Parkinson's disease (PD) is a progressive, multisystem neurodegenerative disorder characterized by motor and nonmotor symptoms [1]. Owing to the progressive nature of the disease, health-related quality of life (HRQoL) is an essential focus when treating PD. Numerous studies have shown the contribution of nonmotor symptoms to the deterioration of patients' quality of life [2–11]. However, nonmotor symptoms are often poorly recognized [2].

HRQoL is a multidimensional concept that is commonly used to examine the impact of health status on the quality of life. It usually includes physical, mental, and social domains of health [12]. The Parkinson´s Disease Questionnaire 39 (PDQ-39) is the most thoroughly tested and frequently applied questionnaire [13]. It is a disease-specific and self-rated questionnaire that detects minor changes in HRQoL [14,15]. The 39 items included in the

PDQ-39 are grouped into eight domains and their respective subscales, the mean value of which determines the summary index. However, as mentioned above, HRQoL is a multidimensional concept, and using the summary index of the PDQ-39 instead of the eight subscales does not adequately account for its complexity [16]. Moreover, patients with limitations in the physical domain of HRQoL are expected to require different therapies than those with limitations in the emotional or social domains. Therefore, consideration of the PDQ-39 subscales provides more specific information.

The Nonmotor Symptoms Scale in Parkinson's Disease (NMSS) is frequently used to comprehensively assess a range of nonmotor symptoms in patients with PD [17–19]. The NMSS consists of 30 items. Each item describes a different nonmotor symptom and considers its severity and frequency. Therefore, the NMSS is a suitable tool for detecting and quantifying nonmotor symptoms in patients with PD. Accordingly, many original studies have used the scale as a clinical outcome measure of nonmotor symptoms [19]. However, owing to the variety of nonmotor symptoms, the total score or domain structure of the NMSS is usually used for statistical analysis. Taking into account the known shortcomings of the NMSS and the limited internal consistency of the domain structure [17,18,20], the consideration of nonmotor symptoms on a single-item level seems advantageous. However, this generally requires more patients, which limits its applicability.

Although previous studies have examined the association between the NMSS and PDQ-39 [7,9,11], the particular symptoms that are most commonly associated with decreased HRQoL have not been clarified, considering the complex interacting network of all nonmotor symptoms. However, due to the variety of nonmotor symptoms, it is important to uncover how these symptoms are linked to HRQoL and to reveal which nonmotor symptoms impact HRQoL. Therefore, we considered both the PDQ-39 summary index and the eight PDQ-39 subscales. Identifying the most important factors that determine HRQoL would allow the prioritization of interventions [21], providing the basis for the improved holistic treatment of patients with PD.

Network analysis is an appropriate tool for gaining these insights, considering all relevant associations between different variables. Accordingly, the present study aimed to reveal (1) the structure of the complex interacting networks of various nonmotor symptoms and HRQoL in PD, (2) the proportion of the HRQoL variance that can be explained by nonmotor symptoms, and (3) which nonmotor symptoms primarily affect HRQoL. This knowledge is crucial as it represents a promising way to improve HRQoL in patients with PD.

2. Materials and Methods

2.1. Study Design

Data were extracted from the Cohort of Patients with Parkinson's Disease in Spain (COPPADIS) study, a national, multicenter, longitudinal study [22]. PD patients aged between 30 and 75 years without dementia were initially recruited from 35 centers in Spain from January 2016 to November 2017. Detailed information on the study design is provided in the COPPADIS study protocol [22].

2.2. Participants

In this study, we included patients with PD whose NMSS and PDQ-39 scores were obtained at the baseline evaluation, resulting in a sample of 689 patients.

2.3. Variables

The NMSS was used to assess nonmotor symptoms. The scale comprises 30 items that describe different nonmotor symptoms experienced during the previous month. The score for each item is calculated by multiplying the severity (0 = none, 1 = mild, 2 = moderate, 3 = severe) and frequency (1 = rarely, 2 = often, 3 = frequent, 4 = very frequent), ranging from 0 to 12 points. The total NMSS score ranges from 0 to 360 points. Theoretically, items are assigned to nine different domains: cardiovascular (domain 1; items 1 and 2), sleep/fatigue (domain 2; items 3, 4, 5, and 6), mood/cognition (domain 3; items 7, 8, 9, 10, 11, and 12), perceptual problems (domain 4; items 13, 14, and 15), attention/memory (domain 5; items 16, 17, and 18), the gastrointestinal tract (domain 6; items 19, 20, and 21), urinary (domain 7; items 22, 23, and 24), sexual function (domain 8; items 25 and 26), and miscellaneous (domain 9; items 27, 28, 29, and 30) [17]. However, for the network analyses, we considered all 30 items.

To assess HRQoL, the subscales and summary indices of the PDQ-39 were considered. The PDQ-39 is a self-rated questionnaire consisting of 39 items divided into eight subscales: mobility (MOB, 10 items), activities of daily living (ADL, 6 items), emotional well-being (EMO, 6 items), stigma (STI, 4 items), social support (SOC, 3 items), cognition (COG, 4 items), communication (COM, 3 items), and bodily discomfort (BOD, 3 items). There are five possible answers for each item: never, occasionally, sometimes, often, and always. Each subscale is converted into a score ranging from 0 to 100 (higher values indicate worse HRQoL). The PDQ-39 summary index is calculated as the mean of the eight subscales and may represent a single value for assessing patients' overall HRQoL. Details of the scoring system for the PDQ-39 can be found in the PDQ user manual [23].

In addition, the following variables were extracted: patient age, sex, Hoehn and Yahr stage [24], and Unified Parkinson's Disease Rating Scale (UPDRS) part III [25].

2.4. Statistical Analysis

For descriptive statistics, normality was tested using the Shapiro–Wilk test. The results are reported as numbers and percentages for categorical variables and the median and interquartile range (IQR) for non-normally distributed continuous variables. The statistical significance for all tests was set at $p < 0.05$ (two-tailed).

Network analyses based on partial correlations were conducted to explore the associations between the 30 NMSS items and HRQoL. In this network approach, the individual nonmotor symptoms and HRQoL measures are seen as complex interacting systems. Therefore, partial correlations refer to associations between two random variables, taking into account other confounding variables related to both variables of interest. Accordingly, the overall pattern of connections is considered to understand interactions, rather than looking at individual correlations that do not take into account whether there is another variable causing that relationship. To precisely assess the influence of nonmotor symptoms on HRQoL, the latter was considered first as the PDQ-39 summary index; second, each of the eight PDQ-39 subscales were considered separately; and third, all subscales were included. This approach was used to identify individual nonmotor symptoms and HRQoL measures.

In general, networks contain two fundamental components: nodes, representing the variables entered into the model, and edges, displaying the correlations between the nodes. Edge thickness reflects the intensity of the connection. Moreover, every node is positioned using the Fruchterman–Reingold algorithm based on the strength of the connections between nodes using pseudorandom numbers [26]. However, instead of relying on simple correlations, a regularization technique, which takes the model complexity into account, is frequently used to prevent overfitting of the partial correlation network structure by reducing the number of spurious correlations between variables [27]. In this study, we used the extended Bayesian information criterion (EBIC) [28,29] with the least absolute shrinkage and selection operator (LASSO) [30]. For more sensitive and specific network analysis, the EBICglasso tuning parameter was set to 0.5, resulting in a sparse network. Nonparanormal transformation (npn) was conducted to generate a normal distribution of non-normally distributed data.

In addition to the layout of the nodes and their edges, centrality measures can be used to assess the variables' influences and their connections statistically. The strength centrality measure was determined for each node using standardized values. Therefore, the strength of a node corresponds to the sum of the absolute edge weights associated with that node [31] and, accordingly, describes the direct connections to other nodes [31–33]. In clinical practice, a node with a high-strength centrality measure can be a potential therapeutic target, because a change in the value of this node can rapidly influence other nodes within the network. In addition, the nodewise predictability was determined to quantify how well a given node (i.e., PDQ) can be predicted by all other nodes connected in the network (i.e., associated nonmotor symptoms) [34]. The determined explained variance R^2 can range from 0 to 1, and values ≥ 0.13 are considered moderate and values ≥ 0.26 are considered high [35].

To identify nonmotor symptoms with the greatest impacts on the eight PDQ-39 subscales, the bridge strength was calculated. The bridge strength is defined as the sum of the absolute values of all edges that exist between a node of a community (i.e., a nonmotor symptom) and all nodes from another community (i.e., PDQ-39 subscales) [36]. Accordingly, a nonmotor symptom with a high bridge strength substantially impacts all PDQ-39 subscales compared with other nonmotor symptoms within the network.

To demonstrate the network's stability, the correlation stability (CS) coefficient was estimated using a case-dropping bootstrap procedure (number of bootstraps = 1000). The CS coefficient quantifies the proportion of cases that can be dropped to retain a correlation with an original strength of at least 0.7 in at least 95% of the samples [33]. To confirm that the network structure was stable, the CS coefficient should preferably exceed 0.5 [33].

Statistical analyses were performed using SPSS (IBM SPSS Statistics 27, IBM, Armonk, NY, USA), R (version 4.2.1, R Foundation for Statistical Computing, Vienna, Austria), and JASP (version 0.15, JASP Team, Amsterdam, The Netherlands) software.

3. Results

3.1. Descriptive Analysis

Of the 689 patients with PD, 414 (60.1%) were male, and 275 (39.9%) were female. The median patient age was 64 years (IQR = 57–70 years). Most patients presented with a disease stage of bilateral involvement (Hoehn and Yahr stage ≥ 2) and moderate motor impairment (median UPDRS III: 21 points, IQR = 14–30). According to the PDQ-39, the patients rated their HRQoL with a median summary index of 12.8 points (IQR = 7.7–24.4). Patients assessed their HRQoL as particularly poor in terms of the bodily discomfort (median value: 25.0, IQR = 8.3–41.6), cognition (median value: 18.7, IQR = 6.3–31.2), and emotional well-being subscales (median value: 16.6, IQR = 4.2–33.3). Patients reported nonmotor symptoms with a median NMSS total score of 35 points (IQR = 19–61). The descriptive statistics of the study population are presented in Table 1.

Table 1. Descriptive statistics.

	Study Population
N	689
Sex	
Male	414 (60.1)
Female	275 (39.9)
Age	64 (57–70)
HY off	2 (2–2)
UPDRS III off	21 (14–30)
PDQ-39 summary index	12.8 (7.7–24.4)
Mobility, MOB	10.0 (2.5–25.0)
Activities of daily living, ADL	12.5 (4.2–25.0)
Emotional well-being, EMO	16.6 (4.2–33.3)
Stigma, STI	0.0 (0.0–25.0)
Social support, SOC	0.0 (0.0–8.3)
Cognition, COG	18.7 (6.3–31.2)
Communication, COM	0.0 (0.0–16.6)
Bodily discomfort, BOD	25.0 (8.3–41.6)
NMSS, total score	35 (19–61)

Table 1. *Cont.*

	Study Population
Cardiovascular (domain 1)	0 (0–2)
1. Light headedness	0 (0–2)
2. Fainting	0 (0–0)
Sleep/fatigue (domain 2)	6 (2–12)
3. Daytime sleepiness	1 (0–3)
4. Fatigue	1 (0–4)
5. Sleep initiation	0 (0–2)
6. Restless legs	0 (0–2)
Mood/apathy (domain 3)	3 (0–11)
7. Loss of interest	0 (0–1)
8. Lack of motivation	0 (0–1)
9. Feeling nervous	0 (0–2)
10. Feeling sad	0 (0–2)
11. Flat mood	0 (0–1)
12. Anhedonia	0 (0–2)
Perceptual (domain 4)	0 (0–1)
13. Hallucinations	0 (0–0)
14. Delusions	0 (0–0)
15. Diplopia	0 (0–0)
Attention/memory (domain 5)	2 (0–5)
16. Concentration	0 (0–2)
17. Forgetfulness	0 (0–2)
18. Forget to do things	0 (0–1)
Gastrointestinal (domain 6)	2 (0–5)
19. Sialorrhea	0 (0–1)
20. Dysphagia	0 (0–0)
21. Constipation	0 (0–2)
Urinary (domain 7)	6 (1.5–12)
22. Urgency	1 (0–6)
23. Frequency	1 (0–4)
24. Nocturia	1 (0–4)
Sexual dysfunction (domain 8)	1 (0–8)
25. Interest	0 (0–4)
26. Problems having sex	0 (0–4)
Miscellaneous (domain 9)	5 (1–12)
27. Pain	0 (0–1)
28. Taste/smell	2 (0–6)
29. Weight change	0 (0–0)
30. Hyperhidrosis	0 (0–1)

The number of participants is given in absolute values; categorical parameters are given as absolute values and percentages; other values are given as medians and interquartile ranges. HY, Hoehn and Yahr stage; N, number of participants; NMSS, Nonmotor Symptoms Scale in Parkinson's disease; PDQ-39, Parkinson's Disease Questionnaire 39; UPDRS, Unified Parkinson's Disease Rating Scale.

3.2. Network Structure

3.2.1. PDQ-39 Summary Index

The network structure between nonmotor symptoms and the PDQ-39 summary index is shown in Figure 1. The white node displays the PDQ-39 summary index (PDQ), and the colored nodes display the NMSS items (i1–i30). Therefore, the color assignment of the nodes corresponds to the distribution of items in the domain structure of the NMSS.

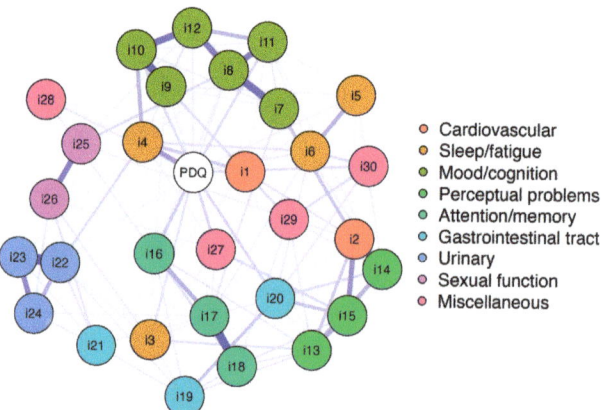

Figure 1. Network structure of the Nonmotor Symptoms Scale in Parkinson's disease (NMSS) and Parkinson's Disease Questionnaire 39 (PDQ-39) summary index. The node *PDQ* displays the PDQ-39 summary index, and nodes *i1–i30* display the items included in the NMSS. The thickness of the edges indicates the strength of the correlations between these nodes. Color coding represents the assignment of the items to the nine domains of the NMSS: cardiovascular (domain 1; items 1 and 2); sleep/fatigue (domain 2; items 3, 4, 5, and 6); mood/cognition (domain 3; items 7, 8, 9, 10, 11, and 12); perceptual problems (domain 4; items 13, 14, and 15); attention/memory (domain 5; items 16, 17, and 18); gastrointestinal tract (domain 6; items 19, 20, and 21); urinary (domain 7; items 22, 23, and 24); sexual function (domain 8; items 25 and 26); and miscellaneous (domain 9; items 27, 28, 29, and 30). Item 1: light headedness; item 2: fainting; item 3: daytime sleepiness; item 4: fatigue; item 5: sleep initiation; item 6: restless legs; item 7: loss of interest; item 8: lack of motivation; item 9: feeling nervous; item 10: feeling sad; item 11: flat mood; item 12: anhedonia; item 13: hallucinations; item 14: delusions; item 15: diplopia; item 16: concentration; item 17: forgetfulness; item 18: forget to do things; item 19: sialorrhea; item 20: dysphagia; item 21: constipation; item 22: urgency; item 23: frequency; item 24: nocturia; item 25: interest; item 26: problems having sex; item 27: pain; item 28: taste/smell; item 29: weight change; and item 30: hyperhidrosis.

On a global level, the network analysis revealed a well-connected network (229 of 465 nonzero edges). None of the 31 nodes were separated entirely. The pre-existing structure of the NMSS based on the nine domains cannot be visually delimited owing to the numerous associations of items from different domains. While items of all the NMSS domains were associated with *PDQ*, the edge between item 4 (*fatigue*) and *PDQ* had the highest weight (edge weight 0.184, as shown in Table S1).

In addition, the strength centrality measure of each node was determined. These values are shown in Figure 2 (and tabulated in Table S1). *PDQ* was determined to have the greatest strength. Accordingly, this node had the highest input weights from being directly connected other items. Respectively, the PDQ-39 summary index is of central importance to the complex interacting network of nonmotor symptoms of the NMSS. The nodewise predictability results revealed that 52.8% of the variance in the PDQ-39 summary index could be explained by the connected NMSS items (see Table S1).

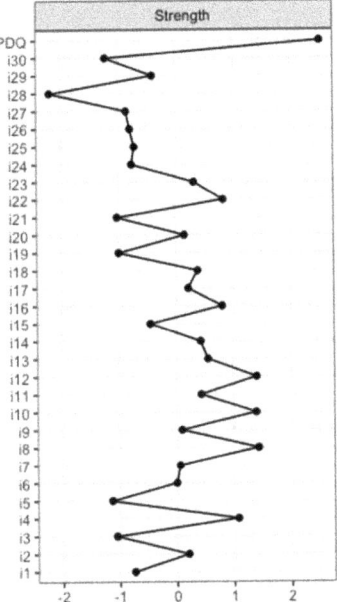

Figure 2. Node strength of the NMSS and PDQ-39 summary index. The strength centrality measures of PDQ-39 summary index (*PDQ*) and the items of the NMSS (*i1–i30*) are given in standardized values. Item 1: light headedness; item 2: fainting; item 3: daytime sleepiness; item 4: fatigue; item 5: sleep initiation; item 6: restless legs; item 7: loss of interest; item 8: lack of motivation; item 9: feeling nervous; item 10: feeling sad; item 11: flat mood; item 12: anhedonia; item 13: hallucinations; item 14: delusions; item 15: diplopia; item 16: concentration; item 17: forgetfulness; item 18: forget to do things; item 19: sialorrhea; item 20: dysphagia; item 21: constipation; item 22: urgency; item 23: frequency; item 24: nocturia; item 25: interest; item 26: problems having sex; item 27: pain; item 28: taste/smell; item 29: weight change; and item 30: hyperhidrosis. NMSS: Nonmotor Symptoms Scale in Parkinson´s disease. PDQ-39: Parkinson´s Disease Questionnaire 39.

The case-dropping bootstrapped procedure revealed that the centrality measure strength remained high (CS (cor = 0.7) = 0.67; Figure S1), and accordingly, the network can be considered stable.

3.2.2. PDQ-39 Subscales

In addition to the aforementioned analysis of the PDQ-39 summary index, we conducted separate network analyses of the eight PDQ-39 subscales (MOB, ADL, EMO, STI, SOC, COG, COM, and BOD). The network structures between the nonmotor symptoms and each of the eight PDQ-39 subscales are shown in Figures S2–S9. The white node displays the PDQ-39 subscale (*MOB, ADL, EMO, STI, SOC, COG, COM,* or *BOD*), and the orange nodes display the items of the NMSS (*i1–i30*).

In general, all eight networks were found to be well-connected without isolated nodes. As revealed by the nodewise predictability analyses, the explained variances of the MOB, EMO, COG, and BOD subscales were high (R^2: 38.5–52.7%) (see Table S2).

Moreover, strength centrality measures for each node within the eight networks were determined (Table S3). The COG subscale had the highest strength within its network and a high impact from directly connected nonmotor symptoms. We also examined the edge weights of each network (Table S3). It became apparent that different items of the NMSS are most highly associated with individual subscale measures. Within the "mobility" and "activities of daily living" network, the highest associations of the nodes *MOB* and *ADL* are with item 4 (*fatigue*) (edge weights 0.251 and 0.121). *Feeling sad* (item 10) is most highly associated with the node *EMO* (edge weights 0.276) in the "emotional well-being" network. Within the "stigma" network, the edge weight between *STI* and item 13 (*hallucinations*) is the highest (0.067), but it is still relatively low in comparison with the other subscales. *Loss of interest* (item 7) is highly connected to *SOC* ("social support" network) with an edge weight of 0.157. Regarding the "cognition" network, edge weight analyses two highly connected items were revealed: the edge weights between *COG* and both *impaired concentration* (item 16) and *daytime sleepiness* (item 3) were very high (edge weights 0.336 and 0.293, respectively). *Daytime sleepiness* (item 3) was also the item with the highest edge weight to *COM* in the "communication" network (edge weight 0.091). Finally, *hyperhidrosis* (item 30) seems to have the most significant influence on *BOD* in the "bodily discomfort" network with an edge weight of 0.220.

Case-dropping bootstrapped procedures revealed that the centrality measure strength remained high for every subscale network (CS (cor = 0.7) > 0.5), and accordingly, the networks can be considered stable (see Table S2).

3.2.3. Bridge Strength

We identified nonmotor symptoms associated with the PDQ-39 summary index and particular subscales of the PDQ-39. However, it is particularly interesting to identify the nonmotor symptoms most associated with all eight PDQ-39 subscales. In this regard, the bridge strength of the NMSS items was determined.

Therefore, we conducted a network analysis including the 30 NMSS items and eight PDQ-39 subscales (MOB, ADL, EMO, STI, SOC, COG, COM, BOD). The network structure is shown in Figure 3. The blue nodes display the PDQ-39 subscales (*MOB, ADL, EMO, STI, SOC, COG, COM,* or *BOD*), and the orange nodes display the NMSS items (*i1–i30*).

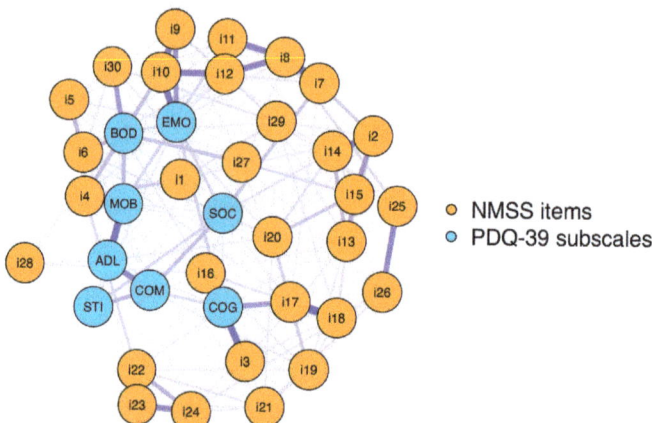

Figure 3. Network structure of the NMSS and PDQ-39 subscales. The blue nodes display the PDQ-39 subscales (*MOB, ADL, EMO, STI, SOC, COG, COM,* and *BOD*), and the orange nodes display the items included in the NMSS (*i1–i30*). The thickness of the edges indicates the strength of the correlations between these nodes. Item 1: light headedness; item 2: fainting; item 3: daytime sleepiness; item 4: fatigue; item 5: sleep initiation; item 6: restless legs; item 7: loss of interest; item 8: lack of motivation; item 9: feeling nervous; item 10: feeling sad; item 11: flat mood; item 12: anhedonia; item 13: hallucinations; item 14: delusions; item 15: diplopia; item 16: concentration; item 17: forgetfulness; item 18: forget to do things; item 19: sialorrhea; item 20: dysphagia; item 21: constipation; item 22: urgency; item 23: frequency; item 24: nocturia; item 25: interest; item 26: problems having sex; item 27: pain; item 28: taste/smell; item 29: weight change; and item 30: hyperhidrosis. PDQ-39 subscale coding: MOB, mobility; ADL, activities of daily living; EMO, emotional well-being; STI, stigma; SOC, social support; COG, cognition; COM, communication; BOD, bodily discomfort. NMSS: Nonmotor Symptoms Scale in Parkinson´s disease. PDQ-39: Parkinson´s Disease Questionnaire 39.

The network analysis revealed a well-connected network (290 of 703 nonzero edges) without isolated nodes. The bridge strength centrality measures are shown in Figure 4. Accordingly, consideration of the community of NMSS items revealed that items 30 (*hyperhidrosis*), 16 (*concentration*), and 3 (*daytime sleepiness*) had the highest bridge strengths. These items are, in turn, associated with the subscales "bodily discomfort" (*hyperhidrosis*) and "cognition" (*concentration* and *daytime sleepiness*).

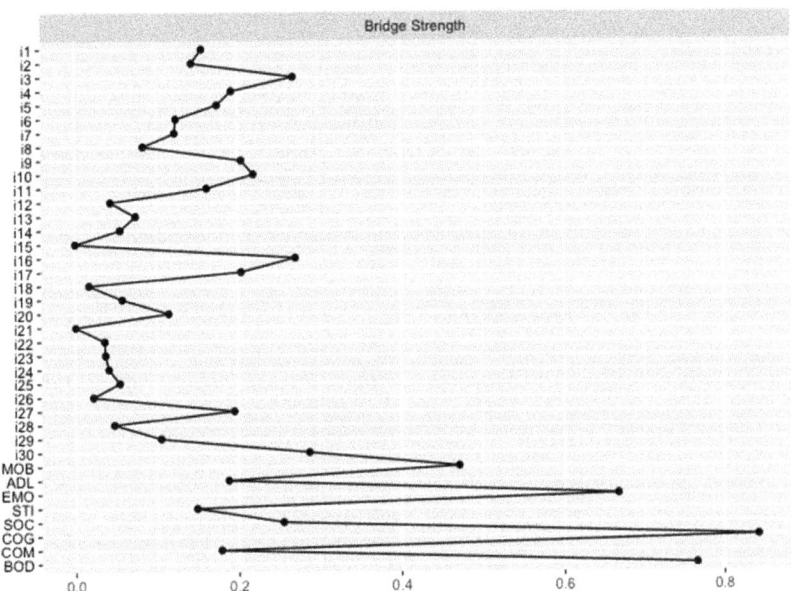

Figure 4. Bridge strengths of the NMSS and PDQ-39 subscales. The bridge strength indicates the sum of the values of all edges that exist between a node of one community and all nodes from another community. Bridge strength values are given for the nodes of the NMSS (*i1–i30*) and PDQ-39 subscales (*MOB, ADL, EMO, STI, SOC, COG, COM,* and *BOD*). Item 1: light headedness; item 2: fainting; item 3: daytime sleepiness; item 4: fatigue; item 5: sleep initiation; item 6: restless legs; item 7: loss of interest; item 8: lack of motivation; item 9: feeling nervous; item 10: feeling sad; item 11: flat mood; item 12: anhedonia; item 13: hallucinations; item 14: delusions; item 15: diplopia; item 16: concentration; item 17: forgetfulness; item 18: forget to do things; item 19: sialorrhea; item 20: dysphagia; item 21: constipation; item 22: urgency; item 23: frequency; item 24: nocturia; item 25: interest; item 26: problems having sex; item 27: pain; item 28: taste/smell; item 29: weight change; and item 30: hyperhidrosis. PDQ-39 subscale coding: MOB, mobility; ADL, activities of daily living; EMO, emotional well-being; STI, stigma; SOC, social support; COG, cognition; COM, communication; BOD, bodily discomfort. NMSS: Nonmotor Symptoms Scale in Parkinson´s disease. PDQ-39: Parkinson´s Disease Questionnaire 39.

The case-dropping bootstrapped procedure confirms that the network can be considered stable because the CS coefficient of the bridge strength remains high (CS (cor = 0.7) = 0.67) (see Figure S10).

4. Discussion

Our study used network analyses to reveal the overall pattern of connections and, accordingly, the complex interactions between nonmotor symptoms and HRQoL in PD patients. We were able to demonstrate that the 30 items of the NMSS mainly influence the MOB, EMO, COG, and BOD subscales of the PDQ-39 due to the high predictability of these subscales. Moreover, considering the variety of other confounding nonmotor symptoms and HRQoL measures, we identified symptoms that were positively associated with overall HRQoL and symptoms that affect specific domains of HRQoL.

In summary, network analyses indicated that *fatigue, feeling sad, hyperhidrosis*, impaired *concentration*, and *daytime sleepiness* are the most influential nonmotor symptoms related to HRQoL. *Loss of interest* and *hallucinations* are also relevant, although their impacts are less pronounced because of the lower predictability of the STI and SOC subscales by the NMSS.

The effect of fatigue on HRQoL can be interpreted in line with previous research. It is already known that fatigue is an early symptom of PD [37,38] that has a negative impact on quality of life [39–41]. Our study confirmed that *fatigue* is of central importance to the PDQ-39 summary index, and particularly for the MOB subscale. Accordingly, fatigue can be considered an influential nonmotor symptom. Therefore, identifying and subsequently treating fatigue in PD patients may be a promising way to improve HRQoL. However, evidence-based treatment strategies for fatigue remain limited [39]. As fatigue is correlated with depression in PD patients [41], treating any associated depressive symptoms may have a positive effect.

Previous studies have revealed that depression is a strong determinant of a low HRQoL [42,43]. In addition, it was recently shown that depressive symptoms, particularly feelings of sadness, are of major importance within the complex network of nonmotor symptoms in PD [20]. However, until now, it has not been clarified whether depressive symptoms, even in the absence of depression, are also important for HRQoL, considering their complex interactions. In this study, we found that feeling sad had the greatest impact on the EMO subscale of the PDQ-39 and may represent a potential therapeutic target for improving HRQoL. Accordingly, close attention should be paid to depressive symptoms when treating patients with PD, especially because they are often heterogeneous and under-recognized [44,45].

Sweating disturbances are common in PD [46]. Axial hyperhidrosis may compensate for reduced sympathetic function in the extremities [47]. Our study demonstrates that *hyperhidrosis* primarily affects the BOD subscale of the PDQ-39 and has the highest bridge strength. Accordingly, hyperhidrosis was shown to have a meaningful impact on all eight subscales of the PDQ-39, which was not directly visible when looking at the network structure of the NMSS items and the PDQ-39 subscales (Figure 3). Nevertheless, this complex effect can be explained by the known relationship between hyperhidrosis and various other autonomic symptoms [48,49]. In general, our data suggest that the consideration of hyperhidrosis is beneficial, as it is a simple clinical screening tool to identify PD patients with autonomic symptoms [48] and could be used to uncover a possible therapeutic target to improve HRQoL.

Excessive daytime sleepiness is a frequent problem in patients with PD [50]. Its pathophysiology is multifactorial and is caused by the degeneration of neurons controlling wakefulness, medications and their side effects, and even poor nocturnal sleep [51]. A previous study showed that PD patients with excessive daytime sleepiness had more severe nonmotor symptoms and a lower PDQ-39 summary index than those without excessive daytime sleepiness [52]. Moreover, excessive daytime sleepiness has been shown to be associated with cognitive impairment [51]. Our study strengthened this finding and showed that *daytime sleepiness* is strongly related to the COG subscale of the PDQ-39 and is a bridge symptom of HRQoL.

Furthermore, our study demonstrated that impaired *concentration* is strongly related to the COG subscale of the PDQ-39 and represents a bridge symptom of HRQoL. Although the high impact of *concentration* on the cognition domain of HRQoL is not surprising, our study revealed a broader influence of *concentration* on all eight subscales of the PDQ-39 and, thus, a multidimensional impact on HRQoL.

Our study provides new insights into the complex interacting network of nonmotor symptoms on HRQoL in PD patients. Nevertheless, our study has several limitations. First, the generated data are not fully representative of the PD population due to the inclusion and exclusion criteria used (i.e., age limit, no dementia, no severe comorbidities, and no second-line therapies) [22]. Accordingly, the results apply to the studied cohort only. However, the estimation of a stable network usually requires a larger sample size, which limits its applicability to smaller local cohorts. Second, nonmotor symptoms were recorded on a scale, and perceptions of nonmotor symptoms may have depended on the participants' mood and motivation. In this regard, nonmotor fluctuations were not considered. Finally, network analysis remains an exploratory approach that cannot be used to determine causality. Thus, further research is needed to confirm whether influencing nonmotor symptoms with the highest impacts positively improve HRQoL.

5. Conclusions

The network analysis revealed complex interactions between nonmotor symptoms and HRQoL in PD patients. *Fatigue, feeling sad, hyperhidrosis,* impaired *concentration,* and *daytime sleepiness* were shown to be the most influential nonmotor symptoms. Further research is needed to confirm whether influencing these nonmotor symptoms could improve HRQoL.

Supplementary Materials: The following supporting information can be downloaded at: https://www.mdpi.com/article/10.3390/jcm12072573/s1, Figure S1: Case-dropping bootstrap strength of the Nonmotor Symptoms Scale in Parkinson's disease (NMSS) and Parkinson´s Disease Questionnaire 39 (PDQ-39) summary index; Figure S2: Network structure of the NMSS and MOB; Figure S3: Network structure of the NMSS and ADL; Figure S4: Network structure of the NMSS and EMO; Figure S5: Network structure of the NMSS and STI; Figure S6: Network structure of the NMSS and SOC; Figure S7: Network structure of the NMSS and COG; Figure S8: Network structure of the NMSS and COM; Figure S9: Network structure of the NMSS and BOD; Figure S10: Case-dropping bootstrap bridge strength of the NMSS and PDQ-39 subscales; Table S1: Network analysis of the PDQ-39 summary index; Table S2: Network characteristics of the PDQ-39 subscales; Table S3: Network analyses of the PDQ-39 subscales. Table S4: Affiliations of the collaborators of the COPPADIS Study Group.

Author Contributions: Conceptualization, K.G.H. and T.P.; Methodology, K.G.H. and T.P.; Formal Analysis, K.G.H.; Data Curation, COPPADIS Study Group; Writing—Original Draft Preparation, K.G.H.; Writing—Review & Editing, A.S., D.S.-G., P.M. and T.P. All authors have read and agreed to the published version of the manuscript.

Funding: Funding to K.G.H. was provided by the Deutsche Forschungsgemeinschaft (DFG, German Research Foundation) as part of the Clinician Scientist-Program OrganAge, funding number 413668513. In addition, K.G.H. received funding from a Bundesministerium für Bildung und Forschung (BMBF, Federal Ministry of Education and Research) grant (01GY1804). T.P. received funding from a Bundesministerium für Bildung und Forschung (BMBF, Federal Ministry of Education and Research) grant (01GY2301).

Institutional Review Board Statement: The study was conducted in accordance with the guidelines of the Declaration of Helsinki and approved by Comité de Ética de la Investigación Clínica de Galicia from Spain (2014/534; 2/DEC/2014). Written informed consent was obtained from all participants in this study before the start of the study.

Informed Consent Statement: Informed consent was obtained from all subjects involved in the study.

Data Availability Statement: The data presented in this study are available on request from D.S.-G. on behalf of the COPPADIS Study Group.

Acknowledgments: We thank the COPPADIS Study Group for their thorough data acquisition and management. A full list of the collaborators of the COPPADIS Study Group is provided in Appendix A, and their affiliations are presented in Table S4.

Conflicts of Interest: The authors declare no conflict of interest. The funders had no role in the design of the study; in the collection, analyses, or interpretation of data; in the writing of the manuscript; or in the decision to publish the results.

Appendix A

The Collaborators of the COPPADIS Study Group (affiliations are shown in Table S4): Adarmes, A.D.; Almeria, M.; Alonso Losada, M.G.; Alonso Cánovas, A.; Alonso Frech, F.;

Alonso Redondo, R.; Álvarez, I.; Álvarez Sauco, M.; Aneiros Díaz, A.; Arnáiz, S.; Arribas, S.; Ascunce Vidondo, A.; Aguilar, M.; Ávila, M.A.; Bernardo Lambrich, N.; Bejr-Kasem, H.; Blázquez Estrada, M.; Botí, M.; Borrue, C.; Buongiorno, M.T.; Cabello González, C.; Cabo López, I.; Caballol, N.; Cámara Lorenzo, A.; Canfield Medina, H.; Carrillo, F.; Carrillo Padilla, F.J.; Casas, E.; Catalán, M.J.; Clavero, P.; Cortina Fernández, A.; Cosgaya, M.; Cots Foraster, A.; Crespo Cuevas, A.; Cubo, E.; de Deus Fonticoba, T.; de Fábregues-Boixar, O.; Díez-Fairen, M.; Dotor García-Soto, J.; Erro, E.; Escalante, S.; Estelrich Peyret, E.; Fernández Guillán, N.; Gámez, P.; Gallego, M.; García Caldentey, J.; García Campos, C.; García Díez, C.; García Moreno, J.M.; Gastón, I.; Gómez Garre, M.P.; Gómez Mayordomo, V.; González Aloy, J.; González-Aramburu, I.; González Ardura, J.; González García, B.; González Palmás, M.J.; González Toledo, G.R.; Golpe Díaz, A.; Grau Solá, M.; Guardia, G.; Hernández Vara, J.; Horta-Barba, A.; Idoate Calderón, D.; Infante, J.; Jesús, S.; Kulisevsky, J.; Kurtis, M.; Labandeira, C.; Labrador, M.A.; Lacruz, F.; Lage Castro, M.; Lastres Gómez, S.; Legarda, I.; López Ariztegui, N.; López Díaz, L.M.; López Domínguez, D.; López Manzanares, L.; López Seoane, B.; Lucas del Pozo, S.; Macías, Y.; Mata, M.; Martí Andres, G.; Martí, M.J.; Martínez Castrillo, J.C.; Martinez-Martin, P.; McAfee, D.; Meitín, M.T.; Mendoza Plasencia, Z.; Menéndez González, M.; Méndez del Barrio, C.; Mir, P.; Miranda Santiago, J.; Morales Casado, M.I.; Moreno Diéguez, A.; Nogueira, V.; Novo Amado, A.; Novo Ponte, S.; Ordás, C.; Pagonabarraga, J.; Pareés, I.; Pascual-Sedano, B.; Pastor, P.; Pérez Fuertes, A.; Pérez Noguera, R.; Planas-Ballvé, A.; Planellas, L.; Prats, M.A.; Prieto Jurczynska, C.; Puente, V.; Pueyo Morlans, M.; Puig Daví, A.; Redondo Rafales, N.; Rodríguez Méndez, L.; Rodríguez Pérez, A.B.; Roldán, F.; Ruíz De Arcos, M.; Ruíz Martínez, J.; Sánchez Alonso, P.; Sánchez-Carpintero, M.; Sánchez Díez, G.; Sánchez Rodríguez, A.; Santacruz, P.; Santos García, D.; Segundo Rodríguez, J.C.; Seijo, M.; Sierra Peña, M.; Solano Vila, B.; Suárez Castro, E.; Tartari, J.P.; Valero, C.; Vargas, L.; Vela, L.; Villanueva, C.; Vives, B.

References

1. Titova, N.; Qamar, M.A.; Chaudhuri, K.R. The Nonmotor Features of Parkinson's Disease. *Int. Rev. Neurobiol.* **2017**, *132*, 33–54. [CrossRef] [PubMed]
2. Chaudhuri, K.R.; Healy, D.G.; Schapira, A.H. Non-motor symptoms of Parkinson's disease: Diagnosis and management. *Lancet Neurol.* **2006**, *5*, 235–245. [CrossRef] [PubMed]
3. Barone, P.; Antonini, A.; Colosimo, C.; Marconi, R.; Morgante, L.; Avarello, T.P.; Bottacchi, E.; Cannas, A.; Ceravolo, G.; Ceravolo, R.; et al. The PRIAMO study: A multicenter assessment of nonmotor symptoms and their impact on quality of life in Parkinson's disease. *Mov. Disord.* **2009**, *24*, 1641–1649. [CrossRef] [PubMed]
4. Barone, P.; Erro, R.; Picillo, M. Quality of Life and Nonmotor Symptoms in Parkinson's Disease. *Int. Rev. Neurobiol.* **2017**, *133*, 499–516. [CrossRef]
5. Duncan, G.W.; Khoo, T.K.; Yarnall, A.J.; O'Brien, J.T.; Coleman, S.Y.; Brooks, D.J.; Barker, R.A.; Burn, D.J. Health-related quality of life in early Parkinson's disease: The impact of nonmotor symptoms. *Mov. Disord.* **2014**, *29*, 195–202. [CrossRef] [PubMed]
6. Rahman, S.; Griffin, H.J.; Quinn, N.P.; Jahanshahi, M. Quality of life in Parkinson's disease: The relative importance of the symptoms. *Mov. Disord.* **2008**, *23*, 1428–1434. [CrossRef]
7. Martinez-Martin, P.; Rodriguez-Blazquez, C.; Kurtis, M.M.; Chaudhuri, K.R. The impact of non-motor symptoms on health-related quality of life of patients with Parkinson's disease. *Mov. Disord.* **2011**, *26*, 399–406. [CrossRef]
8. Santos-García, D.; de la Fuente-Fernández, R. Impact of non-motor symptoms on health-related and perceived quality of life in Parkinson's disease. *J. Neurol. Sci.* **2013**, *332*, 136–140. [CrossRef]
9. Santos García, D.; de Deus Fonticoba, T.; Suárez Castro, E.; Borrué, C.; Mata, M.; Solano Vila, B.; Cots Foraster, A.; Álvarez Sauco, M.; Rodríguez Pérez, A.B.; Vela, L.; et al. Non-motor symptoms burden, mood, and gait problems are the most significant factors contributing to a poor quality of life in non-demented Parkinson's disease patients: Results from the COPPADIS Study Cohort. *Park. Relat. Disord.* **2019**, *66*, 151–157. [CrossRef]
10. Prakash, K.M.; Nadkarni, N.V.; Lye, W.K.; Yong, M.H.; Tan, E.K. The impact of non-motor symptoms on the quality of life of Parkinson's disease patients: A longitudinal study. *Eur. J. Neurol.* **2016**, *23*, 854–860. [CrossRef]
11. Song, W.; Guo, X.; Chen, K.; Chen, X.; Cao, B.; Wei, Q.; Huang, R.; Zhao, B.; Wu, Y.; Shang, H.F. The impact of non-motor symptoms on the Health-Related Quality of Life of Parkinson's disease patients from Southwest China. *Park. Relat. Disord.* **2014**, *20*, 149–152. [CrossRef] [PubMed]
12. Karimi, M.; Brazier, J. Health, Health-Related Quality of Life, and Quality of Life: What is the Difference? *Pharmacoeconomics* **2016**, *34*, 645–649. [CrossRef] [PubMed]

13. Martinez-Martin, P.; Jeukens-Visser, M.; Lyons, K.E.; Rodriguez-Blazquez, C.; Selai, C.; Siderowf, A.; Welsh, M.; Poewe, W.; Rascol, O.; Sampaio, C.; et al. Health-related quality-of-life scales in Parkinson's disease: Critique and recommendations. *Mov. Disord.* **2011**, *26*, 2371–2380. [CrossRef] [PubMed]
14. Jenkinson, C.; Fitzpatrick, R.; Peto, V.; Greenhall, R.; Hyman, N. The Parkinson's Disease Questionnaire (PDQ-39): Development and validation of a Parkinson's disease summary index score. *Age Ageing* **1997**, *26*, 353–357. [CrossRef] [PubMed]
15. Zhao, N.; Yang, Y.; Zhang, L.; Zhang, Q.; Balbuena, L.; Ungvari, G.S.; Zang, Y.F.; Xiang, Y.T. Quality of life in Parkinson's disease: A systematic review and meta-analysis of comparative studies. *CNS Neurosci. Ther.* **2021**, *27*, 270–279. [CrossRef] [PubMed]
16. Hagell, P.; Nilsson, M.H. The 39-Item Parkinson's Disease Questionnaire (PDQ-39): Is it a Unidimensional Construct? *Ther. Adv. Neurol. Disord.* **2009**, *2*, 205–214. [CrossRef] [PubMed]
17. Chaudhuri, K.R.; Martinez-Martin, P.; Brown, R.G.; Sethi, K.; Stocchi, F.; Odin, P.; Ondo, W.; Abe, K.; Macphee, G.; Macmahon, D.; et al. The metric properties of a novel non-motor symptoms scale for Parkinson's disease: Results from an international pilot study. *Mov. Disord.* **2007**, *22*, 1901–1911. [CrossRef]
18. Martinez-Martin, P.; Rodriguez-Blazquez, C.; Abe, K.; Bhattacharyya, K.B.; Bloem, B.R.; Carod-Artal, F.J.; Prakash, R.; Esselink, R.A.; Falup-Pecurariu, C.; Gallardo, M.; et al. International study on the psychometric attributes of the non-motor symptoms scale in Parkinson disease. *Neurology* **2009**, *73*, 1584–1591. [CrossRef]
19. van Wamelen, D.J.; Martinez-Martin, P.; Weintraub, D.; Schrag, A.; Antonini, A.; Falup-Pecurariu, C.; Odin, P.; Ray Chaudhuri, K. The Non-Motor Symptoms Scale in Parkinson's disease: Validation and use. *Acta Neurol. Scand.* **2021**, *143*, 3–12. [CrossRef]
20. Heimrich, K.G.; Schönenberg, A.; Mühlhammer, H.M.; Mendorf, S.; Santos-García, D.; Prell, T. Longitudinal analysis of the Non-Motor Symptoms Scale in Parkinson's Disease (NMSS): An exploratory network analysis approach. *Front. Neurol.* **2023**, *14*, 972210. [CrossRef]
21. Martinez-Martin, P. What is quality of life and how do we measure it? Relevance to Parkinson's disease and movement disorders. *Mov. Disord.* **2017**, *32*, 382–392. [CrossRef]
22. Santos-García, D.; Mir, P.; Cubo, E.; Vela, L.; Rodríguez-Oroz, M.C.; Martí, M.J.; Arbelo, J.M.; Infante, J.; Kulisevsky, J.; Martínez-Martín, P.; et al. COPPADIS-2015 (COhort of Patients with PArkinson's DIsease in Spain, 2015), a global-clinical evaluations, serum biomarkers, genetic studies and neuroimaging-prospective, multicenter, non-interventional, long-term study on Parkinson's disease progression. *BMC Neurol.* **2016**, *16*, 26. [CrossRef]
23. Jenkinson, C.; Fitzpatrick, R.; Peto, V.; Harris, R.; Saunders, P. PDQ-39 user manual (including PDQ-8 and PDQ summary index). *Park. Dis. Quest.* **2008**, *2*, 1–11.
24. Hoehn, M.M.; Yahr, M.D. Parkinsonism: Onset, progression and mortality. *Neurology* **1967**, *17*, 427–442. [CrossRef] [PubMed]
25. Fahn, S.; Elton, R. Recent developments in Parkinson's disease. *Macmillan Health Care Inf.* **1987**, *2*, 293–304.
26. Fruchterman, T.M.; Reingold, E.M. Graph drawing by force-directed placement. *Softw. Pract. And. Exp.* **1991**, *21*, 1129–1164. [CrossRef]
27. Hevey, D. Network analysis: A brief overview and tutorial. *Health Psychol. Behav. Med.* **2018**, *6*, 301–328. [CrossRef]
28. Foygel, R.; Drton, M. Extended Bayesian information criteria for Gaussian graphical models. *arXiv* **2010**, arXiv:1011.6640.
29. Chen, J.; Chen, Z. Extended Bayesian information criteria for model selection with large model spaces. *Biometrika* **2008**, *95*, 759–771. [CrossRef]
30. Friedman, J.; Hastie, T.; Tibshirani, R. Sparse inverse covariance estimation with the graphical lasso. *Biostatistics* **2008**, *9*, 432–441. [CrossRef]
31. Epskamp, S.; Fried, E.I. A tutorial on regularized partial correlation networks. *Psychol. Methods* **2018**, *23*, 617–634. [CrossRef] [PubMed]
32. Opsahl, T.; Agneessens, F.; Skvoretz, J. Node centrality in weighted networks: Generalizing degree and shortest paths. *Soc. Netw.* **2010**, *32*, 245–251. [CrossRef]
33. Epskamp, S.; Borsboom, D.; Fried, E.I. Estimating psychological networks and their accuracy: A tutorial paper. *Behav. Res. Methods* **2018**, *50*, 195–212. [CrossRef]
34. Haslbeck, J.M.B.; Waldorp, L.J. How well do network models predict observations? On the importance of predictability in network models. *Behav. Res. Methods* **2018**, *50*, 853–861. [CrossRef] [PubMed]
35. Cohen, J. *Statistical Power Analysis for the Behavioral Sciences*, 2nd ed.; Erlbaum: Hillsdale, NJ, USA, 1988.
36. Jones, P.J.; Ma, R.; McNally, R.J. Bridge Centrality: A Network Approach to Understanding Comorbidity. *Multivar. Behav. Res.* **2021**, *56*, 353–367. [CrossRef] [PubMed]
37. Kostić, V.S.; Tomić, A.; Ječmenica-Lukić, M. The Pathophysiology of Fatigue in Parkinson's Disease and its Pragmatic Management. *Mov. Disord. Clin. Pract.* **2016**, *3*, 323–330. [CrossRef]
38. Müller, B.; Assmus, J.; Herlofson, K.; Larsen, J.P.; Tysnes, O.B. Importance of motor vs. non-motor symptoms for health-related quality of life in early Parkinson's disease. *Park. Relat. Disord.* **2013**, *19*, 1027–1032. [CrossRef]
39. Lazcano-Ocampo, C.; Wan, Y.M.; van Wamelen, D.J.; Batzu, L.; Boura, I.; Titova, N.; Leta, V.; Qamar, M.; Martinez-Martin, P.; Ray Chaudhuri, K. Identifying and responding to fatigue and apathy in Parkinson's disease: A review of current practice. *Expert Rev. Neurother.* **2020**, *20*, 477–495. [CrossRef]
40. Mantri, S.; Chahine, L.M.; Nabieva, K.; Feldman, R.; Althouse, A.; Torsney, B.; Albert, S.M.; Kopil, C.; Marras, C. Demographic Influences on the Relationship Between Fatigue and Quality of Life in Parkinson's Disease. *Mov. Disord. Clin. Pract.* **2022**, *9*, 76–81. [CrossRef]

41. Béreau, M.; Castrioto, A.; Lhommée, E.; Maillet, A.; Gérazime, A.; Bichon, A.; Pélissier, P.; Schmitt, E.; Klinger, H.; Longato, N.; et al. Fatigue in de novo Parkinson's Disease: Expanding the Neuropsychiatric Triad? *J. Park. Dis.* **2022**, *12*, 1329–1337. [CrossRef]
42. Schrag, A.; Jahanshahi, M.; Quinn, N. What contributes to quality of life in patients with Parkinson's disease? *J. Neurol. Neurosurg. Psychiatry* **2000**, *69*, 308–312. [CrossRef] [PubMed]
43. Kadastik-Eerme, L.; Rosenthal, M.; Paju, T.; Muldmaa, M.; Taba, P. Health-related quality of life in Parkinson's disease: A cross-sectional study focusing on non-motor symptoms. *Health Qual. Life Outcomes* **2015**, *13*, 83. [CrossRef] [PubMed]
44. Ray, S.; Agarwal, P. Depression and Anxiety in Parkinson Disease. *Clin. Geriatr. Med.* **2020**, *36*, 93–104. [CrossRef] [PubMed]
45. Shulman, L.M.; Taback, R.L.; Rabinstein, A.A.; Weiner, W.J. Non-recognition of depression and other non-motor symptoms in Parkinson's disease. *Park. Relat. Disord.* **2002**, *8*, 193–197. [CrossRef]
46. Swinn, L.; Schrag, A.; Viswanathan, R.; Bloem, B.R.; Lees, A.; Quinn, N. Sweating dysfunction in Parkinson's disease. *Mov. Disord.* **2003**, *18*, 1459–1463. [CrossRef]
47. Schestatsky, P.; Valls-Solé, J.; Ehlers, J.A.; Rieder, C.R.; Gomes, I. Hyperhidrosis in Parkinson's disease. *Mov. Disord.* **2006**, *21*, 1744–1748. [CrossRef]
48. van Wamelen, D.J.; Leta, V.; Podlewska, A.M.; Wan, Y.M.; Krbot, K.; Jaakkola, E.; Martinez-Martin, P.; Rizos, A.; Parry, M.; Metta, V.; et al. Exploring hyperhidrosis and related thermoregulatory symptoms as a possible clinical identifier for the dysautonomic subtype of Parkinson's disease. *J. Neurol.* **2019**, *266*, 1736–1742. [CrossRef]
49. Lin, J.; Ou, R.; Wei, Q.; Cao, B.; Li, C.; Hou, Y.; Zhang, L.; Liu, K.; Shang, H. Hyperhidrosis in Parkinson's disease: A 3-year prospective cohort study. *J. Eur. Acad. Dermatol. Venereol.* **2022**, *36*, 1104–1112. [CrossRef]
50. Gjerstad, M.D.; Alves, G.; Wentzel-Larsen, T.; Aarsland, D.; Larsen, J.P. Excessive daytime sleepiness in Parkinson disease: Is it the drugs or the disease? *Neurology* **2006**, *67*, 853–858. [CrossRef]
51. Shen, Y.; Huang, J.Y.; Li, J.; Liu, C.F. Excessive Daytime Sleepiness in Parkinson's Disease: Clinical Implications and Management. *Chin. Med. J. (Engl.)* **2018**, *131*, 974–981. [CrossRef]
52. Yoo, S.W.; Kim, J.S.; Oh, Y.S.; Ryu, D.W.; Lee, K.S. Excessive daytime sleepiness and its impact on quality of life in de novo Parkinson's disease. *Neurol. Sci.* **2019**, *40*, 1151–1156. [CrossRef] [PubMed]

Disclaimer/Publisher's Note: The statements, opinions and data contained in all publications are solely those of the individual author(s) and contributor(s) and not of MDPI and/or the editor(s). MDPI and/or the editor(s) disclaim responsibility for any injury to people or property resulting from any ideas, methods, instructions or products referred to in the content.

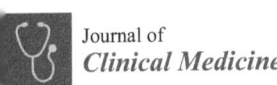

Article

Quantitative High Density EEG Brain Connectivity Evaluation in Parkinson's Disease: The Phase Locking Value (PLV)

Lazzaro di Biase [1,2,3,*], Lorenzo Ricci [1,2], Maria Letizia Caminiti [1,2], Pasquale Maria Pecoraro [1,2], Simona Paola Carbone [1,2] and Vincenzo Di Lazzaro [1,2]

1. Unit of Neurology, Neurophysiology, Neurobiology and Psichiatry, Department of Medicine and Surgery, Università Campus Bio-Medico di Roma, Via Alvaro del Portillo, 21, 00128 Rome, Italy
2. Neurology Unit, Fondazione Policlinico Universitario Campus Bio-Medico, Via Alvaro del Portillo, 200, 00128 Rome, Italy
3. Brain Innovations Lab, Università Campus Bio-Medico di Roma, Via Álvaro del Portillo 21, 00128 Rome, Italy
* Correspondence: l.dibiase@policlinicocampus.it or lazzaro.dibiase@gmail.com; Tel.: +39-06225411220

Abstract: Introduction: The present study explores brain connectivity in Parkinson's disease (PD) and in age matched healthy controls (HC), using quantitative EEG analysis, at rest and during a motor tasks. We also evaluated the diagnostic performance of the phase locking value (PLV), a measure of functional connectivity, in differentiating PD patients from HCs. Methods: High-density, 64-channels, EEG data from 26 PD patients and 13 HC were analyzed. EEG signals were recorded at rest and during a motor task. Phase locking value (PLV), as a measure of functional connectivity, was evaluated for each group in a resting state and during a motor task for the following frequency bands: (i) delta: 2–4 Hz; (ii) theta: 5–7 Hz; (iii) alpha: 8–12 Hz; beta: 13–29 Hz; and gamma: 30–60 Hz. The diagnostic performance in PD vs. HC discrimination was evaluated. Results: Results showed no significant differences in PLV connectivity between the two groups during the resting state, but a higher PLV connectivity in the delta band during the motor task, in HC compared to PD. Comparing the resting state versus the motor task for each group, only HCs showed a higher PLV connectivity in the delta band during motor task. A ROC curve analysis for HC vs. PD discrimination, showed an area under the ROC curve (AUC) of 0.75, a sensitivity of 100%, and a negative predictive value (NPV) of 100%. Conclusions: The present study evaluated the brain connectivity through quantitative EEG analysis in Parkinson's disease versus healthy controls, showing a higher PLV connectivity in the delta band during the motor task, in HC compared to PD. This neurophysiology biomarkers showed the potentiality to be explored in future studies as a potential screening biomarker for PD patients.

Keywords: quantitative EEG analysis; high density EEG; brain connectivity; phase locking value (PLV); Parkinson's disease; biomarkers

1. Introduction

The diagnosis of Parkinson's disease (PD) is currently based on the clinical evaluation Poewe, et al. [1] of the cardinal motor symptoms, bradykinesia, rest tremor, and rigidity, which represent the hallmarks for the in vivo diagnosis [2] according to the current diagnostic criteria for PD [3]. Different strategies have been explored to characterize PD features in a non-invasive way. One first approach is to follow the clinical diagnostic pathway trying to make clinical evaluations of motor symptoms more objective and quantitative, through a motion analysis technique able to characterize PD motor symptoms [4–6], such as bradykinesia [7–9], tremors [10–13], rigidity [9,14–16], and axial symptoms, such as gait, balance, and postural issues [17–22], also with the support of machine learning algorithms [23–27]. Another possible approach is to explore the brain activities that underlay and determine the PD symptoms, which are characterized by pathological oscillatory activities [28,29] and have been widely used to manage therapy, such as deep brain stimulation [30,31], but can be used also as a proxy for PD neurophysiology biomarkers identification.

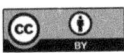

In this context, neurophysiological tests may help to better understand the pathophysiology of PD, and their low cost, brief execution times, and the wide diffusion among hospitals represent a competitive advantage in respect to other techniques to support PD biomarkers identification in clinical practice.

Brain connectivity is a method to explore the way how different brain regions interact and communicate with each other. The degeneration of nigrostriatal dopaminergic neurons, which is the hallmark of the pathophysiology of PD, leads to the dysfunction of the basal ganglia–thalamo-cortical pathway, which underlies the PD motor symptoms [32].

Resting state functional MRI (RS-fMRI) can be used to study the connectivity among different brain areas in PD patients. A meta-analysis of RS-fMRI connectivity studies in PD patients [33], showed a decreased functional connectivity within the posterior putamen. The functional network involving this area and its cortical projections can be modulated by levodopa administration [32–34].

Among the neurophysiological techniques, electroencephalogram (EEG) is one of the most versatile and widely available techniques, it offers good balance between the temporal and spatial resolution, meaning that this technology is most frequently used in studies on PD biomarkers.

In de novo PD patients, compared to controls, a reduced coherence in α-β EEG frequency bands and a hyperconnectivity in γ band were observed [35].

Exploring dynamic networks between neuronal populations in a quantitative way, by noninvasive electrophysiological mapping with EEG, could unveil crucial information about brain connectivity in PD and subsequently, improve the diagnostic process.

Nonlinear and nonstationary systems may be analyzed with the phase locking methodology [36]. Indeed, the brain can be compared to a nonlinear dynamic system and, as such, the phase locking approach can be used for the scope [36–38]. Phase locking value (PLV) is a non-linear measure of pairwise functional connectivity (Lee, Liu et al., 2019), used to quantify the phase coupling between two biological nonlinear signals in a time-series, such as electroencephalographic signals [39]. A high PLV between two brain regions indicates a high synchrony [40].

The present study aims at investigating brain connectivity, through quantitative EEG analysis in Parkinson's disease versus healthy controls, at rest and during a motor task, exploring the performance of the phase locking value (PLV) in discriminating the two study groups.

2. Methods

2.1. Patients and Data Collection

The database and EEG data utilized in this study were obtained from the University of Iowa Hospitals & Clinics (UIHC) Movement Disorders Clinics [41]. The database contains high-density EEG (HD-EEG) [42] data from 26 patients with PD and 13 demographically matched healthy controls (HCs). All patients in the experiment met the UK Parkinson's Disease Brain Bank criteria for the diagnosis of idiopathic PD [43]. All patients underwent neuropsychological evaluation using the Montreal cognitive assessment (MOCA), EEG signals were recorded at rest and during a specific lower-limb pedaling motor task [41] using a customized 64-channels cap (EASYCAP GmbHAm Anger, 582237 Woerthsee-Etterschlag, Germany) with a high-pass filter of 0.1 Hz and a sampling rate of 500 Hz (Brain Products). Online reference and ground channels were Pz and FPz, respectively. Patients and HCs were both instructed to perform a lower-limb motor task during the EEG recording. Therefore, for each subject we analyzed the EEG recorded in both conditions (i.e., Resting State and Motor Task).

2.2. Quantitative EEG Analysis

Quantitative EEG analysis was performed using the Brainstorm Toolbox for MATLAB (Tadel et al., 2011) (The Math Works Inc., Natick, MA, USA), and in home MATLAB code. Offline data pre-processing was performed using Brainstorm and included: (i) DC removal;

(ii) 60-Hz notch filter; (iii) bandpass filter between 1 and 70 Hz (linear phase finite impulse response filter); (iv) EEG re-reference to average; (v) and correction for pulse and eye-blink artifacts using independent component analysis [44,45].

2.3. EEG Connectivity Analysis

To assess the differences in brain networks among PD and HCs we performed a measure of EEG functional connectivity. We selected a total of 180 s continuous epoch from the EEG recordings free from relevant artifacts for further analysis [46,47]. As a measure of connectivity, we computed the phase locking value (PLV). PLV is an important measure of synchronization when studying bio-signals and especially electrical brain activities. It is a measure of non-directional frequency-specific synchronization reflecting long-range integrations and it assesses the extent to which the phase difference between two signals changes over time [36,37,48].

Taking into account the lack of consensus in the classification of frequency bands for quantitative EEG analysis [47], starting from the most recent International Pharmaco-EEG Society (IPEG; [49]) recommendations, also endorsed by the International Federation of Clinical Neurophysiology recommendations on frequency and a topographic analysis of resting state EEG rhythms [47], the final frequency band selected for the phase locking value connectivity analysis was based on the frequency band employed in several previous studies [45,46,48] in which, with respect to the IPEG recommendation, was selected the fastest delta band 2–4 Hz and a restricted theta band 5–7 Hz. We measured the PLV for all possible channel combinations and averaged to obtain a measure of global connectivity [46,48] for the following frequency bands: delta: 2–4 Hz; theta: 5–7 Hz; alpha: 8–12 Hz; beta: 13–29 Hz; and gamma: 30–60 Hz. Connectivity analysis was performed separately for the resting state EEG and for the EEG recorded during the lower limb pedaling motor task.

2.4. Statistical Analysis

Statistical analysis was performed using the R statistical package [50] and MATLAB (Mathworks). Data distribution was checked by means of a Kolmogorov–Smirnov test. The differences in Global Connectivity among PD and HCs was tested using a three-way aligned rank transformed (ART) ANOVA for non-parametric factorial three-way designs [51] with Frequency (five levels: delta, theta, alpha, beta, gamma), Group (two levels: PD and HCs) and Condition (two levels: resting state and motor task) as within the subject factor. A Bonferroni correction was used for post-hoc tests of multiple comparisons when needed.

To estimate the clinical value of EEG connectivity for differentiating between PD and HCs, we built receiver operating characteristic (ROC) curves on the PLV connectivity values for each frequency band and for each condition (i.e., resting state and motor task).

The following performance metrics were estimated in terms of outcome prediction: (i) sensitivity (ii) specificity, (iii) positive predictive value, (iv) negative predictive value; and (v) accuracy. The ROC curve point showing the highest combination of predictive values was selected as the optimum cut-off value to differentiate PD vs. HCs. Finally, we built non-parametric ROC curves to estimate 95% confidence intervals (CIs) for the area under the curve (AUC), sensitivity, specificity, positive predictive value (PPV), negative predictive value (NPV), and accuracy. CIs were validated using 10,000 stratified bootstrap replicates [52]. Moreover, a Spearman correlation test was used to assess the correlation between MOCA scores and the PLV in each frequency band. Significance level was set at $p < 0.05$. Results are reported as the mean ± standard deviation unless differently stated.

3. Results

3.1. Patient Cohort and Control Group

PD patients (nine females and 17 males) had a mean disease duration of 6.2 years (SD: ±3.7), a mean age of 67.3 years (SD: ±9.2), a UPDRS III score of 14.8 (SD: ±7.1), and a MOCA score of 23.3 (SD: ±3.9). The healthy controls (five females and eight males) had a mean age of 68.9 years (SD: ±8.2) [41].

3.2. Comparison between PD and Control Groups

3.2.1. EEG Connectivity

The comparison between PD and HCs revealed no significant differences between groups (factor *group*: $F_{(1,370)} = 0.76$, $p = 0.38$), but a significant group by frequency interaction ($F_{(4,370)} = 3.62$, $p < 0.005$; Figure 1), related to a higher connectivity in the delta frequency band for HCs compared to PD (Bonferroni corrected $p = 0.04$; Figure 2). We also found lower connectivity values in the gamma frequency band for HCs compared to PD, although with a borderline level of significance (Bonferroni corrected $p = 0.05$; Figure 2).

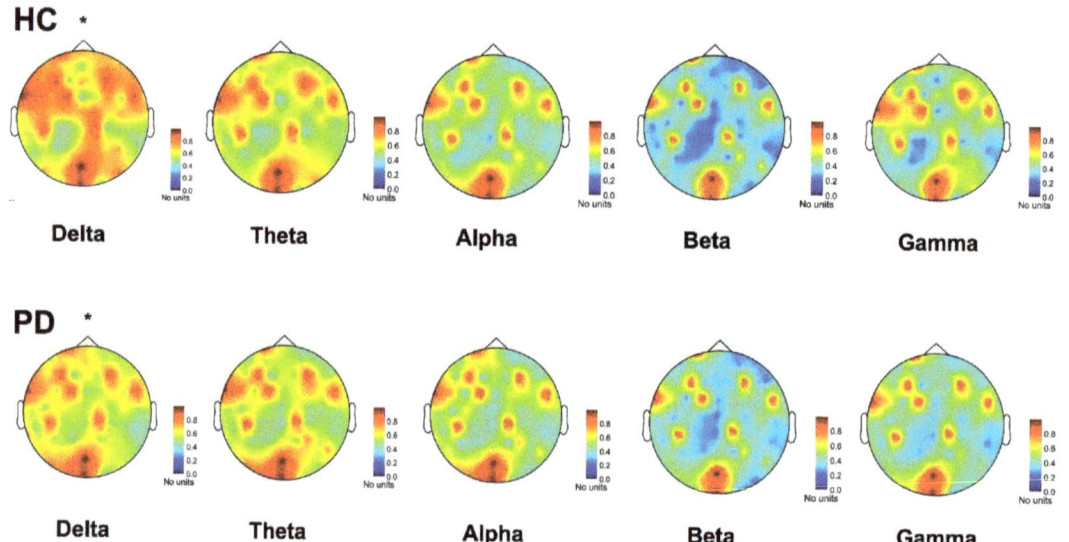

Figure 1. Phase locking value (PLV) connectivity topoplot and comparison between Parkinson Disease (PD) and Healthy Control (HC). PLV is expressed as the average across channels to obtain a measure of global connectivity. Notice how PLV in the delta range is higher in HC compared to PD. *: $p < 0.05$.

The ART ANOVA considering *condition* and *frequency*, as within the subject factor, showed a significant *condition* effect ($F_{(1,370)} = 10.77$, $p = 0.001$), related to higher global connectivity values during the motor task compared to the resting state. A significant *group* by *condition* interaction was also found ($F_{(1,370)} = 5.33$, $p = 0.02$). Post-hoc tests revealed a significant difference in connectivity values during the motor task compared to the resting state in HCs (Bonferroni corrected $p = 0.004$; Figure 3), as opposed to PD patients who did not reach the statistical significance ($p = 0.18$). We also found a significant *condition* by *frequency* interaction ($F_{(4,370)} = 3.48$, $p = 0.008$; Figure 3), related to higher delta connectivity values during the motor task, as opposed to the resting state (Bonferroni corrected $p = 0.03$; see Figure 3). Finally, we found no correlation between the PLV connectivity values and MOCA scores in each frequency band ($p > 0.05$).

3.2.2. ROC Curve Analysis

The ROC curve analysis showed that the PLV connectivity analysis in the delta frequency band during the motor task band was able to differentiate HC from PD (Figure 4) with an area under the curve (AUC) of 0.75 (95% CI, 0.58–0.89), a sensitivity of 100% (95% CI, 100–100%), a specificity of 50% (95% CI, 31–69%), a PPV of 50% (95% CI, 42–62%), an NPV of 100% (95% CI, 100–100%), and an accuracy of 66.7% (95% CI, 54–79%).

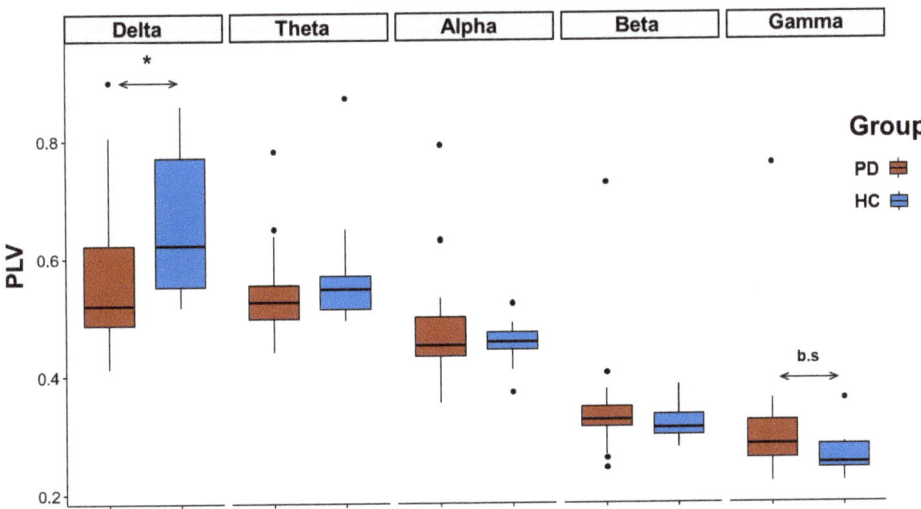

Figure 2. Boxplot distribution of the phase locking value (PLV) connectivity values between Parkinson disease (PD, red) and healthy control (HC, blue) across different frequency bands during the motor task. Black lines represent median values. Dots denote values that are farther than 1.5 interquartile ranges. Notice how PD subjects present a lower delta connectivity ($p = 0.04$) and a higher gamma connectivity, although with a borderline level of significance ($p = 0.05$). *: $p < 0.05$.

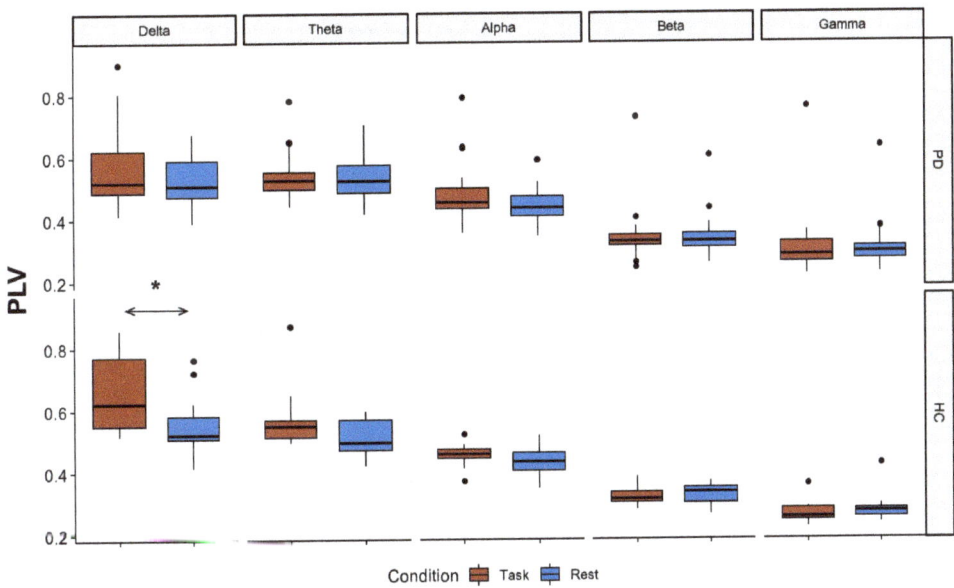

Figure 3. Boxplot distributions of the phase locking value (PLV) mean connectivity values. Boxplot distributions of the mean PLV values for different frequency bands across Groups: Parkinson disease (PD) vs. healthy control (HC) and conditions: motor task (red) vs. resting state (blue). Black lines represent median values. Dots denote values that are farther than 1.5 interquartile ranges. Connectivity values were significantly higher during the motor task compared to the resting state in HC ($p = 0.004$), as opposed to PD ($p = 0.18$). *: $p < 0.05$.

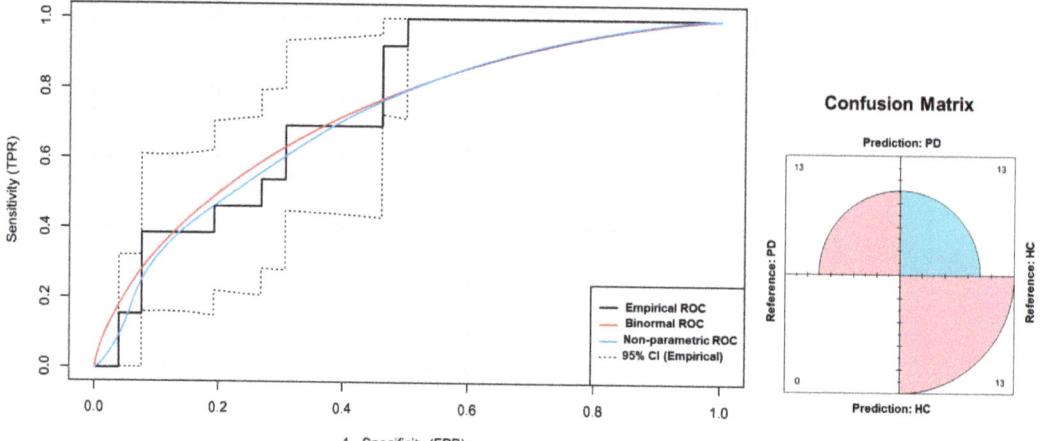

Figure 4. Receiver operating characteristic (ROC) curve (black line) (left image) and confusion matrix (right image) of the phase locking value (PLV) in the delta frequency band during the motor task for the classification of healthy controls (HCs) and Parkinson disease (PD) patients in our cohort. Non-parametric ROC curve (blue line), binormal ROC curve (red line) and 95% confidence interval (C.I.; dotted lines) are shown. AUC = area under the curve. CI = confidence interval. TPR = true positive ratio; FPR = false positive ratio.

4. Discussion

In the present study, we evaluated brain connectivity through a quantitative EEG analysis in Parkinson's disease versus healthy controls, at rest and during a pedaling motor task, exploring the diagnostic performance of the phase locking value (PLV) in discriminating the two study groups.

In the literature, few studies explored the PLV analysis in the PD population. Bertrand, McIntosh, Postuma, Kovacevic, Latreille, Panisset, Chouinard and Gagnon [40] compared the baseline resting state EEG of healthy subjects and PD patients, and after a follow-up classified the PD patients who developed dementia and patients who did not developed dementia. The results were assessed in terms of both signal synchrony and variability at different timescales, respectively, and statistically expressed by the PLV and multiscale entropy (MSE). In the delta frequencies, the PLV was lower in the PD who developed dementia compared to the PD without dementia and controls, while, for the beta and gamma frequencies, the PD-dementia patients showed a higher PLV when compared with the PD-non dementia patients, and both groups showed a higher PLV when compared to the controls. Conversely, the signal variability was lower at the higher frequencies and higher at the lower ones.

The main hypothesis in Gerardo Sánchez-Dinorín et al.'s [53] research was that functional connectivity abnormalities could predict cognitive decline in Parkinson's disease. The study showed that the increased synchrony of frontal slow waves predicts cognitive decline in PD patients after less than a decade with the illness [53].

In Soojin Lee et al.'s [54] study, the PLV was employed to evaluate the effect of dopaminergic medication and electrical vestibular stimulation (EVS) in Parkinson's disease. While levodopa medication was effective in normalizing the mean PLV only, all EVS stimuli normalized the mean, variability, and entropy of the PLV in the PD subject, demonstrating both low- and high-frequency EVS exert widespread influences on cortico-cortical connectivity [54].

In the present study, the results showed no significant differences in the PLV connectivity between the two groups (PD vs. HCs) during the resting state, but a higher PLV connectivity in the delta band during the motor task in the HCs compared to PD. In addition, comparing the resting state versus motor task for each group, only in the HC results showed a higher PLV connectivity in the delta band during the motor task. These results showed a deficit for the PD subjects in modulating the delta band PLV brain synchrony during movement, in contrast with the healthy controls. In addition, in our study the PLV connectivity was not correlated with cognitive performance.

These preliminary results also show that the higher value of the PLV during the motor task could be a potential useful tool as a neurophysiological connectivity biomarker for PD. Considering the ROC AUC of 0.75, which indicates a good discrimination performance, the sensitivity of 100%, indicating the ability to identify a high number of patients potentially affected by PD, and a NPV of 100% indicating the ability to exclude only truly HCs, combined with its lower specificity and PPV, leads this predictor to be the candidate as a screening biomarker.

The main limitations of the study are the small number of the sample, the type of motor task which was not compared to different motor tasks of lower limbs or tasks of upper limbs, and in line with the lack of consensus in the classification of frequency bands for the quantitative EEG analysis [47], the specific band selected for the present study can be a limitation, therefore further studies are needed to confirm the results and the proposed applications.

5. Conclusions

The present study evaluated the brain connectivity through a quantitative EEG analysis in Parkinson's disease versus healthy controls, showing a higher PLV connectivity in the delta band during the motor task in the HCs compared to PD. This neurophysiology biomarker showed the potentiality to be explored in future studies as a potential screening biomarker for PD patients.

Author Contributions: Conceptualization, L.d.B.; writing—original draft preparation, L.d.B., L.R., M.L.C., P.M.P. and S.P.C.; writing—review and editing, L.d.B., L.R. and V.D.L.; supervision, V.D.L. All authors have read and agreed to the published version of the manuscript.

Funding: This research received no external funding.

Institutional Review Board Statement: The study of the original dataset was approved by the University of Iowa Office of the Institutional Review Board (IRB). In addition, the present study was approved with a notification by the local ethics committee of the University Campus Bio-Medico of Rome.

Informed Consent Statement: Informed consent was obtained from all subjects involved in the original dataset studies.

Data Availability Statement: The data presented in this study are openly available in http://www.predictsite.com/ (accessed on 1 January 2022) [42].

Conflicts of Interest: The authors declare no conflict of interest.

References

1. Poewe, W.; Seppi, K.; Tanner, C.M.; Halliday, G.M.; Brundin, P.; Volkmann, J.; Schrag, A.-E.; Lang, A.E. Parkinson disease. *Nat. Rev. Dis. Prim.* **2017**, *3*, 1–21. [CrossRef] [PubMed]
2. Rizzo, G.; Copetti, M.; Arcuti, S.; Martino, D.; Fontana, A.; Logroscino, G. Accuracy of clinical diagnosis of Parkinson disease: A systematic review and meta-analysis. *Neurology* **2016**, *86*, 566–576. [CrossRef] [PubMed]
3. Gibb, W.; Lees, A. The relevance of the Lewy body to the pathogenesis of idiopathic Parkinson's disease. *J. Neurol. Neurosurg. Psychiatry.* **1988**, *51*, 745–752. [CrossRef] [PubMed]
4. Sanchez-Ferro, A.; Elshehabi, M.; Godinho, C.; Salkovic, D.; Hobert, M.A.; Domingos, J.; van Uem, J.M.; Ferreira, J.J.; Maetzler, W. New methods for the assessment of Parkinson's disease (2005 to 2015): A systematic review. *Mov. Disord.* **2016**, *31*, 1283–1292. [CrossRef] [PubMed]
5. di Biase, L.; Pecoraro, P.M.; Pecoraro, G.; Caminiti, M.L.; Di Lazzaro, V. Markerless Radio Frequency Indoor Monitoring for Telemedicine: Gait Analysis, Indoor Positioning, Fall Detection, Tremor Analysis, Vital Signs and Sleep Monitoring. *Sensors* **2022**, *22*, 8486. [CrossRef]

6. d'Angelis, O.; Di Biase, L.; Vollero, L.; Merone, M. IoT architecture for continuous long term monitoring: Parkinson's Disease case study. *Internet Things* **2022**, *20*, 100614. [CrossRef]
7. Stamatakis, J.; Ambroise, J.; Cremers, J.; Sharei, H.; Delvaux, V.; Macq, B.; Garraux, G. Finger tapping clinimetric score prediction in Parkinson's disease using low-cost accelerometers. *Comput. Intell. Neurosci.* **2013**, *2013*, 717853. [CrossRef]
8. Summa, S.; Tosi, J.; Taffoni, F.; Di Biase, L.; Marano, M.; Rizzo, A.C.; Tombini, M.; Di Pino, G.; Formica, D. Assessing bradykinesia in Parkinson's disease using gyroscope signals. In Proceedings of the 2017 international conference on rehabilitation robotics (ICORR), London, UK, 17–20 July 2017; pp. 1556–1561.
9. di Biase, L.; Summa, S.; Tosi, J.; Taffoni, F.; Marano, M.; Cascio Rizzo, A.; Vecchio, F.; Formica, D.; Di Lazzaro, V.; Di Pino, G.; et al. Quantitative Analysis of Bradykinesia and Rigidity in Parkinson's Disease. *Front. Neurol.* **2018**, *9*, 121. [CrossRef]
10. Deuschl, G.; Krack, P.; Lauk, M.; Timmer, J. Clinical neurophysiology of tremor. *J. Clin. Neurophysiol.* **1996**, *13*, 110–121. [CrossRef]
11. Di Pino, G.; Formica, D.; Melgari, J.-M.; Taffoni, F.; Salomone, G.; di Biase, L.; Caimo, E.; Vernieri, F.; Guglielmelli, E. Neurophysiological bases of tremors and accelerometric parameters analysis. In Proceedings of the 2012 4th IEEE RAS & EMBS International Conference on Biomedical Robotics and Biomechatronics (BioRob), Rome, Italy, 24–27 June 2012; pp. 1820–1825.
12. di Biase, L.; Brittain, J.S.; Shah, S.A.; Pedrosa, D.J.; Cagnan, H.; Mathy, A.; Chen, C.C.; Martin-Rodriguez, J.F.; Mir, P.; Timmerman, L.; et al. Tremor stability index: A new tool for differential diagnosis in tremor syndromes. *Brain* **2017**, *140*, 1977–1986. [CrossRef]
13. di Biase, L.; Brittain, J.S.; Peter, B.; Di Lazzaro, V.; Shah, S.A. Methods and System for Characterising Tremors. US20200046259A1, 5 January 2023. Filed 17 January 2018 and issued 26 July 2018.
14. Endo, T.; Okuno, R.; Yokoe, M.; Akazawa, K.; Sakoda, S. A novel method for systematic analysis of rigidity in Parkinson's disease. *Mov. Disord. Off. J. Mov. Disord. Soc.* **2009**, *24*, 2218–2224. [CrossRef]
15. Kwon, Y.; Park, S.H.; Kim, J.W.; Ho, Y.; Jeon, H.M.; Bang, M.J.; Koh, S.B.; Kim, J.H.; Eom, G.M. Quantitative evaluation of parkinsonian rigidity during intra-operative deep brain stimulation. *Bio-Medical Mater. Eng.* **2014**, *24*, 2273–2281. [CrossRef] [PubMed]
16. Raiano, L.; Di Pino, G.; Di Biase, L.; Tombini, M.; Tagliamonte, N.L.; Formica, D. PDMeter: A Wrist Wearable Device for an at-home Assessment of the Parkinson's Disease Rigidity. *IEEE Trans. Neural Syst. Rehabil. Eng.* **2020**, *28*, 1325–1333. [CrossRef]
17. Moore, S.T.; MacDougall, H.G.; Gracies, J.M.; Cohen, H.S.; Ondo, W.G. Long-term monitoring of gait in Parkinson's disease. *Gait Posture* **2007**, *26*, 200–207. [CrossRef] [PubMed]
18. Schlachetzki, J.C.M.; Barth, J.; Marxreiter, F.; Gossler, J.; Kohl, Z.; Reinfelder, S.; Gassner, H.; Aminian, K.; Eskofier, B.M.; Winkler, J.; et al. Wearable sensors objectively measure gait parameters in Parkinson's disease. *PLoS ONE* **2017**, *12*, e0183989. [CrossRef] [PubMed]
19. Tosi, J.; Summa, S.; Taffoni, F.; Biase, L.d.; Marano, M.; Rizzo, A.C.; Tombini, M.; Schena, E.; Formica, D.; Pino, G.D. Feature Extraction in Sit-to-Stand Task Using M-IMU Sensors and Evaluatiton in Parkinson's Disease. In Proceedings of the 2018 IEEE International Symposium on Medical Measurements and Applications (MeMeA), Rome, Italy, 11–13 June 2018; pp. 1–6. [CrossRef]
20. Suppa, A.; Kita, A.; Leodori, G.; Zampogna, A.; Nicolini, E.; Lorenzi, P.; Rao, R.; Irrera, F. L-DOPA and freezing of gait in Parkinson's disease: Objective assessment through a wearable wireless system. *Front. Neurol.* **2017**, *8*, 406. [CrossRef]
21. di Biase, L.; Di Santo, A.; Caminiti, M.L.; De Liso, A.; Shah, S.A.; Ricci, L.; Di Lazzaro, V. Gait analysis in Parkinson's disease: An overview of the most accurate markers for diagnosis and symptoms monitoring. *Sensors* **2020**, *20*, 3529. [CrossRef]
22. di Biase, L.; Raiano, L.; Caminiti, M.L.; Pecoraro, P.M.; Di Lazzaro, V. Parkinson's Disease Wearable Gait Analysis: Kinematic and Dynamic Markers for Diagnosis. *Sensors* **2022**, *22*, 8773. [CrossRef]
23. Alam, M.N.; Garg, A.; Munia, T.T.K.; Fazel-Rezai, R.; Tavakolian, K. Vertical ground reaction force marker for Parkinson's disease. *PLoS ONE* **2017**, *12*, e0175951. [CrossRef]
24. Cavallo, F.; Moschetti, A.; Esposito, D.; Maremmani, C.; Rovini, E. Upper limb motor pre-clinical assessment in Parkinson's disease using machine learning. *Park. Relat. Disord.* **2019**, *63*, 111–116. [CrossRef]
25. Xu, S.; Pan, Z. A novel ensemble of random forest for assisting diagnosis of Parkinson's disease on small handwritten dynamics dataset. *Int. J. Med. Inform.* **2020**, *144*, 104283. [CrossRef]
26. di Biase, L.; Raiano, L.; Caminiti, M.L.; Pecoraro, P.M.; Di Lazzaro, V. Artificial intelligence in Parkinson's disease—Symptoms identification and monitoring. In *Augmenting Neurological Disorder Prediction and Rehabilitation Using Artificial Intelligence*; Elsevier: Amsterdam, The Netherlands, 2022; pp. 35–52.
27. di Biase, L.; Tinkhauser, G.; Martin Moraud, E.; Caminiti, M.L.; Pecoraro, P.M.; Di Lazzaro, V. Adaptive, personalized closed-loop therapy for Parkinson's disease: Biochemical, neurophysiological, and wearable sensing systems. *Expert Rev. Neurother.* **2021**, *21*, 1371–1388. [CrossRef] [PubMed]
28. Assenza, G.; Capone, F.; di Biase, L.; Ferreri, F.; Florio, L.; Guerra, A.; Marano, M.; Paolucci, M.; Ranieri, F.; Salomone, G. Oscillatory activities in neurological disorders of elderly: Biomarkers to target for neuromodulation. *Front. Aging Neurosci.* **2017**, *9*, 189. [CrossRef]
29. Melgari, J.-M.; Curcio, G.; Mastrolilli, F.; Salomone, G.; Trotta, L.; Tombini, M.; Di Biase, L.; Scrascia, F.; Fini, R.; Fabrizio, E. Alpha and beta EEG power reflects L-dopa acute administration in parkinsonian patients. *Front. Aging Neurosci.* **2014**, *6*, 302. [CrossRef]
30. Tinkhauser, G.; Pogosyan, A.; Debove, I.; Nowacki, A.; Shah, S.A.; Seidel, K.; Tan, H.; Brittain, J.S.; Petermann, K.; di Biase, L. Directional local field potentials: A tool to optimize deep brain stimulation. *Mov. Disord.* **2018**, *33*, 159–164. [CrossRef]
31. di Biase, L.; Fasano, A. Low-frequency deep brain stimulation for Parkinson's disease: Great expectation or false hope? *Mov. Disord.* **2016**, *31*, 962–967. [CrossRef] [PubMed]

32. Tessitore, A.; Cirillo, M.; De Micco, R. Functional connectivity signatures of Parkinson's disease. Journal of Parkinson's disease. *J. Park. Dis.* **2019**, *9*, 637–652.
33. Herz, D.M.; Eickhoff, S.B.; Løkkegaard, A.; Siebner, H.R. Functional neuroimaging of motor control in Parkinson's disease: A meta-analysis. *Hum. Brain Mapp.* **2014**, *35*, 3227–3237. [CrossRef]
34. Tahmasian, M.; Bettray, L.M.; van Eimeren, T.; Drzezga, A.; Timmermann, L.; Eickhoff, C.R.; Eickhoff, S.B.; Eggers, C. A systematic review on the applications of resting-state fMRI in Parkinson's disease: Does dopamine replacement therapy play a role? *Cortex* **2015**, *73*, 80–105. [CrossRef]
35. Conti, M.; Bovenzi, R.; Garasto, E.; Schirinzi, T.; Placidi, F.; Mercuri, N.B.; Cerroni, R.; Pierantozzi, M.; Stefani, A. Brain Functional Connectivity in de novo Parkinson's Disease Patients Based on Clinical EEG. *Front. Neurol.* **2022**, *13*, 844745. [CrossRef]
36. Aydore, S.; Pantazis, D.; Leahy, R.M. A note on the phase locking value and its properties. *Neuroimage* **2013**, *74*, 231–244. [CrossRef]
37. Lachaux, J.P.; Rodriguez, E.; Martinerie, J.; Varela, F.J. Measuring phase synchrony in brain signals. *Hum. Brain Mapp.* **1999**, *8*, 194–208. [CrossRef]
38. Mormann, F.; Lehnertz, K.; David, P.; Elger, C.E. Mean phase coherence as a measure for phase synchronization and its application to the EEG of epilepsy patients. *Phys. D Nonlinear Phenom.* **2000**, *144*, 358–369. [CrossRef]
39. Amano, S.; Hong, S.L.; Sage, J.I.; Torres, E.B. Behavioral inflexibility and motor dedifferentiation in persons with Parkinson's disease: Bilateral coordination deficits during a unimanual reaching task. *Neurosci. Lett.* **2015**, *585*, 82–87. [CrossRef]
40. Bertrand, J.-A.; McIntosh, A.R.; Postuma, R.B.; Kovacevic, N.; Latreille, V.; Panisset, M.; Chouinard, S.; Gagnon, J.-F. Brain connectivity alterations are associated with the development of dementia in Parkinson's disease. *Brain Connect.* **2016**, *6*, 216–224. [CrossRef] [PubMed]
41. Singh, A.; Cole, R.C.; Espinoza, A.I.; Brown, D.; Cavanagh, J.F.; Narayanan, N.S. Frontal theta and beta oscillations during lower-limb movement in Parkinson's disease. *Clin. Neurophysiol.* **2020**, *131*, 694–702. [CrossRef] [PubMed]
42. Cavanagh, J.F.; Napolitano, A.; Wu, C.; Mueen, A. The Patient Repository for EEG Data + Computational Tools (PRED+CT). *Front. Neuroinform* **2017**, *11*, 67. [CrossRef] [PubMed]
43. Gibb, W.; Lees, A. A comparison of clinical and pathological features of young-and old-onset Parkinson's disease. *Neurology* **1988**, *38*, 1402. [CrossRef]
44. Ricci, L.; Croce, P.; Lanzone, J.; Boscarino, M.; Zappasodi, F.; Tombini, M.; Di Lazzaro, V.; Assenza, G. Transcutaneous Vagus Nerve Stimulation Modulates EEG Microstates and Delta Activity in Healthy Subjects. *Brain Sci.* **2020**, *10*, 668. [CrossRef]
45. Croce, P.; Ricci, L.; Pulitano, P.; Boscarino, M.; Zappasodi, F.; Lanzone, J.; Narducci, F.; Mecarelli, O.; Di Lazzaro, V.; Tombini, M.; et al. Machine learning for predicting levetiracetam treatment response in temporal lobe epilepsy. *Clin. Neurophysiol.* **2021**, *132*, 3035–3042. [CrossRef]
46. Ricci, L.; Assenza, G.; Pulitano, P.; Simonelli, V.; Vollero, L.; Lanzone, J.; Mecarelli, O.; Di Lazzaro, V.; Tombini, M. Measuring the effects of first antiepileptic medication in Temporal Lobe Epilepsy: Predictive value of quantitative-EEG analysis. *Clin. Neurophysiol.* **2021**, *132*, 25–35. [CrossRef]
47. Babiloni, C.; Barry, R.J.; Başar, E.; Blinowska, K.J.; Cichocki, A.; Drinkenburg, W.; Klimesch, W.; Knight, R.T.; Lopes da Silva, F.; Nunez, P.; et al. International Federation of Clinical Neurophysiology (IFCN)—EEG research workgroup: Recommendations on frequency and topographic analysis of resting state EEG rhythms. Part 1: Applications in clinical research studies. *Clin. Neurophysiol.* **2020**, *131*, 285–307. [CrossRef] [PubMed]
48. Pellegrino, G.; Mecarelli, O.; Pulitano, P.; Tombini, M.; Ricci, L.; Lanzone, J.; Brienza, M.; Davassi, C.; Di Lazzaro, V.; Assenza, G. Eslicarbazepine Acetate Modulates EEG Activity and Connectivity in Focal Epilepsy. *Front. Neurol.* **2018**, *9*, 1054. [CrossRef]
49. Jobert, M.; Wilson, F.J.; Ruigt, G.S.; Brunovsky, M.; Prichep, L.S.; Drinkenburg, W.H.; Committee, I.P.-E.G. Guidelines for the recording and evaluation of pharmaco-EEG data in man: The International Pharmaco-EEG Society (IPEG). *Neuropsychobiology* **2012**, *66*, 201–220. [CrossRef] [PubMed]
50. Team, R.C. R: A Language and Environment for Statistical Computing. R Foundation for Statistical Computing 2018. Available online: https://www.R-project.org/ (accessed on 1 January 2022).
51. Wobbrock, J.O.; Findlater, L.; Gergle, D.; Higgins, J.J. The aligned rank transform for nonparametric factorial analyses using only anova procedures. In Proceedings of the SIGCHI Conference on Human Factors in Computing Systems, Vancouver, BC, Canada, 7–12 May 2011; pp. 143–146.
52. Carpenter, J.; Bithell, J. Bootstrap confidence intervals: When, which, what? A practical guide for medical statisticians. *Stat. Med.* **2000**, *19*, 1141–1164. [CrossRef]
53. Sánchez-Dinorín, G.; Rodríguez-Violante, M.; Cervantes-Arriaga, A.; Navarro-Roa, C.; Ricardo-Garcell, J.; Rodríguez-Camacho, M.; Solís-Vivanco, R. Frontal functional connectivity and disease duration interactively predict cognitive decline in Parkinson's disease. *Clin. Neurophysiol.* **2021**, *132*, 510–519. [CrossRef]
54. Lee, S.; Liu, A.; Wang, Z.J.; McKeown, M.J. Abnormal phase coupling in Parkinson's disease and normalization effects of subthreshold vestibular stimulation. *Front. Hum. Neurosci.* **2019**, *13*, 118. [CrossRef]

Disclaimer/Publisher's Note: The statements, opinions and data contained in all publications are solely those of the individual author(s) and contributor(s) and not of MDPI and/or the editor(s). MDPI and/or the editor(s) disclaim responsibility for any injury to people or property resulting from any ideas, methods, instructions or products referred to in the content.

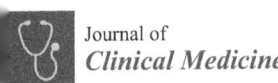

Article

Gait Characterization and Analysis of Hereditary Amyloidosis Associated with Transthyretin Patients: A Case Series

Maria do Carmo Vilas-Boas [1,2,*], Pedro Filipe Pereira Fonseca [3], Inês Martins Sousa [3,4], Márcio Neves Cardoso [1], João Paulo Silva Cunha [2,3] and Teresa Coelho [1]

1. Centro Hospitalar Universitário do Porto, Hospital Santo António, Unidade Corino de Andrade, E.P.E., Largo do Prof. Abel Salazar, 4099-001 Porto, Portugal; marciocardoso.neurofisiologia@chporto.min-saude.pt (M.N.C.); tcoelho@netcabo.pt (T.C.)
2. INESC TEC (Instituto de Engenharia de Sistemas e Computadores, Tecnologia e Ciência), FEUP (Faculdade de Engenharia da Universidade do Porto), University of Porto, R. Dr. Roberto Frias, 4200-465 Porto, Portugal; jpcunha@inesctec.pt
3. LABIOMEP: Porto Biomechanics Laboratory, University of Porto, R. Dr. Plácido de Costa, 91, 4200-450 Porto, Portugal; pedro.labiomep@fade.up.pt (P.F.P.F.); inesmartinsdesousaa@gmail.com (I.M.S.)
4. Escola Superior de Biotecnologia, Universidade Católica Portuguesa Rua de Diogo Botelho, 1327, 4169-005 Porto, Portugal
* Correspondence: carmo.vilas.boas@inesctec.pt; Tel.: +351-22-209-4000

Abstract: Hereditary amyloidosis associated with transthyretin (ATTRv), is a rare autosomal dominant disease characterized by length-dependent symmetric polyneuropathy that has gait impairment as one of its consequences. The gait pattern of V30M ATTRv amyloidosis patients has been described as similar to that of diabetic neuropathy, associated with steppage, but has never been quantitatively characterized. In this study we aim to characterize the gait pattern of patients with V30M ATTRv amyloidosis, thus providing information for a better understanding and potential for supporting diagnosis and disease progression evaluation. We present a case series in which we conducted two gait analyses, 18 months apart, of five V30M ATTRv amyloidosis patients using a 12-camera, marker based, optical system as well as six force platforms. Linear kinematics, ground reaction forces, and angular kinematics results are analyzed for all patients. All patients, except one, showed a delayed toe-off in the second assessment, as well as excessive pelvic rotation, hip extension and external transverse rotation and knee flexion (in stance and swing phases), along with reduced vertical and mediolateral ground reaction forces. The described gait anomalies are not clinically quantified; thus, gait analysis may contribute to the assessment of possible disease progression along with the clinical evaluation.

Keywords: ATTRv amyloidosis; clinical neurology; peripheral neuropathy; gait analysis; movement quantification; Familial Amyloid Polyneuropathy

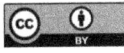

1. Introduction

Hereditary amyloidosis associated with transthyretin (ATTRv amyloidosis), once known as Familial Amyloid Polyneuropathy, is a rare autosomal dominant disease characterized by polyneuropathy due to amyloid deposition in the peripheral nerves and major organs [1]. More than 120-point mutations related to ATTRv amyloidosis and nerve degeneration have been identified, with the most common cases linked to the replacement of valine by methionine at position 30 of the TTR protein (V30M). This has led to the current designation of this condition as V30M ATTRv amyloidosis.

V30M ATTRv amyloidosis is a highly disabling multisystemic disorder with variable onset and penetration worldwide [2]. The global prevalence has been recently estimated by Schmidt et al. [2] to be around 10,000 persons, although considerable uncertainty exists (range 5526–38,468). In Northern Portugal, where this pathology is endemic, the latest epidemiologic study reported a prevalence of 163.1 per 100,000 adult inhabitants [2]. A prevalence increase of 16% was reported for the Portuguese cities with the highest prevalence (Vila do Conde and Póvoa de Varzim) in the last 21 years [3]. In other countries, the reported prevalence was 104 per 100,000 inhabitants in the northern region of Sweden in 2018 [2]; 1.1–1.55 per 100,000 inhabitants in Nagano (Japan), in 2005 [4]; and 3.72 per 100,000 in Cyprus, in 2003 [5].

The disease presents itself as a nerve length-dependent symmetric polyneuropathy that typically starts at the feet with loss of temperature and pain sensations. It is associated with life-threatening autonomic dysfunction, leading to cachexia and death within 7.3 to 11 years from onset, if left untreated [6]. The natural course of this condition is classified into three stages: I—patients are ambulatory, have mostly mild sensory, motor, and autonomic neuropathy in the lower limbs; II—patients are still ambulatory but require assistance and have mostly moderate impairment progression in the lower limbs, upper limbs, and trunk; and III—patients are bedridden or wheelchair bound and present severe sensory, motor, and autonomic involvement of all limbs [7].

Regarding treatment, liver transplantation has often been the only option for these patients. In recent decades, however, other therapeutic strategies have been developed, such as TTR stabilizers (e.g., tafamidis, indicated for stage I patients, especially for women with slow disease progression [8]), small interfering RNAs (e.g., Patisiran, indicated for stage II, which is intravenous and not indicated for patients with prevalent cardiac involvement [9]) and antisense oligonucleotides (e.g., Inotersen, also indicated for stage II, which affects the kidney and platelets volume [10]). However, liver transplantation is still the most effective and affordable option for V30M ATTRv amyloidosis patients, as management strategies lack cohesion and patients experience years of misdiagnosis and negligible treatment [11].

Motor function of V30M ATTRv amyloidosis patients is currently evaluated with a comprehensive neurological examination, which may include nerve conduction studies with sympathetic skin response (SSR), quantitative sensory testing [12] and self-report questionnaires, such as the Norfolk Quality of Life—Diabetic Neuropathy (QoL-DN) questionnaire [13]. Direct observation followed by a qualitative assessment of movement-associated symptoms based on rating scales is also an approach frequently used [14,15]. The gait pattern of V30M ATTRv amyloidosis patients has been described as similar to that of diabetic neuropathy, associated with steppage gait, loss of dorsiflexion and consequent foot drop and high lifting of the leg [1,16]. On visual inspection, patients spread the legs to improve balance, exaggerating knee and hip flexion and "throwing" the feet forward, as a compensatory strategy in order to improve ground clearance.

There are several different ways of performing gait analysis, with the optic camera-based systems being described as highly accurate [17]. These systems determine a point-position of specific anatomical landmarks on the subject's body, with a high time and spatial resolution. Multiple infrared cameras can be used to compute a 3D trajectory [18], but other than some markers placed directly to the skin, there are no more constraints to the patient's movement [18]. Despite the advantages of the quantification of gait characteristics with the use of motion capture technology, this is still relatively rare in neurological conditions [14], and an exploratory subject with patients with V30M ATTRv amyloidosis [19].

The objective of this study is to quantitatively characterize the gait pattern of patients with V30M ATTRv amyloidosis, thus providing information for a better understanding of the loss of function and with potential for supporting diagnosis and progression evaluation. To the best of our knowledge this analysis has not yet been reported with patients suffering of V30M ATTRv amyloidosis, with only one study reporting a selection of spatiotemporal and angular parameters obtained with a RGB-D camera [20] and another using a machine learning model to distinguish between healthy and V30M ATTRv amyloidosis mutation carriers (with or without symptoms), also using gait information recorded with a RGB-D system [21].

Due to the lack of information in the scientific literature [20], this study's objective is to present an ATTRv V30M amyloidosis patients' gait quantitative characterization over a period of 18 months. Since this is a rare disease, this study is structured as a case series reporting the gait pattern of five V30M ATTRv amyloidosis patients.

2. Materials and Methods

2.1. Participants

A group of five patients from the V30M ATTRv amyloidosis unit of the Hospital Santo António—Centro Hospitalar Universitário do Porto (Porto, Portugal) were invited to participate in this study. All the participants had the V30M mutation, although presenting different impairments, such as gait abnormalities, muscular weakness, pain, thermal or tactile anesthesia, or reduced proprioception.

The exclusion criteria were defined and assessed by a neurologist as the presence of orthopaedic, musculoskeletal, rheumatically or cardiovascular constraints that might impair locomotion, and other neurological conditions not associated to the pathology under study. Gait analysis of this group was performed twice: at an initial assessment (T0) and at a second assessment 18 months later (T1). The participants' demographic and clinical data can be consulted in Table 1.

Table 1. Demographics and clinical data for each patient that participated in the experiment. All data reports to the time of the first gait analysis, while BMI variation represents the change between analysis periods.

Patient	Gender [1]	Height (m)	Weight (kg)	Age (Years)	BMI (kg/m^2)	BMI Variation (kg/m^2)	Years of Disease Progression	Years since Diagnosis
P1	M	1.72	72.0	34	24.34	0.0	9	8
P2	M	1.73	58.5	33	19.55	1.5	8	8
P3	F	1.68	63.8	48	22.60	0.6	5	2
P4	F	1.48	61.5	54	28.08	−1.4	18	17
P5	M	1.71	53.0	52	18.13	0.9	13	13

[1] Gender is expressed as male (M) and female (F). BMI stands for body mass index.

This study was authorized by the Centro Hospitalar Universitário do Porto Ethics Committee with the protocol number 2014/167(119-DEFI/149-CES), in accordance with the Declaration of Helsinki. All participants read and signed an informed consent form prior to any data collection.

2.2. Clinical Assessment

The Medical Research Council Scale (MRC) was applied to the patients by a neurologist in order to assess the state of each analyzed movement: (0) no contraction, (1) flicker or trace of contraction, (2) active movement with gravity eliminated, (3) active movement against gravity, (4) active movement against gravity and resistance, and (5) normal strength [22]. A minus (−) or plus (+) sign was introduced to characterize the movement against a smaller or stronger resistance exerted by a physician, respectively.

Additionally, the Polyneuropathy Disability score (PND) was applied as: (0) no impairment, (I) sensory disturbances in extremities but preserved walking capacity, (II) difficulties in walking but without the need for a walking stick, (IIIa) one stick or one crutch required for walking, (IIIb) two sticks or two crutches required for walking and (IV) patient confined to a wheelchair or bed [23].

The Transthyretin Familial Amyloid Polyneuropathy (TTR-FAP) score was applied as: (Stage 0) asymptomatic; (Stage I) mild, ambulatory, symptoms at lower limbs limited; (Stage II) moderate, further neuropathic deterioration, ambulatory but requires assistance; (Stage III) severe, bedridden/wheelchair bound with generalized weakness.

2.3. Experimental Setup

Kinematic data was recorded using a 11-camera Oqus system (Qualisys AB, Gotenburg, Sweden) operating at a sampling frequency of 200 Hz. Prior to each session the camera system was calibrated with a maximum acceptable error of 0.7 mm. Ground reaction forces were collected with five resistive (Bertec, Columbus, OH, USA) and one piezoelectric (Kistler, Winterthur, Switzerland) force platforms, operating at a sampling frequency of 2000 Hz, and in synchrony with the motion capture system. The force platforms occupied an area of 2.4 m by 0.9 m.

The gait analysis area was defined as a region of 7.0 m length and 1.0 m width, with the first pair of force platforms placed at its midpoint, and delimited by a pair of signaling cones, as depicted in Figure 1. This region coincided with the motion capture system calibrated volume.

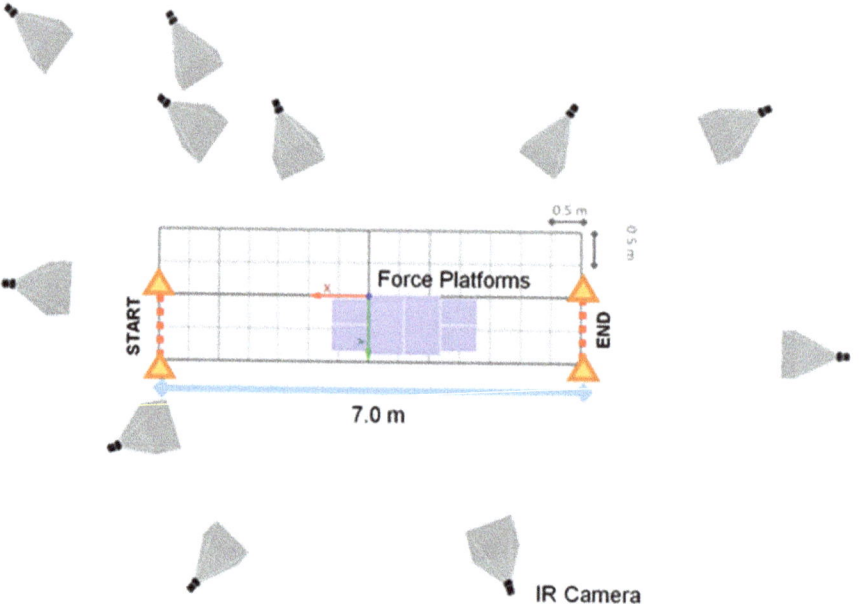

Figure 1. Representation of the gait analysis path with its dimension and limits. The setup of the motion capture cameras is represented by their viewing cones, and the purple squares represent the force platforms.

2.4. Marker Setup and Biomechanical Model

A lower-limb marker setup was used, comprising thirty-two passive retro-reflective markers placed over relevant anatomical landmarks. Markers were placed on the right and left anterior and posterior iliac spines, at the right and left trochanter, on the right and left lateral and medial femur epicondyles, on the right and left tibial tuberosity, on the right and left head of the fibula, on the right and left lateral prominence of the lateral and medial malleolus, on the right and left distal end of the posterior aspect of the calcaneus, on the right and left lateral aspect of the first and fifth metatarsal head, and on the dorsal aspect of the second metatarsal head. Additionally, four-marker clusters were positioned on right and left thighs and shanks, according to the CAST marker set [24,25].

2.5. Experimental Procedures

Participants were instructed to walk naturally and barefoot at a comfortable self-selected pace, back and forth, along the analysis path. At least 10 valid trials were performed by each participant.

Patients who normally used walking aids or splints did not use them for this experiment. Additionally, a research assistant accompanied the participant along the path and was prepared to help in case of difficulties during the task.

2.6. Data Processing

After data collection, the Qualisys Track Manager (Qualisys AB, Gotenburg, Sweden) software was used to review and identify each marker trajectory, and trajectory gaps were interpolated using the built-in polynomial calculations. The resulting processed data was then exported to the Visual3D software (C-Motion, Inc., Germantown, MD, USA) for further processing and analysis, including trajectory filtration with a 6 Hz bidirectional low-pass Butterworth filter and the creation of a six degrees of freedom anatomical model. A global and local coordinate system (for each segment) has been defined in which the X axis corresponds to the lateral (+) and medial (−) directions, the Y axis corresponds to the anterior (+) and posterior (−) directions, and the Z axis corresponds to the cephalic (+) and caudal (−) directions [26]. Gait events were calculated automatically with the appropriate Visual3D built-in routine, and included heel strike (HS), midstance (MS) and toe off (TO). Joint angles were calculated using the rotation order of the distal segment with respect to the proximal segment, applying each segment's local coordinate system [26]. Lower-limb angles were assigned with three rotational degrees of freedom and calculated using an XYZ Cardan sequence of rotations, which are equivalent to flexion/extension, abduction/adduction and axial rotation, respectively. Hip flexion, knee flexion, and ankle dorsiflexion were displayed as positive angular displacement.

Linear and angular kinematics, as well as the corresponding ground reaction forces were retrieved. Linear kinematics included gait speed, stride length and width, step length, cadence (steps/minute), as well as gait cycle, stance, swing and double limb support duration. Angular metrics were extracted at the instant of left and right heel strike (HS), midstance (MD) and toe-off (TO).

Angular kinematics were time-normalized to the gait cycle (heel strike to heel strike), while ground reaction forces were normalized to the stance duration (heel strike to toe off). Ground reaction forces were also amplitude-normalized and expressed as a percentage of the participant's body weight (BW). Events were calculated for the characterizing points in the anterior-posterior (FAP), medial-lateral (FML) and vertical (FV) force vectors, and numbered consecutively, according to [25].

The reference gait data for non-pathological individuals used as comparison in this study were retrieved from the Qualisys Clinical Gait Plug-In analysis module.

2.7. Statistical Analysis

Data normality was assessed using the Kolmogorov–Smirnov test for variables over 50 data points, or the Shapiro–Wilk test when less than 50 data points were available. For parametric data, a paired sample t-test and effect size calculation was performed between T0 and T1. Effect size was evaluated according to the η_ρ^2 value [27]. Results were interpreted as small (0.01), moderate (0.06) or large (0.14) [27]. For non-parametric data, the Wilcoxon signed rank test was performed and effect size calculated as Cohen's d, and interpreted as small (0.1), moderate (0.3) or large (0.5) [27]. Descriptive statistics were computed for each subject and are presented as mean (standard deviation) or median [interquartile range] for parametric and non-parametric variables, respectively.

All statistical procedures were performed using SPSS 26 (IBM, New York, NY, USA) and a significance level of $\alpha = 0.05$ was used.

3. Results

3.1. Clinical Assessment

The results from the clinical assessment of each participant revealed different scores, indicating distinct progression and manifestation of the pathology. These results are presented in Table 2.

Table 2. Clinical evolution of the ATTRv V30M patients based on the Medical Research Council (MRC) Scale. The Polyneuropathy disability (PND) and TTR-FAP scores are also indicated.

Patient	MRC [1] Scores at T0	MRC [1] Scores at T1	PND Score [2],*	TTR-FAP Score [2],*	Treatment at T0
P1	Dorsiflexion deficit (4), minor vibration anesthesia on the hallux	Dorsiflexion deficit (4−), minor vibration anesthesia on the hallux	II	I	Transplant 6 years ago
P2	Dorsiflexion (0), plantar-flexion (1), knee flexion and extension (4), sensory ataxia and high steppage	Dorsiflexion (0), plantar-flexion (0), knee flexion and extension (4), sensory ataxia and high steppage	II	I	Tafamidis for 3.5 years
P3	Only vibration anesthesia on the hallux, minor difficulties on heels or tip toes gait	Only vibration anesthesia on the hallux, minor difficulties on heels or tip toes gait	II	I	Tafamidis for 1 year
P4	Dorsiflexion (4), plantar-flexion (4), sensory ataxia, low steppage	Dorsiflexion (3), plantar-flexion (4), sensory ataxia, steppage	II	I	Transplant 12 years ago
P5	Dorsiflexion and plantar-flexion (2), sensory ataxia and high steppage	Dorsiflexion (0), plantar-flexion (1), sensory ataxia and high steppage	II	I	Transplant 18 years ago

[1] MRC scores range from 0 (worst result) to 5 (best result). [2] PND and TTR-FAP range from I (*sensory disturbances in extremities but preserved walking capacity and mild, ambulatory, symptoms at lower limbs limited*) to IV (*patient confined to a wheelchair or bed*) or III (*severe, bedridden/wheelchair bound with generalized weakness*), respectively. * PND and TTR-FAP scores were the same in both evaluation periods.

They also presented some degree of motor deficit at the lower limbs: one patient had no strength deficit but had slight difficulty in walking on heels (P3), while the others had ankle dorsiflexion strength from 4/5 to 0/5, in the MRC scale [22], and ankle plantar-flexion from 4/5 to 1/5. All patients had normal knee segmental force (5/5), except P2 which had knee flexion and extension 4/5. All patients had flexion/extension of the toes between 0 and 3, and absent Achilles reflexes in both T0 and T1. Overall, patients presented sensory ataxia and steppage gait with different instability and movement coordination degrees during stride. They presented heterogeneous gait, although the clinical perception is that all alterations resulted from the sensory-motor polyneuropathy caused by the disease.

3.2. Summary of Results

Complete results are shown in Appendix A: Linear Kinematics, Appendix B: Ground Reaction Forces, and Appendix C: Angular Kinematics.

3.2.1. Linear Kinematics

A significant decrease in gait speed (P1: −13.51%, P2: −16.53%, P5: −5.62%) was observed at T1, associated with a shortening of the step length (but not stride width or length) and a lower cadence. These alterations also affected the gait cycle duration, which increased, along with the stance phase duration. In general, V30M ATTRv amyloidosis patients show longer gait cycles, associated with longer double limb support and shorter steps. There is no significant increase in step width, as one would expect, at least for P4 which went from "very low steppage", at T0 to formal "steppage" at T1. The patient P3 shows the least changes between sessions.

3.2.2. Ground Reaction Forces

The ground reaction forces recorded at T0 and T1 for the left (LLL) and right (RLL) lower limbs were recorded and compared. Figure 2 shows a representation of the (a) anterior-posterior, (b) medial-lateral and (c) vertical ground reaction forces produced by each subject at T1 as a function of the values recorded at T0. A full description of the ground reaction values can be consulted in Appendix B.

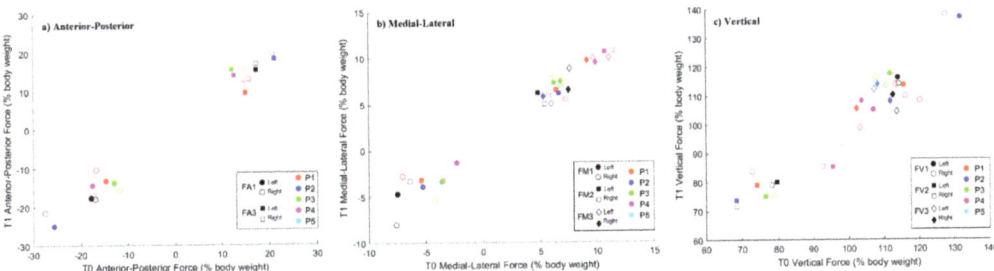

Figure 2. Scatterplot of the ground reaction force (% body weight) produced by each subject and limb at T1 in respect to T0 in the (**a**) anterior-posterior, (**b**) medial-lateral and (**c**) vertical directions, at the respective force characterizing events. FA1: maximum posterior loading force; FA3: maximum anterior thrusting force; FM1: first maximum lateral force; FM3: second maximum medial force; FV1: first maximum vertical loading force; FV2: dip trough force; FV3: second maximum vertical thrusting force.

Between evaluation sessions, significant alterations occurred in the ground reaction forces generated during gait, which were more expressive in the RLL (P1 and P4). Significant differences with moderate to large effect size were found for both limbs at maximum anterior thrusting force (FA3) for both patients, at the first maximum lateral force (FM1) for P1, and at the dip trough and second maximum vertical forces, FV2 and FV3, respectively, for P4. P5 showed significant alterations (with large effect size) in the FA3 and FM1 ground reaction forces generated during gait. From Figure 2 it is possible to see that FM1, FM3 and also FV3 are the force peaks that, in general, show the most prominent changes from T0 to T1.

P2 and P3 did not show significant alterations in the ground reaction forces generated during gait between T0 and T1. For P2, effect size was generally higher for RLL and at FV1 and FM1 for both limbs, and the patient shows lower FA1/FV2 and higher FA3/FV1. For P3, only the FV2 of the left limbs showed high effect size.

Regarding the healthy values described in the literature [28], P1, along with P3 and P4, show a lower maximum posterior loading force (FA1) than the mean reference value (20% body weight). P3 and P4 have a lower first maximum medial force (FM1, between 5 and 10% body weight). With regards to the first maximum vertical force (FV1) P1 shows a lowering in RLL cycles at T0, P2 shows a higher peak and all other patients show a lower value than normal (around 120% body weight). Minimum vertical force (FV2) is higher than normal (around 70% body weight) for P1, at T1, and for both lower limbs cycles for P3, P4 and P5. The maximum vertical force (FV3) is lower than usual (around 120% body weight) for all patients.

3.2.3. Angular Kinematics

A detailed description of each participant's joint angles at the analyzed gait events, as well as a representation of the joint angles during the gait cycle can be consulted in Appendix C.

In the three analyzed planes (sagittal, frontal and transverse), P1 showed a statistically significant difference with a large effect size in heel strike (HS) from T0 to T1 (27 of the 42 registered instances, 15 in the left and 12 in the right lower limb). Midstance (MD) and toe-off (TO) showed statistically significant differences in 20 and 22 moments, respectively (12 left and 8 and 10 right, each phase). P2 showed a statistically significant difference with a large effect size from T0 to T1 for 30 of the 42 HS analyzed (18 left and 12 right), 28 MD (14 left and 14 right) and 30 TO (16 left and 14 right). For P3, 22 HS (10 left and 12 right), 19 MD (11 left and 8 right) and 17 TO (8 left and 9 right) presented statistically significant differences from T0 to T1, along with a large effect size. P4 showed the following differences between assessments with 25 HS (12 left and 13 right), 22 MD (10 left and 12 right), and 21 TO (12 left and 9 right). P5 has the higher amount of differences between assessments 35 HS (16 left and 19 right), 35 MD (17 left and 18 right), and 37 TO (18 left and 19 right).

With regards to angular kinematics, graphical representation of the pelvis, hip, knees and ankles is presented in Appendix C. Statistical difference was explored for the different moments (T0 and T1), limbs (right and left) and between patients and reference gait data mean values for the three planes sagittal, frontal and transverse.

In summary, the results show that there is a general tendency to delay the toe-off at T1 (P1, P2, P3 and P5). All patients show a more retroverted pelvis than the reference data. P1, P2, and P4 show more prominent left and right pelvic rotation at T1 than T0. P1, P2, P3 and P5 show higher hip extension than the reference gait data. Excessive transverse rotation is also observed for the same participants. For all patients the knee flexion of the stance and swing phases (before and after the toe-off mark) is higher at T1 than T0 and also than the reference data. For P1, P2, P3 and P4, the transverse plane shows a tendency for the right lower limb cycles to show a more external rotation of the knee and the left lower limb cycles a more internal rotation. The ankle angle shows a higher dorsiflexion than the reference gait data before the toe-off for all participants, as well as higher ankle plantar-flexion immediately after the initial contact. In the transverse plane, P1, P2 and P3 show a generally more prominent internal rotation of the ankle than in the reference gait data.

4. Discussion

The goal of this study was to quantitatively characterize the gait pattern of patients with V30M ATTRv amyloidosis, thus providing information for a better understanding and potential for supporting disease progression. Laboratory gait analysis is an important part of the clinical evaluation of patients with complex locomotor disability and is claimed to improve the clinical outcomes [17].

We assessed five V30M ATTRv amyloidosis patients twice (18 months apart), using a 12-camera, marker-based, optical system as well as six force platforms. Linear kinematics, ground reaction forces, and angular kinematics results are analyzed for all patients. All patients, except one, showed a delayed toe-off in the second assessment, as well as excessive pelvic rotation, hip extension and external transverse rotation and knee flexion (in stance and swing phases), along with reduced vertical and medial-lateral ground reaction forces.

Our findings reveal that in general, V30M ATTRv amyloidosis patients show longer gait cycles, associated to longer double limb support time and shorter steps. In diabetic neuropathy, these alterations have been associated with decreased muscle strength of the ankle dorsiflexors and plantar-flexors [29]. All except one patient showed a delayed toe-off between assessments, increasing the stance phase and overall cycle time. All patients show a more retroverted pelvis than the reference data. Pelvic rotation was higher than for the reference healthy population for the majority of the patients, some even with a higher angular variation which denotes pelvic instability. On the contrary, P3 who is the patient with the minimal clinical abnormalities, shows a minimal pelvic rotation (around 1 degree, in the transverse plane) at T1. The normal rotation of about 4 degrees on either side of the central axis has the effect of smoothing the vertical dislocation of the center of mass and reducing the impact at foot strike [28], which may be difficult for the referred patient.

Our results show that the hip flexion-extension active range of motion, in the sagittal plane, is more prominent in ATTRv V30M amyloidosis patients (50 to 60 degrees) than in the reference population (around 45 degrees). Adduction and transverse external rotation are also more present in the pathological group, in different gait cycle phases, than in the reference data. Abnormal hip rotation may result from a compensatory movement. External rotation, in particular, may be used to facilitate hip flexion, using adductors as flexors [17].

Regarding the stance phase knee flexion, it is shown to be higher for patients than for the reference gait data and increases from one assessment (T0) to the other (T1). The same happens to the swing phase knee flexion. Excessive knee flexion usually follows abnormal initial contact, occurring to compensate for excessive plantar-flexion, without which the foot would drag. For a diabetic neuropathy group described in the literature, compared with reference group values, the maximum knee joint angle was smaller, in the sagittal plane [30]. A significantly reduced level of peak torques at the ankle and knee in a diabetic polyneuropathy group was also reported [31]. Steppage, which is present in P2, P3, P4 and P5, is a swing phase alteration consisting of exaggerated knee and hip flexion, to lift the foot higher than usual, for increased ground clearance. Usually patients present steppage to compensate for an excessive plantar-flexion—"foot drop"—due to inadequate dorsiflexion control.

All patients in this study show higher ankle plantar-flexion than the reference data immediately after the initial contact. This excessive ankle plantar-flexion during stance has a primary functional penalty which is loss of progression and leads to the shortening of the stride length and reduced gait speed. It also affects stability through the difficulty in maintaining the upright posture. It may be caused by weakness of the pretibial muscles (e.g., the tibialis anterior) which fail to produce an adequate dorsiflexion, allowing the foot to fall in an uncontrolled manner and therefore possibly hampering shock absorption [32]. In this study, patients also presented a higher dorsiflexion during midstance. This may be caused by prolonged heel contact and weakness or impaired control of the soleus which fails to stabilize the tibia, causing a sustained knee flexion. Without a stable foot base, the quadriceps are not able to extend the knee. A higher dorsiflexion may be caused by lack of feet stabilization. Concomitantly, knee flexion may besustained to lower the center of gravity and increase stabilization, or due to the lack of subclinical strength in knee extension (except in the case of P2 that has MRC 4 for knee strength). P3, although exhibiting a close to normal neurological examination, shows an interesting almost permanent dorsiflexion, which has been described as being associated with an inefficient push-off [28]. Excessive dorsiflexion at the time the heel contacts the floor is rare, and translates a position of instability [32]. The correct foot placement in stance and the adequate clearance of the ground in the swing phase are important requisites for safe walking.

With the GRF analysis, we find that FM1, FM3 and also FV3 are the force peaks that, in general, show the most prominent changes from T0 to T1. With regard to the FMs, these are the most variable of the three components of force and can be easily affected. The second vertical force peak (FV3), in which all patients had a performance lower than the values in the literature [28], relates to the amount of vertical propulsive force, which drives the person upwards. A low peak is associated with a poor ability to push off. Causes for insufficient push off may be associated, among other factors, with the triceps suræ weakness, that in these series was observed in P2, P4 and P5, or pain under the forefoot. Patients with V30M ATTRv amyloidosis may experience foot pain throughout the natural history of the disease [23]. The first peak of vertical force relates to the amount of loading the person is putting onto the front foot. In patients with diabetic neuropathy, the maximum values of the vertical component of GRF were found to be lower than in two control groups [30].

Reduced FA3 (P1, P3, P4 and P5) also shows that the person is not propelling the body forward efficiently. The maximum value of the anteroposterior forces was also found to be higher in a control group than in a diabetic neuropathy group [30]. A reduced loading, as was the observed with most of the ATTRv V30M amyloidosis patients, could relate to the presence of pain, discomfort, poor functional movement of lower limb joints or slow walking speed. Karmakar et al. [33], reported, regarding neuropathic pain, that it influenced gait stability and its potential relief using pharmacotherapy did not improve gait dysfunction.

With regard to disease modifying treatments, P1, P4 and P5 underwent orthotopic liver transplantation (LT), 6, 12 and 18 years before, and they presented 9, 18 and 13 years of disease progression. LT removes the main source of the circulating mutated TTR (over 90%), reduces the rate of axonal degeneration, and was the first available treatment of V30M ATTRv amyloidosis. It is an invasive surgical procedure, with long-term risks and morbidity. Nevertheless, early LT is reported to improve the course of the neuropathy [34,35] and to slow disease progression relative to the natural history of this disease [36]. After the first few years following LT, patients they are considered to be in a phase of almost no progression of the neuropathy due to a reduction of nerve loss in transplanted patients [34]. Clinically, the observed patients have a similar profile at T0 and T1 with only a small worsening (see Table 2), which may be attributed to slight clinical subjective impressions between the two clinical consultations. Furthermore, patients may complain of limb weakness, extreme fatigue, postural hypotension and cardiac involvement that are not generally protected/treated by LT [34]. These too can contribute to some gait changes, which may justify several statistically significant differences between both gait assessments, in the patients of this series. More studies are needed to understand the impact of these variables on gait abnormalities.

P2 and P3 have been taking tafamidis, a TTR stabilizer, for 3.5 years and 1 year, with 8 and 5 years of disease progression, respectively. Tafamidis has been reported as having a protective effect of a few years on those who take the medication from the beginning of the disease onset in contrast to those who started it later [37]. P3 started treatment at year 4 of disease progression and P2 at year 4.5 years. There was practically no clinical evolution between T0 and T1 for either P2 or P3: P2 is in a more advanced moment of disease progression with clear steppage, and P3 showed only a mild sensitive neuropathy, with vibration anesthesia on the hallux and minor difficulties on heels or tip toes gait, in both clinical observations. Nevertheless, they exhibited some of the same gait alterations as the other patients between gait assessments, such as the delayed toe-off, hip extension and knee flexion, which may suggest a slight worsening of the clinical condition, not detected on the clinical evaluation, despite the treatment with tafamidis. Non-responders to this medication have been described in the literature [38].

This study shows gait abnormalities that vary in time and that, nowadays, are not clinically quantified. Gait analysis is an important complement to the clinical assessment to the extent that it shows the overall effects that disease progression is having in daily life. Therefore, this assessment may contribute to and complement the current clinical analysis.

Since this is a rare disease, and our sample includes only a small number of patients, we structured this study as a case series, which seemed to be more useful. Although a case series is frequently incomplete and biased, it may enlighten future study strategies [39], and avoid the effects of data heterogeneity. Group analysis has been described as possibly having a negative impact on understanding the pathophysiology and management of rare diseases, since it may not reflect exactly what happens in individual patients [39]. Nevertheless, individual measurements may not always correspond to average reference values not only because of the disease but also because of the normal variability between individuals.

Adding to the small number of participants, this study has some other limitations including a longer, and single time between assessments, and the heterogenicity of the participants' clinical condition/disease progression/treatment. Nevertheless, a valuable insight into the problems related to V30M ATTRv amyloidosis characteristic gait pattern has been obtained.

Although V30M ATTRv amyloidosis is a degenerative disease, and patients suffer from muscle weakness, neuralgic pain and sensory loss, all of which contribute to settling into a pathological gait pattern, clinical importance should be given to rehabilitation and maintenance of the functionality of the ankle complex, in order to maintain greater mobility and muscle strength of the ankle for a better gait performance, as suggested for diabetic neuropathy [29]. Further studies are needed, for a more comprehensive assessment of motor control impairment during gait, such as electromyography studies, orthopedic assessment, especially articular, which may also be affected in these patients (e.g., Charcot joint neuroarthropathy). It would also be interesting to specifically design a comparison study with ATTRv amyloidosis and other neuropathies, including the diabetic neuropathy, in order to understand if the different diseases present distinct pathological gait characteristics.

Author Contributions: Conceptualization, M.d.C.V.-B., J.P.S.C. and T.C.; methodology, M.d.C.V.-B.; software, M.d.C.V.-B. and I.M.S.; validation, P.F.P.F., I.M.S. and M.d.C.V.-B.; formal analysis, M.d.C.V.-B. and P.F.P.F.; investigation, M.d.C.V.-B. and P.F.P.F.; resources, M.d.C.V.-B. and P.F.P.F.; data curation, M.d.C.V.-B. and M.N.C.; writing—original draft preparation, M.d.C.V.-B.; writing—review and editing, M.d.C.V.-B., P.F.P.F., M.N.C. and J.P.S.C.; visualization, M.d.C.V.-B.; supervision, T.C. and J.P.S.C.; project administration, M.d.C.V.-B.; funding acquisition, J.P.S.C. and T.C. All authors have read and agreed to the published version of the manuscript.

Funding: This work was supported by the National funding agency, FCT—Fundação para a Ciência e a Tecnologia, in the context of the project [LA/P/0063/2020] and by the Porto University Hospital Center (CHUP) in the context of the scholarship [BI.02/2018/UCA/CHP].

Institutional Review Board Statement: In this section, you should add the Institutional Review Board Statement and approval number, if relevant to your study. You might choose to exclude this statement if the study did not require ethical approval. Please note that the Editorial Office might ask you for further information. Please add "The study was conducted in accordance with the Declaration of Helsinki, and approved by the Ethics Committee of CENTRO HOSPITALAR DO PORTO, HOSPITAL DE SANTO ANTÓNIO (2014/167(119-DEFI/149-CES) for studies involving humans.

Informed Consent Statement: Informed consent was obtained from all subjects involved in the study.

Data Availability Statement: Not applicable.

Acknowledgments: The authors would like to thank Daria Rudnik, Ana Patricia Rocha, Hugo Miguel Pereira Choupina and Ricardo Sebastião for their contribution to data collection and processing.

Conflicts of Interest: The authors declare no conflict of interest. The funders had no role in the design of the study; in the collection, analyses, or interpretation of data; in the writing of the manuscript, or in the decision to publish the results.

Appendix A. Spatiotemporal Analysis

Appendix A.1. Participant 1

Table A1. Spatiotemporal gait parameters results for T0 and T1, left (LLL) and right (RLL) lower limbs.

Parameter	T0		T1	
	LLL	RLL	LLL	RLL
Speed (m/s)	0.955		0.826	
Stride width (m)	0.156 ± 0.021		0.156 ± 0.025	
Stride length (m)	1.088 ± 0.034		0.995 ± 0.038	
Step length (m)	0.529 ± 0.023	0.559 ± 0.019	0.487 ± 0.029	0.503 ± 0.020
Double Limb Support (s)	0.158 ± 0.026	0.157 ± 0.013	0.160 ± 0.016	0.172 ± 0.027
Cycle Time (s)	1.137 ± 0.053	1.143 ± 0.084	1.183 ± 0.04	1.225 ± 0.071
Stance Time (%)	63.6	64.3	66.3	69.3
Swing Time (%)	36.3	36.2	37.7	38.4
Cadence (steps/min)	104.163 ± 5.926	106.346 ± 6.943	97.782 ± 7.512	100.591 ± 5.446

Appendix A.2. Participant 2

Table A2. Spatiotemporal gait parameters results for T0 and T1, left (LLL) and right (RLL) lower limbs.

Parameter	T0		T1	
	LLL	RLL	LLL	RLL
Speed (m/s)	0.944		0.788	
Stride width (m)	0.093 ± 0.046		0.108 ± 0.045	
Stride length (m)	1.166 ± 0.047		1.01 ± 0.046	
Step length (m)	0.523 ± 0.022	0.634 ± 0.038	0.476 ± 0.033	0.524 ± 0.031
Double Limb Support (s)	0.129 ± 0.014	0.122 ± 0.016	0.166 ± 0.021	0.161 ± 0.025
Cycle Time (s)	1.239 ± 0.047	1.228 ± 0.047	1.28 ± 0.044	1.281 ± 0.057
Stance Time (%)	61.4	59.5	61.9	62.7
Swing Time (%)	38.6	40.6	38.1	37.4
Cadence (steps/min)	99.813 ± 4.258	93.951 ± 5.085	93.245 ± 5.459	93.089 ± 4.858

Appendix A.3. Participant 3

Table A3. Spatiotemporal gait parameters results for T0 and T1, left (LLL) and right (RLL) lower limbs.

Parameter	T0		T1	
	LLL	RLL	LLL	RLL
Speed (m/s)	0.854		0.860	
Stride width (m)	0.104 ± 0.019		0.121 ± 0.022	
Stride length (m)	0.959 ± 0.038		0.926 ± 0.100	
Step length (m)	0.463 ± 0.024	0.493 ± 0.024	0.431 ± 0.108	0.482 ± 0.043
Double Limb Support (s)	0.151 ± 0.025	0.154 ± 0.030	0.169 ± 0.044	0.149 ± 0.025
Cycle Time (s)	1.128 ± 0.072	1.119 ± 0.053	1.079 ± 0.167	1.074 ± 0.050
Stance Time (%)	67.5	65.2	73.4	74.8
Swing Time (%)	42.4	44.6	45.2	44.6
Cadence (steps/min)	105.897 ± 6.684	107.852 ± 7.452	116.099 ± 28.739	107.825 ± 11.058

Appendix A.4. Participant 4

Table A4. Spatiotemporal gait parameters results for T0 and T1, left (LLL) and right (RLL) lower limbs.

Parameter	T0		T1	
	LLL	RLL	LLL	RLL
Speed (m/s)	0.669		0.757	
Stride width (m)	0.177 ± 0.026		0.165 ± 0.030	
Stride length (m)	0.769 ± 0.046		0.845 ± 0.112	
Step length (m)	0.371 ± 0.033	0.396 ± 0.030	0.416 ± 0.036	0.434 ± 0.019
Double Limb Support (s)	0.158 ± 0.025	0.167 ± 0.041	0.161 ± 0.025	0.159 ± 0.036
Cycle Time (s)	1.148 ± 0.078	1.151 ± 0.070	1.134 ± 0.054	1.103 ± 0.197
Stance Time (%)	65.5	64.0	63.6	65.8
Swing Time (%)	36.9	36.0	36.4	37.0
Cadence (steps/min)	102.715 ± 8.615	105.822 ± 8.256	106.139 ± 8.520	105.713 ± 7.669

Appendix A.5. Participant 5

Table A5. Spatiotemporal gait parameters results for T0 and T1, left (LLL) and right (RLL) lower limbs.

Parameter	T0		T1	
	LLL	RLL	LLL	RLL
Speed (m/s)	0.995		0.939	
Stride width (m)	0.093 ± 0.022		0.117 ± 0.026	
Stride length (m)	1.160 ± 0.032		1.167 ± 0.064	
Step length (m)	0.593 ± 0.016	0.561 ± 0.027	0.574 ± 0.059	0.585 ± 0.027
Double Limb Support (s)	0.089 ± 0.024	0.117 ± 0.013	0.123 ± 0.030	0.157 ± 0.026

Table A5. Cont.

Parameter	T0		T1	
	LLL	RLL	LLL	RLL
Cycle Time (s)	1.157 ± 0.033	1.170 ± 0.025	1.222 ± 0.053	1.254 ± 0.061
Stance Time (%)	58.1	59.2	61.8	61.2
Swing Time (%)	41.9	40.8	38.2	38.8
Cadence (steps/min)	98.711 ± 3.223	106.280 ± 4.570	93.612 ± 7.640	98.656 ± 4.491

Appendix B. Ground Reaction Forces

Appendix B.1. Participant 1

Table A6. Mean and standard deviation of ground reaction forces in different gait cycle events at T0 and T1 for the left (LLL) and right (RLL) lower limbs, presented as % of body weight. * indicates a statistically significant difference ($p < 0.05$) between T0 and T1.

Parameter (% Body Weight)	T0		T1		Effect Size	
	LLL	RLL	LLL	RLL	LLL	RLL
FA1	−14.67 ± 2.26	−16.76 ± 1.96	−13.32 ± 1.35	−10.42 ± 1.73	0.27	0.83 *
FA3	14.96 ± 2.06	15.67 ± 1.82	9.58 ± 1.58	13.04 ± 1.66	0.83 *	0.69 *
FM1	−5.41 ± 1.77	−7.06 ± 1.84	−3.25 ± 1.27	−2.84 ± 1.06	0.50 *	0.76 *
FM2	6.38 ± 1.43	7.22 ± 0.66	6.49 ± 1.38	5.43 ± 1.46	0.08	0.54 *
FM3	9.13 ± 1.62	11.09 ± 0.87	9.66 ± 1.31	9.94 ± 3.22	0.01	0.20
FV1	115.49 ± 6.12	120.25 ± 4.67	113.45 ± 5.64	108.17 ± 5.54	0.08	0.72 *
FV2	74.15 ± 6.63	72.83 ± 4.98	78.86 ± 4.15	83.6 ± 2.77	0.24	0.77 *
FV3	102.34 ± 7.55	113.24 ± 3.69	105.43 ± 3.18	113.74 ± 3.92	0.60 *	0.00

Appendix B.2. Participant 2

Table A7. Mean and standard deviation of ground reaction forces in different gait cycle events at T0 and T1 for the left (LLL) and right (RLL) lower limbs, presented as % of body weight. * indicates a statistically significant difference ($p < 0.05$) between T0 and T1.

Parameter (% Body Weight)	T0		T1		Effect Size	
	LLL	RLL	LLL	RLL	LLL	RLL
FA1	−25.64 ± 6.3	−27.48 ± 5.38	−25.01 ± 3.27	−21.52 ± 4.06	0.10	0.60 *
FA3	21.12 ± 1.64	20.75 ± 1.74	18.25 ± 1.15	19.57 ± 0.8	0.03 *	0.10
FM1	−5.29 ± 1.97	−6.4 ± 2.61	−3.94 ± 2.02	−3.33 ± 1.73	0.34	0.50 *
FM2	6.66 ± 3.53	5.78 ± 2.48	6.1 ± 3.22	5.88 ± 2.85	0.10	0.00
FM3	5.28 ± 1.56	5.99 ± 1.77	5.78 ± 2.58	4.98 ± 1.65	0.00	0.13
FV1	131.65 ± 4.32	127.51 ± 8.19	136.91 ± 4.76	138.01 ± 6.49	0.34	0.40 *
FV2	68.47 ± 5.82	68.56 ± 6.82	73.63 ± 5.93	71.6 ± 7.95	0.33	0.06
FV3	111.74 ± 7.44	107.22 ± 6.04	107.93 ± 2.59	112.05 ± 3.16	0.04	0.06

Appendix B.3. Participant 3

Table A8. Mean and standard deviation of ground reaction forces in different gait cycle events at T0 and T1 for the left (LLL) and right (RLL) lower limbs, presented as % of body weight. * indicates a statistically significant difference ($p < 0.05$) between T0 and T1.

Parameter (% Body Weight)	T0		T1		Effect Size	
	LLL	RLL	LLL	RLL	LLL	RLL
FA1	−12.9 ± 1.9	−11.8 ± 1.6	−13.9 ± 2.3	−15.8 ± 2.9	0.1	0.1
FA3	12.1 ± 2.1	14.6 ± 2.6	15.5 ± 1.6	15.8 ± 1.2	0.0	0.0
FM1	−3.6 ± 1.3	−4.2 ± 1.7	−3.4 ± 1.5	−5.4 ± 1.1	0.3	0.2
FM2	6.2 ± 1.3	6.0 ± 1.1	7.2 ± 1.5	7.7 ± 1.7	0.1	0.1

Table A8. Cont.

Parameter (% Body Weight)	T0 LLL	T0 RLL	T1 LLL	T1 RLL	Effect Size LLL	Effect Size RLL
FM3	6.8 ± 1.0	6.8 ± 0.9	7.4 ± 1.2	7.0 ± 1.4	0.3 *	0.1
FV1	111.6 ± 4.9	107.8 ± 4.5	117.4 ± 5.7	116.9 ± 5.1	0.3 *	0.1
FV2	76.5 ± 4.3	78.6 ± 2.7	75.0 ± 2.7	75.6 ± 3.7	0.5 *	0.3
FV3	108.2 ± 3.2	110.6 ± 4.1	113.7 ± 5.1	113.3 ± 5.5	0.8 *	0.3

Appendix B.4. Participant 4

Table A9. Mean and standard deviation of ground reaction forces in different gait cycle events at T0 and T1 for the left (LLL) and right (RLL) lower limbs, presented as % of body weight. * indicates a statistically significant difference ($p < 0.05$) between T0 and T1.

Parameter (% body weight)	T0 LLL	T0 RLL	T1 LLL	T1 RLL	Effect Size LLL	Effect Size RLL
FA1	−17.5 ± 4.4	−17.2 ± 3.2	−14.5 ± 3.2	−17.1 ± 2.0	0.16	0.00
FA3	12.6 ± 2.4	14.6 ± 1.9	14.0 ± 1.3	11.9 ± 1.6	0.29	0.56 *
FM1	−2.3 ± 3.7	−3.5 ± 1.3	−1.4 ± 1.4	−3.33 ± 1.7	0.00	0.00
FM2	10.7 ± 1.4	11.4 ± 1.4	10.6 ± 1.3	10.7 ± 2.9	0.04	0.05
FM3	9.9 ± 1.6	9.7 ± 1.3	9.4 ± 1.5	9.9 ± 1.7	0.06	0.03
FV1	107.0 ± 10.1	116.0 ± 3.9	105.0 ± 5.0	109.7 ± 4.4	0.00	0.54 *
FV2	95.6 ± 6.2	92.7 ± 4.1	85.2 ± 2.6	85.3 ± 3.7	0.69 *	0.66 *
FV3	103.7 ± 5.9	103.3 ± 3.5	108.1 ± 4.6	98.8 ± 6.6	−0.40	−0.50 *

Appendix B.5. Participant 5

Table A10. Mean and standard deviation of ground reaction forces in different gait cycle events at T0 and T1 for the left (LLL) and right (RLL) lower limbs, presented as % of body weight. * indicates a statistically significant difference ($p < 0.05$) between T0 and T1.

Parameter (% Body Weight)	T0 LLL	T0 RLL	T1 LLL	T1 RLL	Effect Size LLL	Effect Size RLL
FA1	−17.8 ± 4.8	−16.9 ± 3.3	−17.6 ± 2.0	−17.9 ± 3.6	0.02	0.03
FA3	17.3 ± 1.8	17.3 ± 2.7	15.0 ± 1.5	17.0 ± 0.9	0.61 *	0.00
FM1	−7.5 ± 2.3	−7.6 ± 2.8	−4.7 ± 1.2	−8.0 ± 2.2	−0.58 *	0.03
FM2	4.8 ± 1.4	5.4 ± 1.5	6.2 ± 1.0	5.0 ± 1.1	0.29 *	0.03
FM3	7.5 ± 1.9	7.6 ± 1.9	6.5 ± 0.9	8.8 ± 1.1	0.21	0.25
FV1	113.9 ± 4.2	114.2 ± 4.8	114.0 ± 4.1	116.2 ± 3.7	0.00	0.17
FV2	79.6 ± 4.1	78.2 ± 4.3	80.1 ± 4.1	79.1 ± 2.9	0.03	0.03
FV3	112.4 ± 8.2	113.6 ± 6.3	110.2 ± 5.1	104.5 ± 35.9	−0.24	−0.16

Appendix C. Angular Kinematics

Appendix C.1. Participant 1

Table A11. Sagittal plane mean and standard deviation angles of different joints (hip, pelvis, knee and ankle), at T0 and T1, at the heel strike (HS), mid stance (MD), and toe off (TO), for both lower limbs, along with the *p*-value between both assessment periods. The effect size is presented as large ([a]), moderate ([b]) or small ([c]).

Joint Angle (Degrees)	Time of Assessment	Left Lower Limb HS	Left Lower Limb MD	Left Lower Limb TO	Right Lower Limb HS	Right Lower Limb MD	Right Lower Limb TO
Pelvis	T0	4.07 ± 0.86	−0.55 ± 0.83	6.57 ± 0.64	−2.08 ± 1.02	1.31 ± 1.06	−4.85 ± 0.76
	T1	3.62 ± 1.15	0.57 ± 0.49	6.83 ± 0.78	0.26 ± 1.55	1.16 ± 0.84	−3.78 ± 0.80
	p-value	0.016 [a]	0.011 [a]	0.213 [b]	0.000 [a]	0.305 [c]	0.003 [a]

Table A11. Cont.

Joint Angle (Degrees)	Time of Assessment	Left Lower Limb			Right Lower Limb		
		HS	MD	TO	HS	MD	TO
Left Hip	T0	20.31 ± 1.98	1.26 ± 1.87	−5.11 ± 2.44	−11.56 ± 1.21	21.09 ± 7.36	19.98 ± 2.08
	T1	21.36 ± 2.10	0.23 ± 1.58	−2.98 ± 2.95	−10.38 ± 2.20	24.98 ± 1.65	17.91 ± 3.05
	p-value	0.083 [a]	0.083 [a]	0.022 [a]	0.134 [b]	0.000 [a]	0.011 [a]
Right Hip	T0	−9.83 ± 1.36	21.55 ± 1.97	21.47 ± 2.33	25.93 ± 1.28	3.98 ± 5.54	−4.28 ± 1.9
	T1	−11.09 ± 1.45	20.76 ± 2.90	17.81 ± 3.39	24.43 ± 3.20	−0.46 ± 1.76	−5.17 ± 2.23
	p-value	0.025 [b]	0.334 [c]	0.001 [a]	0.016 [b]	0.000 [a]	0.691 [c]
Left Knee	T0	7.31 ± 1.47	12.4 ± 1.9	43.56 ± 3.83	10.15 ± 0.48	59.47 ± 11.38	22.08 ± 3.77
	T1	7.60 ± 1.50	8.05 ± 2.32	40.56 ± 4.44	7.11 ± 1.33	60.85 ± 2.03	17.84 ± 3.31
	p-value	0.697 [c]	0.000 [a]	0.008 [b]	0.000 [a]	0.741 [c]	0.001 [a]
Right Knee	T0	15.09 ± 1.58	53.61 ± 1.42	25.47 ± 2.99	12.52 ± 1.38	16.85 ± 3.05	40.46 ± 5.38
	T1	9.01 ± 0.84	51.67 ± 4.96	18.4 ± 4.26	10.58 ± 3.32	8.81 ± 1.93	35.48 ± 5.14
	p-value	0.000 [a]	0.460 [c]	0.000 [a]	0.030 [b]	0.000 [a]	0.639 [c]
Left Ankle	T0	−3.86 ± 0.97	8.56 ± 0.91	7.08 ± 3.31	20.2 ± 0.74	−2.45 ± 5.37	1.69 ± 1.76
	T1	−3.31 ± 1.53	9.57 ± 1.10	8.74 ± 2.53	21.58 ± 1.05	−1.89 ± 1.50	2.42 ± 1.70
	p-value	0.247 [c]	0.000 [a]	0.068 [b]	0.017 [b]	0.073 [b]	0.017 [b]
Right Ankle	T0	22.7 ± 1.87	7.19 ± 0.59	3.34 ± 1.55	3.37 ± 0.79	10.21 ± 2.05	12.01 ± 2.84
	T1	20.45 ± 1.68	6.54 ± 1.30	2.78 ± 2.29	0.26 ± 1.68	8.5 ± 1.72	12.63 ± 2.10
	p-value	0.000 [a]	0.053 [a]	0.768 [c]	0.000 [a]	0.006 [b]	0.427 [c]

Table A12. Frontal plane mean and standard deviation angles of different joints (hip, pelvis, knee and ankle), at T0 and T1, at the heel strike (HS), mid stance (MD), and toe off (TO), for both lower limbs, along with the p-value between both assessment periods. The effect size is presented as large ([a]), moderate ([b]) or small ([c]).

Joint Angle (Degrees)	Time of Assessment	Left Lower Limb			Right Lower Limb		
		HS	MD	TO	HS	MD	TO
Pelvis	T0	−2.07 ± 1.17	−2.48 ± 1.73	−2.96 ± 1.34	0.23 ± 1.02	−4.57 ± 1.98	−1.62 ± 1.51
	T1	−0.01 ± 1.31	−0.48 ± 1.21	0.19 ± 2.78	2.59 ± 1.75	−2.24 ± 1.87	0.24 ± 1.82
	p-value	0.000 [a]	0.001 [a]	0.000 [a]	0.000 [a]	0.002 [b]	0.047 [b]
Left Hip	T0	−8.80 ± 1.30	1.37 ± 0.98	−11.91 ± 1.02	−0.28 ± 1	−7.28 ± 2.07	1.71 ± 1.62
	T1	−7.61 ± 1.49	0.73 ± 0.98	−12.27 ± 1.49	−1.34 ± 1.59	−7.41 ± 1.13	2.20 ± 1.36
	p-value	0.000 [a]	0.234 [a]	0.147 [a]	0.009 [b]	0.244 [a]	0.338 [b]
Right Hip	T0	6.57 ± 1.05	−0.70 ± 1.04	7.99 ± 1.54	−4.97 ± 1.90	6.06 ± 3.15	−2.99 ± 1.06
	T1	5.51 ± 1.53	−2.25 ± 1.16	6.96 ± 1.35	−4.66 ± 2.01	4.36 ± 1.62	−4.39 ± 1.32
	p-value	0.007 [a]	0.003 [c]	0.042 [b]	0.715 [c]	0.006 [c]	0.046 [a]
Left Knee	T0	0.60 ± 0.47	−0.27 ± 0.48	−8.66 ± 1.08	−1.01 ± 0.69	−5.76 ± 1.76	1.95 ± 2.43
	T1	1.13 ± 0.60	0.77 ± 0.55	−3.08 ± 1.18	0.46 ± 0.40	2.13 ± 1.74	1.50 ± 1.10
	p-value	0.001 [a]	0.000 [a]	0.254 [a]	0.000 [a]	0.254 [a]	0.733 [c]
Right Knee	T0	2.98 ± 1.41	4.07 ± 2.26	2.36 ± 2.05	−1.67 ± 0.89	−0.56 ± 1.06	−2.40 ± 2.18
	T1	−1.22 ± 0.67	0.38 ± 1.54	−0.89 ± 1.06	−0.79 ± 1.82	−0.71 ± 0.63	−3.48 ± 1.03
	p-value	0.254 [a]	0.001 [a]	0.000 [a]	0.217 [c]	0.099 [c]	0.069 [b]
Left Ankle	T0	7.71 ± 1.04	1.62 ± 1.04	9.07 ± 1.21	7.85 ± 0.95	7.40 ± 0.72	−1.74 ± 0.51
	T1	6.65 ± 1.05	−0.54 ± 1.67	5.42 ± 1.93	3.41 ± 1.22	6.74 ± 1.04	−3.29 ± 1.31
	p-value	0.002 [a]	0.001 [a]	0.000 [a]	0.000 [a]	0.027 [b]	0.000 [a]
Right Ankle	T0	3.01 ± 1.23	7.19 ± 0.76	−1.77 ± 0.99	6.36 ± 1.05	−0.26 ± 2.13	8.27 ± 1.70
	T1	1.07 ± 1.31	1.43 ± 0.89	−2.66 ± 1.37	5.18 ± 1.37	−1.17 ± 1.32	3.00 ± 1.18
	p-value	0.002 [a]	0.000 [a]	0.130 [b]	0.004 [a]	0.455 [c]	0.000 [a]

Table A13. Transverse plane mean and standard deviation angles of different joints (hip, pelvis, knee and ankle), at T0 and T1, at the heel strike (HS), mid stance (MD), and toe off (TO), for both lower limbs, along with the p-value between both assessment periods. The effect size is presented as large ([a]), moderate ([b]) or small ([c]).

Joint Angle (Degrees)	Time of Assessment	Left Lower Limb			Right Lower Limb		
		HS	MD	TO	HS	MD	TO
Pelvis	T0	80.93 ± 2.86	89.49 ± 1.12	98.11 ± 2.35	100.6 ± 2.45	90.25 ± 3.55	82.35 ± 2.64
	T1	83.66 ± 2.87	89.69 ± 2.64	96.84 ± 3.09	98.55 ± 3.08	91.15 ± 2.88	83.64 ± 2.83
	p-value	0.000 [a]	0.691 [c]	0.050 [b]	0.019 [b]	0.322 [c]	0.360 [b]

Table A13. Cont.

Joint Angle (Degrees)	Time of Assessment	Left Lower Limb			Right Lower Limb		
		HS	MD	TO	HS	MD	TO
Left Hip	T0	−23.28 ± 2.89	−19.29 ± 1.27	−16.00 ± 2.73	−19.69 ± 1.42	−15.07 ± 1.91	−15.77 ± 5.17
	T1	−19.3 ± 2.52	−14.91 ± 2.65	−11.03 ± 2.96	−15.01 ± 2.52	−6.70 ± 2.25	−14.15 ± 2.61
	p-value	0.001 [a]	0.000 [a]	0.000 [a]	0.000 [a]	0.000 [a]	0.434 [b]
Right Hip	T0	−1.85 ± 3.12	−1.30 ± 3.03	−1.29 ± 3.38	−10.04 ± 2.16	−0.45 ± 4.58	−0.58 ± 4.13
	T1	−11.79 ± 2.46	−10.74 ± 3.39	−14.44 ± 2.84	−22.56 ± 3.21	−13.85 ± 2.76	−8.82 ± 2.55
	p-value	0.001 [b]	0.001 [a]	0.000 [a]	0.000 [a]	0.000 [a]	0.003 [a]
Left Knee	T0	−7.00 ± 3.02	2.24 ± 1.69	−4.02 ± 4.30	10.41 ± 3.19	−6.85 ± 4.43	−7.45 ± 3.09
	T1	−3.00 ± 2.52	4.34 ± 3.04	5.29 ± 2.93	9.51 ± 2.32	2.54 ± 1.30	−0.74 ± 2.70
	p-value	0.000 [a]	0.009 [b]	0.000 [a]	0.114 [c]	0.000 [b]	0.001 [a]
Right Knee	T0	15.09 ± 1.58	−25.87 ± 2.23	−22.64 ± 4.00	−16.74 ± 1.99	−12.43 ± 2.75	−18.55 ± 7.88
	T1	7.42 ± 2.14	−0.95 ± 3.71	0.48 ± 3.87	0.21 ± 3.52	4.18 ± 2.18	1.46 ± 2.24
	p-value	0.000 [a]	0.052 [a]	0.000 [a]	0.000 [a]	0.001 [a]	0.001 [b]
Left Ankle	T0	10.81 ± 2.34	7.44 ± 1.98	15.45 ± 2.39	9.9 ± 2.02	16.11 ± 2.14	5.16 ± 2.27
	T1	5.66 ± 1.17	2.59 ± 2.60	4.75 ± 2.04	6.55 ± 1.84	4.91 ± 1.06	−1.14 ± 2.31
	p-value	0.000 [a]	0.001 [a]	0.000 [a]	0.000 [a]	0.000 [a]	0.000 [a]
Right Ankle	T0	−0.85 ± 1.37	10.52 ± 1.85	−1.91 ± 1.46	−0.88 ± 1.18	−3.22 ± 1.56	6.37 ± 5.38
	T1	−12.64 ± 2.96	−13.59 ± 1.73	−18.66 ± 3.13	−9.70 ± 1.89	−15.06 ± 2.78	−13.00 ± 2.27
	p-value	0.000 [a]	0.001 [a]	0.000 [a]	0.000 [a]	0.000 [a]	0.000 [a]

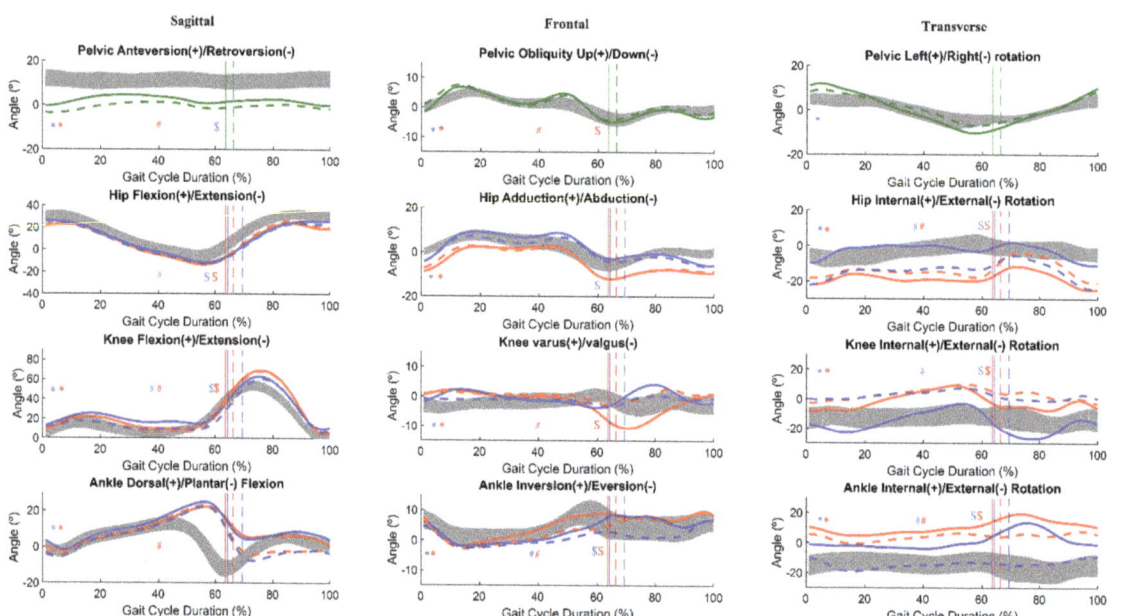

Figure A1. Average pelvis and lower limbs joint angles (in degrees) in the three anatomical planes during a gait cycle of the right (blue), left (red) lower limb and irrespective of the side (green). The joint angles at T0 are denoted by a solid line, while T1 is represented by a dashed line. The reference interval from the healthy gait dataset is shaded grey. A set of symbols are used to denote statistically significant differences, associated with large effect size, between T0 and T1 at the heel strike (*), midstance (#) and toe-off ($), with their color indicating the limb presenting such differences.

P1 shows a more retroverted pelvis than the reference population, although with a normal angle variation during the whole gait cycle. At T1 this angle was lower in general, being even lower than the reference population. In the frontal plane, the pelvic obliquity during the RLL cycle is higher than the reference data. In the transverse plane left and right rotations are more prominent at T1 than T0 and the variation is around −10 to 10 degrees.

P1 also presents a delayed toe-off at T1, more prominent for the right lower limb cycles, as can be seen in the charts showing the angular behavior of the other limbs. The hip angle shows higher extension than the reference population, more abduction (frontal plane) and external rotation (transverse plane) at T1 than T0. It also presents an abduction lower than the reference data for left lower limb cycles, in both assessments, at T1 with a frontal range of motion of 25 degrees. Looking at the transverse plane, all except right lower limb cycles during T0 show more external rotation (up to 15° lower) during the whole gait cycle, than the reference data. The stance phase knee flexion is higher at T1 than T0 and also than the reference. Swing phase knee flexion is higher than the reference gait data and higher at T1 than T0. The knee and ankle rotation are more internal at T1 and the transition from dorsi- to plantar-flexion occurs later than in the reference population. In the transverse plane, knee rotation is in general more internal than the reference data, except for the right lower limb cycles at T0 which is mainly within a normal range. The ankle angle shows a higher dorsiflexion than the reference data, before the toe-off. In the frontal plane, the first eversion is also more prominent than the correspondent for the reference. In the transverse plane it is possible to see that with the exception of right lower limb cycles at T1, all assessments show higher internal rotation of the ankle during the whole gait cycle.

Appendix C.2. Participant 2

Table A14. Sagittal plane mean and standard deviation angles of different joints (hip, pelvis, knee and ankle), at T0 and T1, at the heel strike (HS), mid stance (MD), and toe off (TO), for both lower limbs, along with the *p*-value between both assessment periods. The effect size is presented as large ([a]), moderate ([b]) or small ([c]).

Joint Angle (Degrees)	Time of Assessment	Left Lower Limb			Right Lower Limb		
		HS	MD	TO	HS	MD	TO
Pelvis	T0	6.53 ± 0.98	5.67 ± 0.95	2.80 ± 0.86	−2.10 ± 0.89	−1.43 ± 1.01	0.84 ± 1.35
	T1	5.94 ± 1.01	3.74 ± 0.89	1.74 ± 1.00	−3.77 ± 1.35	−1.55 ± 1.04	−0.07 ± 1.37
	p-value	0.005 [a]	0.000 [a]	0.004 [b]	0.000 [a]	0.943 [c]	0.003 [b]
Left Hip	T0	27.92 ± 1.70	12.99 ± 1.67	−8.20 ± 1.78	−10.18 ± 2.69	40.50 ± 1.85	30.04 ± 2.02
	T1	24.27 ± 2.15	8.75 ± 1.83	−3.89 ± 2.97	−14.68 ± 2.83	35.52 ± 1.92	20.76 ± 5.80
	p-value	0.000 [a]	0.000 [a]	0.000 [a]	0.000 [a]	0.000 [a]	0.000 [a]
Right Hip	T0	−11.71 ± 2.13	37.42 ± 2.64	30.31 ± 2.08	27.06 ± 2.51	9.15 ± 1.82	−4.83 ± 2.17
	T1	−16.24 ± 2.07	33.62 ± 2.43	20.01 ± 2.25	19.29 ± 1.85	4.55 ± 1.58	−3.69 ± 4.28
	p-value	0.000 [a]	0.000 [a]	0.000 [a]	0.000 [a]	0.000 [a]	0.601 [c]
Left Knee	T0	15.81 ± 2.45	23.95 ± 3.40	43.61 ± 4.68	23.63 ± 4.41	77.63 ± 2.23	35.01 ± 2.68
	T1	15.36 ± 3.84	17.80 ± 2.02	47.76 ± 4.34	9.2 ± 3.05	73.84 ± 2.39	31.19 ± 5.12
	p-value	0.493 [c]	0.000 [a]	0.006 [a]	0.000 [a]	0.000 [a]	0.000 [a]
Right Knee	T0	−1.78 ± 0.84	75.87 ± 1.92	34.47 ± 3.29	15.91 ± 2.85	17.54 ± 2.24	37.75 ± 3.02
	T1	1.24 ± 1.95	70.13 ± 3.03	27.99 ± 3.14	10.23 ± 3.00	11.75 ± 2.83	42.93 ± 7.45
	p-value	0.000 [a]	0.000 [a]	0.000 [a]	0.000 [a]	0.000 [a]	0.000 [a]
Left Ankle	T0	1.76 ± 1.75	28.12 ± 2.66	32.94 ± 2.77	47.60 ± 3.26	8.42 ± 2.11	21.92 ± 1.96
	T1	−4.47 ± 2.00	9.01 ± 1.90	6.68 ± 4.32	19.18 ± 2.96	−12.22 ± 3.30	8.97 ± 2.62
	p-value	0.000 [a]	0.000 [a]	0.000 [a]	0.000 [a]	0.000 [a]	0.000 [a]
Right Ankle	T0	20.36 ± 2.28	−13.29 ± 2.48	5.94 ± 1.58	−3.13 ± 1.24	10.61 ± 1.26	16.05 ± 1.83
	T1	16.87 ± 2.72	−11.05 ± 2.40	8.66 ± 2.39	−3.93 ± 1.65	−1.55 ± 1.04	8.36 ± 3.59
	p-value	0.000 [a]	0.001 [a]	0.000 [a]	0.587 [c]	0.000 [a]	0.000 [a]

Table A15. Frontal plane mean and standard deviation angles of different joints (hip, pelvis, knee and ankle), at T0 and T1, at the heel strike (HS), mid stance (MD), and toe off (TO), for both lower limbs, along with the *p*-value between both assessment periods. The effect size is presented as large ([a]), moderate ([b]) or small ([c]).

Joint Angle (Degrees)	Time of Assessment	Left Lower Limb			Right Lower Limb		
		HS	MD	TO	HS	MD	TO
Pelvis	T0	1.12 ± 1.20	0.22 ± 1.61	−1.63 ± 1.11	−1.10 ± 1.07	0.29 ± 1.72	0.28 ± 1.57
	T1	−0.55 ± 0.82	−0.67 ± 1.23	−2.56 ± 1.17	−2.10 ± 0.99	−1.63 ± 1.06	−2.68 ± 0.90
	p-value	0.000 [a]	0.062 [c]	0.088 [c]	0.017 [a]	0.000 [a]	0.000 [a]

Table A15. Cont.

Joint Angle (Degrees)	Time of Assessment	Left Lower Limb			Right Lower Limb		
		HS	MD	TO	HS	MD	TO
Left Hip	T0 T1 p-value	−8.06 ± 1.63 −6.92 ± 2.30 0.011 [a]	−1.96 ± 1.68 −1.90 ± 2.09 0.833 [c]	−2.70 ± 2.23 −3.31 ± 2.21 0.902 [c]	0.68 ± 2.11 1.67 ± 2.71 0.073 [b]	2.87 ± 1.34 0.81 ± 1.95 0.000 [a]	0.75 ± 1.98 1.42 ± 2.08 0.115 [b]
Right Hip	T0 T1 p-value	6.37 ± 2.04 6.60 ± 1.89 0.853 [a]	−0.81 ± 1.02 −1.83 ± 1.53 0.075 [a]	0.63 ± 1.79 −0.54 ± 2.48 0.285 [c]	−7.76 ± 1.83 −8.90 ± 2.25 0.163 [b]	0.94 ± 2.26 −0.41 ± 2.49 0.019 [b]	1.34 ± 1.48 −0.55 ± 2.56 0.001 [b]
Left Knee	T0 T1 p-value	−2.95 ± 1.42 1.34 ± 1.11 0.001 [a]	−3.45 ± 0.96 1.34 ± 1.00 0.000 [a]	−6.57 ± 2.42 −1.58 ± 2.51 0.003 [a]	−3.62 ± 1.73 1.87 ± 0.94 0.000 [a]	−6.39 ± 2.34 9.49 ± 3.96 0.003 [a]	−3.03 ± 1.89 2.80 ± 2.01 0.000 [a]
Right Knee	T0 T1 p-value	−2.53 ± 1.50 4.88 ± 1.40 0.003 [b]	12.12 ± 2.20 12.05 ± 2.66 0.361 [c]	7.41 ± 2.26 5.15 ± 1.96 0.000 [a]	2.34 ± 0.96 2.38 ± 1.09 0.361 [c]	3.69 ± 0.83 4.48 ± 1.11 0.093 [c]	5.99 ± 1.47 6.51 ± 4.41 0.575 [c]
Left Ankle	T0 T1 p-value	1.72 ± 1.81 7.36 ± 1.77 0.000 [a]	−10.04 ± 1.08 4.00 ± 1.01 0.000 [a]	−3.13 ± 1.30 8.75 ± 1.22 0.000 [a]	−7.72 ± 1.63 11.47 ± 1.52 0.000 [a]	−5.15 ± 4.05 5.20 ± 2.69 0.000 [a]	−10.37 ± 1.30 3.50 ± 1.88 0.000 [a]
Right Ankle	T0 T1 p-value	3.83 ± 1.98 5.48 ± 1.88 0.003 [b]	3.12 ± 2.78 7.48 ± 2.76 0.000 [a]	−3.51 ± 1.19 −3.05 ± 1.93 0.463 [c]	5.03 ± 1.82 5.95 ± 2.54 0.009 [a]	−1.98 ± 1.35 −1.63 ± 1.06 0.143 [c]	5.62 ± 0.57 3.39 ± 1.92 0.000 [a]

Table A16. Transverse plane mean and standard deviation angles of different joints (hip, pelvis, knee and ankle), at T0 and T1, at the heel strike (HS), mid stance (MD), and toe off (TO), for both lower limbs, along with the p-value between both assessment periods. The effect size is presented as large ([a]), moderate ([b]) or small ([c]).

Joint Angle (Degrees)	Time of Assessment	Left Lower Limb			Right Lower Limb		
		HS	MD	TO	HS	MD	TO
Pelvis	T0 T1 p-value	80.91 ± 2.70 82.6 ± 2.62 0.001 [b]	92.93 ± 2.71 90.43 ± 2.79 0.009 [c]	100.20 ± 2.53 94.28 ± 2.91 0.000 [a]	106.72 ± 3.43 98.19 ± 3.48 0.000 [a]	94.48 ± 2.71 92.22 ± 3.37 0.004 [b]	85.78 ± 2.60 87.3 ± 2.86 0.029 [a]
Left Hip	T0 T1 p-value	−16.47 ± 4.22 −5.29 ± 3.63 0.000 [a]	−9.95 ± 2.08 −2.9 ± 2.52 0.000 [a]	−5.65 ± 3.27 0.54 ± 2.89 0.000 [a]	−5.51 ± 4.01 2.86 ± 3.82 0.000 [a]	−2.83 ± 2.74 10.58 ± 4.37 0.000 [a]	−9.63 ± 2.45 −2.21 ± 2.62 0.000 [a]
Right Hip	T0 T1 p-value	1.92 ± 4.55 −1.64 ± 3.13 0.001 [b]	3.28 ± 2.70 2.62 ± 2.74 0.072 [c]	−1.59 ± 3.21 −10.83 ± 3.35 0.000 [a]	−9.75 ± 3.28 −22.34 ± 3.15 0.000 [a]	−0.48 ± 3.89 −7.56 ± 3.42 0.000 [a]	1.98 ± 3.18 −1.79 ± 7.59 0.000 [b]
Left Knee	T0 T1 p-value	−1.49 ± 3.35 −34.33 ± 3.53 0.000 [a]	2.65 ± 2.32 −22.25 ± 2.00 0.000 [a]	−4.43 ± 4.59 −26.19 ± 2.37 0.000 [a]	9.53 ± 4.26 −21.55 ± 2.69 0.000 [a]	−10.71 ± 5.35 −29.86 ± 3.74 0.000 [a]	−4.58 ± 3.63 −25.85 ± 2.97 0.000 [a]
Right Knee	T0 T1 p-value	8.29 ± 1.67 −25.11 ± 2.41 0.000 [a]	−18.79 ± 2.99 −25.39 ± 4.18 0.000 [a]	−29.62 ± 3.14 −24.07 ± 2.52 0.000 [a]	−28.71 ± 3.42 −25.85 ± 3.25 0.004 [b]	−23.09 ± 1.9 −25.74 ± 1.61 0.000 [b]	−30.18 ± 3.10 −32.97 ± 7.68 0.067 [c]
Left Ankle	T0 T1 p-value	1.48 ± 1.51 19.63 ± 2.81 0.000 [a]	6.18 ± 1.36 8.91 ± 1.35 0.000 [a]	10.73 ± 1.84 15.81 ± 3.15 0.000 [a]	6.07 ± 1.55 11.73 ± 1.31 0.000 [a]	11.9 ± 4.68 21.33 ± 4.01 0.000 [a]	5.21 ± 2.39 8.16 ± 1.46 0.000 [a]
Right Ankle	T0 T1 p-value	0.14 ± 2.08 0.94 ± 1.46 0.057 [c]	15.31 ± 3.33 12.09 ± 3.81 0.002 [c]	0.95 ± 1.45 −3.02 ± 1.55 0.000 [a]	4.76 ± 1.25 10.3 ± 2.42 0.000 [a]	−2.09 ± 1.32 92.22 ± 3.37 0.000 [a]	5.89 ± 2.80 3.43 ± 2.86 0.001 [a]

P2 also shows a slightly delayed toe-off on the right lower limb cycles, at T1, and a statistically significant higher retroversion of the pelvis at HS at T1. In the frontal plane, the last elevations are higher than the reference data and at T1 they exceed the normal 5 degrees of variation, reaching near 10°. In the transverse plane left and right rotations are more prominent at T1 than T0 and the variation is around −10 to 20 degrees at T0 and lowers to −10 to 10 at T1. The hip is more extended and also more flexed (right after extension) than in the reference population and in the frontal plane shows a range of motion of 20 degrees. In the transverse plane the rotators pattern is closer to the reference values than P1 but with excessive rotation (more than 10 degrees total displacement). The stance phase knee flexion is higher at T1 than T0 and also than the reference population. Swing phase knee flexion is higher than the reference data and higher at T1 than T0 (steppage). In the transverse plane, knee rotation is more external than normal, reaching $-40°$ at some point, except for the left lower limb cycles at T0 in which the knee is more internally rotated. The ankle angle shows a marked asymmetry with the left lower limb cycles, at T0, being more dorsiflexed in general (up to 45°), with a timid plantar-flexion right after toe-off. In the frontal plane it is possible to see that the eversion angles vary from the right limb cycles, and left limb cycles at T0 and T1, but the pattern is similar and the eversion is not marked. The swing phase was different for all the assessments. The transverse plane, as for P1, shows a more internally rotated ankle than the reference population, along the entire gait cycle.

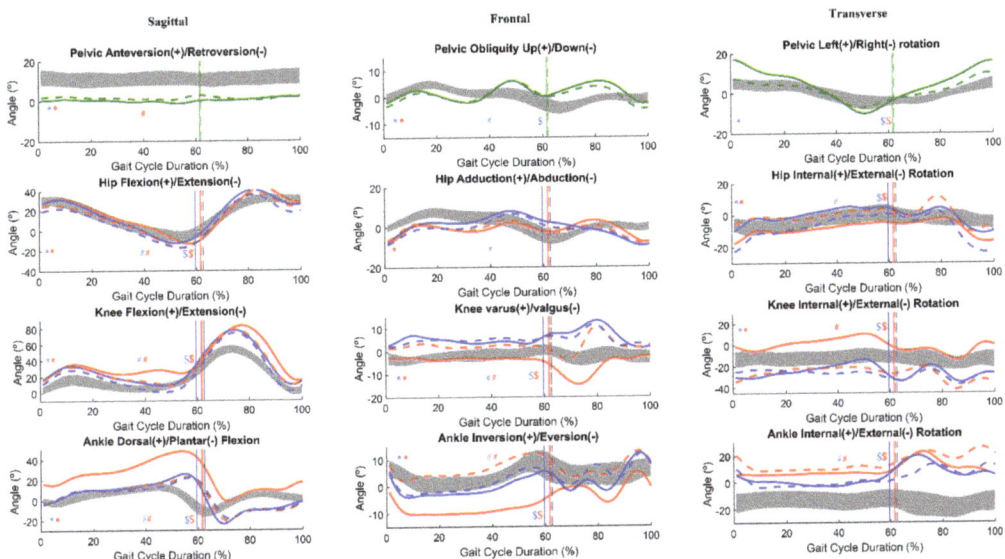

Figure A2. Average pelvis and lower limbs joint angles (in degrees) in the three anatomical planes during a gait cycle of the right (blue), left (red) lower limb and irrespective of the side (green). The joint angles at T0 are denoted by a solid line, while T1 is represented by a dashed line. The reference interval from the healthy gait dataset is shaded grey. A set of symbols are used to denote statistically significant differences, associated with large effect size, between T0 and T1 at the heel strike (*), midstance (#) and toe-off ($), with their color indicating the limb presenting such differences.

Appendix C.3. Participant 3

Table A17. Sagittal plane mean and standard deviation angles of different joints (hip, pelvis, knee and ankle), at T0 and T1, at the heel strike (HS), mid stance (MD), and toe off (TO), for both lower limbs, along with the *p*-value between both assessment periods. The effect size is presented as large ([a]), moderate ([b]) or small ([c]).

Joint Angle (Degrees)	Time of Assessment	Left Lower Limb			Right Lower Limb		
		HS	MD	TO	HS	HS	MD
Pelvis	T0	0.68 ± 0.84	0.28 ± 0.59	5.71 ± 0.69	2.12 ± 0.67	1.82 ± 0.69	−4.31 ± 0.71
	T1	0.60 ± 1.72	−0.79 ± 0.87	6.26 ± 1.13	0.89 ± 1.17	1.64 ± 0.87	−5.30 ± 0.77
	p-value	0.812 [c]	0.000 [a]	0.013 [b]	0.000 [a]	0.480 [c]	0.000 [a]
Left Hip	T0	24.31 ± 1.57	2.80 ± 0.89	−5.20 ± 2.26	−16.05 ± 1.51	23.84 ± 1.49	19.7 ± 3.26
	T1	23.45 ± 4.22	2.43 ± 2.22	−5.02 ± 5.11	−19.19 ± 2.50	22.80 ± 3.48	19.00 ± 3.20
	p-value	0.057 [b]	0.057 [b]	0.657 [c]	0.000 [a]	0.008 [b]	0.302 [c]
Right Hip	T0	−11.48 ± 4.40	25.41 ± 2.31	23.54 ± 2.98	27.85 ± 2.51	6.91 ± 3.45	0.47 ± 3.29
	T1	−18.07 ± 5.30	23.39 ± 2.27	20.85 ± 7.73	25.87 ± 3.12	2.20 ± 2.58	−5.90 ± 2.86
	p-value	0.000 [a]	0.000 [a]	0.004 [b]	0.001 [b]	0.000 [a]	0.000 [a]

Table A17. Cont.

Joint Angle (Degrees)	Time of Assessment	Left Lower Limb			Right Lower Limb		
		HS	MD	TO	HS	HS	MD
Left Knee	T0 T1 p-value	9.81 ± 2.38 12.89 ± 4.21 0.002 [b]	4.35 ± 0.94 8.16 ± 1.55 0.000 [a]	32.07 ± 4.94 34.92 ± 6.12 0.035 [c]	−4.89 ± 2.2 −8.55 ± 2.52 0.000 [a]	46.2 ± 2.64 49.19 ± 5.58 0.001 [b]	17.6 ± 3.92 22.59 ± 2.51 0.000 [a]
Right Knee	T0 T1 p-value	3.77 ± 1.03 −8.02 ± 5.92 0.000 [a]	49.62 ± 3.39 51.14 ± 3.63 0.087 [c]	23.12 ± 3.92 21.04 ± 5.88 0.008 [b]	15.3 ± 3.63 12.4 ± 4.49 0.001 [b]	12.58 ± 5.45 6.88 ± 3.42 0.000 [a]	40.2 ± 5.71 35.76 ± 5.27 0.001 [b]
Left Ankle	T0 T1 p-value	1.21 ± 1.30 −0.90 ± 2.35 0.029 [b]	6.61 ± 1.19 9.03 ± 1.14 0.000 [a]	9.94 ± 3.13 12.8 ± 3.39 0.001 [b]	14.11 ± 2.37 13.17 ± 2.38 0.000 [a]	5.65 ± 0.77 6.97 ± 1.13 0.000 [b]	2.58 ± 1.51 6.08 ± 1.79 0.000 [a]
Right Ankle	T0 T1 p-value	15.55 ± 5.38 11.18 ± 3.08 0.000 [a]	7.45 ± 2.15 8.58 ± 1.25 0.012 [b]	2.77 ± 1.34 3.29 ± 2.38 0.307 [c]	1.81 ± 1.56 −2.13 ± 2.41 0.000 [a]	7.54 ± 1.86 6.83 ± 1.54 0.002 [b]	11.97 ± 4.39 13.70 ± 2.41 0.155 [c]

Table A18. Frontal plane mean and standard deviation angles of different joints (hip, pelvis, knee and ankle), at T0 and T1, at the heel strike (HS), mid stance (MD), and toe off (TO), for both lower limbs, along with the *p*-value between both assessment periods. The effect size is presented as large ([a]), moderate ([b]) or small ([c]).

Joint Angle (Degrees)	Time of Assessment	Left Lower Limb			Right Lower Limb		
		HS	MD	TO	HS	MD	TO
Pelvis	T0 T1 p-value	2.55 ± 0.67 0.37 ± 1.61 0.000 [a]	3.38 ± 0.81 1.49 ± 2.17 0.000 [b]	2.61 ± 0.88 1.80 ± 1.82 0.001 [a]	2.46 ± 1.01 1.47 ± 1.47 0.000 [b]	3.10 ± 0.76 0.98 ± 1.81 0.000 [a]	2.81 ± 0.76 0.20 ± 2.75 0.000 [b]
Left Hip	T0 T1 p-value	1.36 ± 1.32 0.38 ± 2.23 0.088 [a]	6.24 ± 0.70 6.29 ± 1.08 0.044 [b]	−2.41 ± 0.85 −4.07 ± 1.36 0.000 [a]	2.36 ± 0.94 2.62 ± 1.40 0.334 [a]	1.50 ± 0.74 0.36 ± 1.05 0.000 [a]	9.19 ± 1.08 9.28 ± 1.13 0.558 [b]
Right Hip	T0 T1 p-value	5.79 ± 1.84 4.14 ± 1.80 0.000 [b]	1.97 ± 0.79 1.40 ± 1.01 0.018 [c]	10.02 ± 0.91 9.75 ± 1.39 0.088 [b]	4.18 ± 0.92 2.30 ± 1.60 0.000 [a]	8.31 ± 0.66 7.46 ± 1.14 0.001 [b]	−1.12 ± 1.51 −3.07 ± 1.32 0.000 [a]
Left Knee	T0 T1 p-value	−4.33 ± 0.52 −4.15 ± 0.86 0.596 [c]	−4.43 ± 0.39 −3.75 ± 0.69 0.000 [a]	−8.73 ± 0.99 −5.08 ± 0.65 0.000 [a]	−1.95 ± 1.02 −1.40 ± 0.92 0.011 [c]	−9.91 ± 1.07 −2.10 ± 1.05 0.000 [a]	−3.38 ± 1.61 −2.64 ± 1.01 0.046 [c]
Right Knee	T0 T1 p-value	−14.23 ± 3.12 −1.54 ± 1.39 0.000 [a]	5.47 ± 3.00 −3.11 ± 2.01 0.463 [c]	3.11 ± 2.07 −1.66 ± 1.52 0.000 [a]	−0.87 ± 1.48 −3.49 ± 1.64 0.000 [a]	−1.75 ± 1.16 −3.07 ± 1.02 0.075 [b]	5.82 ± 3.69 −2.85 ± 1.82 0.899 [c]
Left Ankle	T0 T1 p-value	1.12 ± 1.11 2.65 ± 1.69 0.973 [c]	−0.95 ± 1.89 −1.26 ± 0.82 0.392 [c]	5.51 ± 1.28 5.78 ± 1.69 0.436 [c]	−0.55 ± 1.37 0.06 ± 0.85 0.044 [b]	3.18 ± 1.09 3.71 ± 1.13 0.026 [c]	−1.68 ± 1.73 −2.12 ± 1.22 0.336 [c]
Right Ankle	T0 T1 p-value	2.41 ± 6.95 1.65 ± 1.65 0.070 [c]	4.00 ± 1.93 1.08 ± 0.83 0.000 [a]	−0.29 ± 2.31 −1.93 ± 1.22 0.000 [b]	3.58 ± 1.47 0.69 ± 1.17 0.000 [a]	0.24 ± 4.80 −1.04 ± 0.95 0.509 [c]	5.82 ± 3.46 3.92 ± 1.02 0.000 [a]

Table A19. Transverse plane mean and standard deviation angles of different joints (hip, pelvis, knee and ankle), at T0 and T1, at the heel strike (HS), mid stance (MD), and toe off (TO), for both lower limbs, along with the *p*-value between both assessment periods. The effect size is presented as large ([a]), moderate ([b]) or small ([c]).

Joint Angle (Degrees)	Time of Assessment	Left Lower Limb			Right Lower Limb		
		HS	MD	TO	HS	MD	TO
Pelvis	T0 T1 p-value	84.81 ± 2.62 84.55 ± 3.14 0.000 [a]	87.49 ± 1.95 85.41 ± 2.11 0.000 [a]	93.89 ± 2.17 92.94 ± 3.45 0.294 [c]	93.89 ± 2.07 92.11 ± 2.30 0.001 [a]	93.51 ± 2.01 92.35 ± 2.71 0.062 [c]	86.01 ± 2.63 84.03 ± 2.16 0.008 [a]
Left Hip	T0 T1 p-value	−14.13 ± 2.01 −13.00 ± 4.62 0.017 [a]	−12.67 ± 0.96 −7.60 ± 1.65 0.000 [a]	−8.90 ± 1.53 −3.13 ± 4.10 0.000 [a]	−10.84 ± 1.36 −5.82 ± 1.81 0.000 [a]	−10.26 ± 1.08 −0.08 ± 1.95 0.000 [a]	−6.94 ± 3.07 −4.76 ± 2.54 0.001 [b]

Table A19. *Cont.*

Joint Angle (Degrees)	Time of Assessment	Left Lower Limb			Right Lower Limb		
		HS	MD	TO	HS	MD	TO
Right Hip	T0	13.18 ± 4.99	8.07 ± 3.79	12.95 ± 4.49	8.91 ± 3.14	11.5 ± 4.79	14.3 ± 4.77
	T1	0.31 ± 4.74	−3.78 ± 3.32	−2.79 ± 2.51	−6.39 ± 5.65	−2.41 ± 2.22	−0.37 ± 3.74
	p-value	0.000 [a]	0.000 [a]	0.000 [a]	0.000 [a]	0.000 [a]	0.000 [a]
Left Knee	T0	−5.54 ± 2.45	2.64 ± 2.19	−7.47 ± 4.13	10.88 ± 2.25	−11.05 ± 1.74	−7.20 ± 2.02
	T1	−15.04 ± 3.10	−8.83 ± 1.86	−11.05 ± 2.27	−3.21 ± 1.83	−15.86 ± 2.11	−15.77 ± 2.36
	p-value	0.000 [a]	0.000 [a]	0.000 [a]	0.000 [a]	0.000 [a]	0.000 [a]
Right Knee	T0	4.22 ± 6.81	−25.63 ± 15.2	−32.39 ± 15.18	−30.58 ± 13.86	−27.93 ± 18.71	−30.00 ± 14.83
	T1	−14.94 ± 7.28	−15.91 ± 2.44	−20.92 ± 2.98	−19.71 ± 2.86	−17.64 ± 3.38	−17.25 ± 2.93
	p-value	0.000 [a]	0.052 [c]	0.000 [c]	0.000 [c]	0.001 [c]	0.001 [b]
Left Ankle	T0	1.47 ± 1.46	−1.54 ± 1.93	5.93 ± 3.94	−6.21 ± 2.30	6.62 ± 1.93	−0.73 ± 2.36
	T1	9.19 ± 1.70	1.09 ± 1.21	4.36 ± 2.70	1.05 ± 1.06	6.34 ± 1.48	0.73 ± 1.26
	p-value	0.000 [a]	0.000 [a]	0.038 [a]	0.000 [a]	0.000 [c]	0.002 [b]
Right Ankle	T0	−13.10 ± 23.26	−1.69 ± 16.01	−9.28 ± 17.48	−6.77 ± 15.44	−9.95 ± 21.76	−3.35 ± 17.26
	T1	5.48 ± 2.22	7.41 ± 1.63	3.17 ± 1.57	9.15 ± 3.21	3.08 ± 1.49	4.52 ± 1.42
	p-value	0.000 [b]	0.000 [b]	0.000 [b]	0.000 [b]	0.000 [b]	0.000 [b]

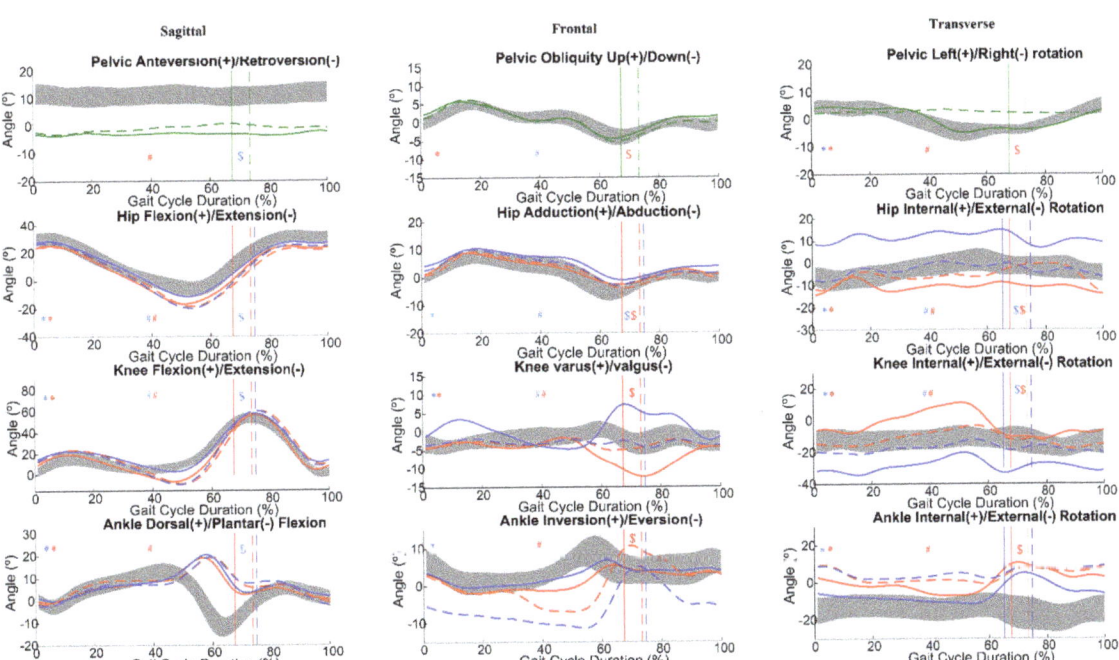

Figure A3. Average pelvis and lower limbs joint angles (in degrees) in the three anatomical planes during a gait cycle of the right (blue), left (red) lower limb and irrespective of the side (green). The joint angles at T0 are denoted by a solid line, while T1 is represented by a dashed line. The reference interval from the healthy gait dataset is shaded grey. A set of symbols are used to denote statistically significant differences, associated with large effect size, between T0 and T1 at the heel strike (*), midstance (#) and toe-off ($), with their color indicating the limb presenting such differences.

P3 shows a clear delayed toe-off for both limbs at T1. It exhibits a generally higher pelvic angle at T1, than T0, both in retroversion when compared with the reference data, but within the normal 5 degrees of range of motion. In the transverse plane it is possible to see that at T1 the rotation is minimal and T0 shows a 10-degree variation. This patient shows a prominent hip extension in comparison to the reference population, although hip flexion remains within reference values. The frontal range of motion is also within reference values. In the transverse plane hip rotation is smooth but more internal for the right lower limb cycles at T0. With regards to the knee angle, the stance phase knee flexion and the following extension are higher than the reference data. The swing phase knee flexion is slightly higher than the reference. The frontal variation of the knee rotation in swing phase is also higher than 10 degrees at T0. The transverse plane shows a tendency for the right lower limb cycles to show a more external rotation of the knee and the left lower limb cycles a more internal rotation. The ankle angle of P3 exhibits an almost permanent dorsiflexion, with a peak higher than the reference gait data. In the frontal plane, eversion/inversion transition is stricter and less regular at T1. The transverse plane, shows a generally more prominent internal rotation of the ankle than in the used reference population.

Appendix C.4. Participant 4

Table A20. Sagittal plane mean and standard deviation angles of different joints (hip, pelvis, knee and ankle), at T0 and T1, at the heel strike (HS), mid stance (MD), and toe off (TO), for both lower limbs, along with the *p*-value between both assessment periods. The effect size is presented as large ([a]), moderate ([b]) or small ([c]).

Joint Angle (Degrees)	Time of Assessment	Left Lower Limb			Right Lower Limb		
		HS	MD	TO	HS	MD	TO
Pelvis	T0	−0.35 ± 1.15	0.36 ± 1.08	−0.06 ± 1.03	−1.55 ± 1.16	−3.60 ± 1.25	−4.80 ± 1.07
	T1	4.89 ± 1.24	3.63 ± 0.60	5.67 ± 0.86	3.25 ± 1.18	3.04 ± 0.87	−0.40 ± 1.16
	p-value	0.000 [a]	0.001 [a]	0.000 [a]	0.000 [a]	0.001 [a]	0.000 [a]
Left Hip	T0	30.09 ± 1.93	7.93 ± 2.89	0.38 ± 6.70	−9.56 ± 5.68	34.19 ± 2.67	23.78 ± 2.61
	T1	24.82 ± 2.39	0.02 ± 0.65	−9.10 ± 3.99	−17.18 ± 1.97	24.8 ± 2.20	16.15 ± 5.72
	p-value	0.000 [a]	0.000 [a]	0.000 [a]	0.000 [a]	0.000 [a]	0.000 [a]
Right Hip	T0	−3.29 ± 3.36	32.03 ± 2.13	27.15 ± 2.28	31.33 ± 1.45	14.25 ± 1.65	0.44 ± 3.10
	T1	−15.27 ± 2.92	23.91 ± 1.26	20.71 ± 2.05	25.20 ± 1.97	5.53 ± 1.48	−9.06 ± 6.02
	p-value	0.000 [a]	0.000 [a]	0.000 [a]	0.000 [a]	0.000 [a]	0.000 [a]
Left Knee	T0	20.48 ± 3.48	18.46 ± 3.54	41.9 ± 5.96	12.61 ± 5.05	65.36 ± 4.20	29.78 ± 2.65
	T1	19.08 ± 3.06	15.91 ± 1.81	38.49 ± 4.20	8.59 ± 3.91	62.45 ± 2.89	28.74 ± 4.86
	p-value	0.024 [c]	0.014 [b]	0.005 [b]	0.000 [b]	0.094 [a]	0.288 [c]
Right Knee	T0	−4.05 ± 2.11	70.39 ± 4.08	35.19 ± 1.94	25.25 ± 1.99	27.48 ± 2.00	45.84 ± 3.07
	T1	5.51 ± 4.50	23.91 ± 1.26	30.65 ± 3.07	18.87 ± 4.57	21.05 ± 1.92	40.81 ± 6.26
	p-value	0.000 [a]	0.000 [a]	0.000 [a]	0.000 [a]	0.001 [b]	0.000 [a]
Left Ankle	T0	3.62 ± 3.58	11.63 ± 3.34	−0.72 ± 2.24	18.67 ± 3.70	−2.96 ± 3.82	6.61 ± 3.54
	T1	−0.77 ± 1.63	9.64 ± 0.86	2.31 ± 3.30	15.85 ± 1.50	−4.55 ± 2.25	6.33 ± 2.05
	p-value	0.800 [c]	0.116 [b]	0.000 [b]	0.312 [c]	0.331 [c]	0.372 [c]
Right Ankle	T0	20.1 ± 2.19	−4.37 ± 2.03	6.23 ± 1.55	−4.74 ± 1.37	12.64 ± 1.37	10.55 ± 2.28
	T1	18.01 ± 2.70	−2.58 ± 2.02	5.97 ± 2.08	−3.27 ± 1.65	12.16 ± 1.72	5.07 ± 3.72
	p-value	0.001 [b]	0.222 [a]	0.545 [c]	0.000 [b]	0.354 [b]	0.000 [a]

Table A21. Frontal plane mean and standard deviation angles of different joints (hip, pelvis, knee and ankle), at T0 and T1, at the heel strike (HS), mid stance (MD), and toe off (TO), for both lower limbs, along with the *p*-value between both assessment periods. The effect size is presented as large ([a]), moderate ([b]) or small ([c]).

Joint Angle (Degrees)	Time of Assessment	Left Lower Limb			Right Lower Limb		
		HS	MD	TO	HS	MD	TO
Pelvis	T0	−0.69 ± 1.66	−3.20 ± 1.95	−2.72 ± 2.4	−3.58 ± 1.86	−1.36 ± 1.84	−2.99 ± 1.88
	T1	−2.89 ± 1.61	−5.32 ± 0.57	−4.70 ± 2.3	−4.58 ± 1.87	−3.72 ± 1.48	−5.44 ± 1.98
	p-value	0.000 [a]	0.037 [a]	0.000 [b]	0.002 [b]	0.024 [a]	0.000 [a]
Left Hip	T0	3.49 ± 3.20	11.28 ± 2.51	5.41 ± 2.16	12.79 ± 2.31	4.36 ± 1.99	12.00 ± 2.12
	T1	0.48 ± 2.40	7.31 ± 1.37	1.29 ± 1.65	7.25 ± 1.86	1.61 ± 1.06	9.26 ± 1.50
	p-value	0.000 [b]	0.028 [a]	0.000 [a]	0.000 [a]	0.002 [a]	0.000 [b]

Table A21. Cont.

Joint Angle (Degrees)	Time of Assessment	Left Lower Limb			Right Lower Limb		
		HS	MD	TO	HS	MD	TO
Right Hip	T0	4.87 ± 1.71	−4.88 ± 1.54	2.27 ± 1.22	−2.54 ± 1.96	2.17 ± 1.29	−7.83 ± 1.53
	T1	10.39 ± 1.93	−0.45 ± 0.59	9.90 ± 1.58	3.52 ± 1.70	9.51 ± 1.63	−1.15 ± 1.36
	p-value	0.000 [b]	0.028 [a]	0.000 [a]	0.000 [a]	0.000 [a]	0.005 [b]
Left Knee	T0	−6.98 ± 6.74	−12.45 ± 4.17	−11.81 ± 10.89	−12.72 ± 8.29	−1.44 ± 9.61	−3.29 ± 6.73
	T1	−9.4 ± 1.05	−9.27 ± 0.35	−0.43 ± 2.30	−11.13 ± 0.81	3.92 ± 1.39	−5.09 ± 2.24
	p-value	0.018 [c]	0.000 [a]	0.000 [b]	0.000 [b]	0.000 [a]	0.196 [c]
Right Knee	T0	−10.36 ± 4.95	3.73 ± 4.66	0.16 ± 2.71	−0.91 ± 2.64	−3.57 ± 2.57	−5.49 ± 3.45
	T1	−10.24 ± 0.81	−0.45 ± 0.59	−6.58 ± 1.24	−7.22 ± 1.53	−7.28 ± 0.64	−5.77 ± 1.54
	p-value	0.000 [a]	0.000 [a]	0.000 [b]	0.000 [b]	0.000 [a]	0.000 [c]
Left Ankle	T0	6.90 ± 6.84	3.08 ± 7.54	−1.86 ± 1.61	6.41 ± 6.41	4.03 ± 7.37	−0.27 ± 7.07
	T1	6.93 ± 1.78	2.99 ± 1.38	7.40 ± 2.95	5.28 ± 1.69	6.98 ± 1.29	1.02 ± 1.35
	p-value	0.186 [c]	0.028 [c]	0.000 [a]	0.918 [c]	0.001 [b]	0.000 [b]
Right Ankle	T0	6.49 ± 1.58	−3.70 ± 1.61	0.73 ± 1.45	3.55 ± 1.58	1.02 ± 1.46	2.22 ± 1.83
	T1	4.71 ± 1.28	−0.19 ± 1.80	0.39 ± 1.43	1.49 ± 2.01	0.83 ± 1.42	2.38 ± 2.23
	p-value	0.000 [a]	0.054 [a]	0.226 [c]	0.000 [a]	0.063 [a]	0.707 [c]

Table A22. Transverse plane mean and standard deviation angles of different joints (hip, pelvis, knee and ankle), at T0 and T1, at the heel strike (HS), mid stance (MD), and toe off (TO), for both lower limbs, along with the p-value between both assessment periods. The effect size is presented as large ([a]), moderate ([b]) or small ([c]).

Joint Angle (Degrees)	Time of Assessment	Left Lower Limb			Right Lower Limb		
		HS	MD	TO	HS	MD	TO
Pelvis	T0	84.10 ± 2.74	86.55 ± 2.16	92.58 ± 2.47	92.06 ± 2.52	91.16 ± 2.52	84.67 ± 2.37
	T1	88.67 ± 2.29	91.79 ± 1.51	93.44 ± 2.43	95.43 ± 2.33	94.31 ± 2.16	89.17 ± 2.43
	p-value	0.000 [a]	0.017 [a]	0.121 [c]	0.000 [a]	0.001 [a]	0.000 [a]
Left Hip	T0	−7.3 ± 9.13	−13.23 ± 6.89	−15.61 ± 11.6	−12.11 ± 18.20	−10.99 ± 10.06	−3.00 ± 9.21
	T1	4.65 ± 3.86	3.21 ± 1.01	5.06 ± 2.58	5.76 ± 2.98	4.38 ± 1.37	5.14 ± 2.33
	p-value	0.000 [a]	0.028 [a]	0.000 [a]	0.000 [a]	0.001 [a]	0.000 [b]
Right Hip	T0	−6.31 ± 3.82	−6.06 ± 4.59	−1.60 ± 3.43	0.05 ± 3.95	−3.72 ± 3.89	−10.28 ± 3.96
	T1	−6.25 ± 2.87	−10.03 ± 2.17	−8.66 ± 2.58	−12.33 ± 5.91	−6.23 ± 3.23	−5.32 ± 3.52
	p-value	0.725 [c]	0.249 [b]	0.000 [a]	0.000 [a]	0.683 [c]	0.000 [a]
Left Knee	T0	−13.98 ± 9.31	−4.46 ± 5.52	−10.22 ± 7.02	0.37 ± 24.10	−18.15 ± 5.28	−16.34 ± 8.27
	T1	−19.26 ± 2.16	−16.13 ± 2.64	−31.03 ± 2.76	−16.47 ± 1.89	−25.14 ± 3.96	−18.35 ± 2.36
	p-value	0.001 [a]	0.096 [c]	0.000 [a]	0.000 [a]	0.003 [a]	0.036 [c]
Right Knee	T0	−3.29 ± 3.36	−8.49 ± 3.60	−13.66 ± 3.53	−18.66 ± 4.47	−10.95 ± 4.33	−4.46 ± 4.38
	T1	6.10 ± 2.03	−10.03 ± 2.17	0.40 ± 1.93	−0.99 ± 1.93	2.06 ± 1.49	−1.52 ± 1.55
	p-value	0.000 [a]	0.052 [a]	0.000 [a]	0.000 [a]	0.001 [a]	0.001 [b]
Left Ankle	T0	4.29 ± 4.25	−29.49 ± 2.14	−0.02 ± 1.87	−29.40 ± 3.66	−27.30 ± 3.78	−30.90 ± 2.87
	T1	−24.37 ± 0.83	−28.99 ± 0.30	−30.84 ± 1.39	−28.51 ± 1.11	−24.47 ± 0.92	−30.25 ± 1.04
	p-value	0.399 [c]	0.046 [a]	0.000 [b]	0.000 [c]	0.000 [c]	0.041 [c]
Right Ankle	T0	−6.65 ± 2.35	−9.04 ± 2.47	−9.11 ± 3.16	−1.70 ± 2.88	−8.20 ± 2.41	−7.32 ± 2.66
	T1	−18.05 ± 1.05	−10.21 ± 0.68	−19.78 ± 1.81	−13.49 ± 1.57	−19.39 ± 1.32	−17.46 ± 2.79
	p-value	0.000 [a]	0.506 [b]	0.000 [a]	0.000 [a]	0.001 [a]	0.000 [a]

P4 shows similar toe-off moments at T0 and T1. The pelvic angle shows a slight retroversion, when compared to the reference data, and a generally lower retroversion at T1, than T0. In the frontal plane, obliquity is within the normal 5° variation, and in the transverse plane left and right rotations are more prominent at T1 than T0 and the variation is around −5 to 5 degrees which is near the reference pattern. P4's hip extension, is more prominent than the reference population. The frontal range of motion is within reference values and, in the transverse plane, an excessive rotation (more than 10 degrees total displacement) is observed at T0. T1, on the contrary, exhibits slightly more external but smoother rotations, than the reference gait data, to sustain body weight. The stance phase knee flexion is higher than the reference population, and the following extension is lower. Swing phase knee flexion is also higher than the reference. In the transverse plane it is possible to see an asymmetry at T1 with the right lower limb cycles presenting a more internal knee rotation and the left lower limb cycles a more external knee rotation throughout the whole gait cycle. The ankle angle shows a higher dorsiflexion (up to 25°) than the reference data. In the frontal plane eversion is less strict than the other patients and within the reference values. The transverse plane shows almost no alterations on ankle rotation during the gait cycle for each assessment, despite right lower limb cycles being more within the normal rotation range and the left lower limb cycles more externally rotated.

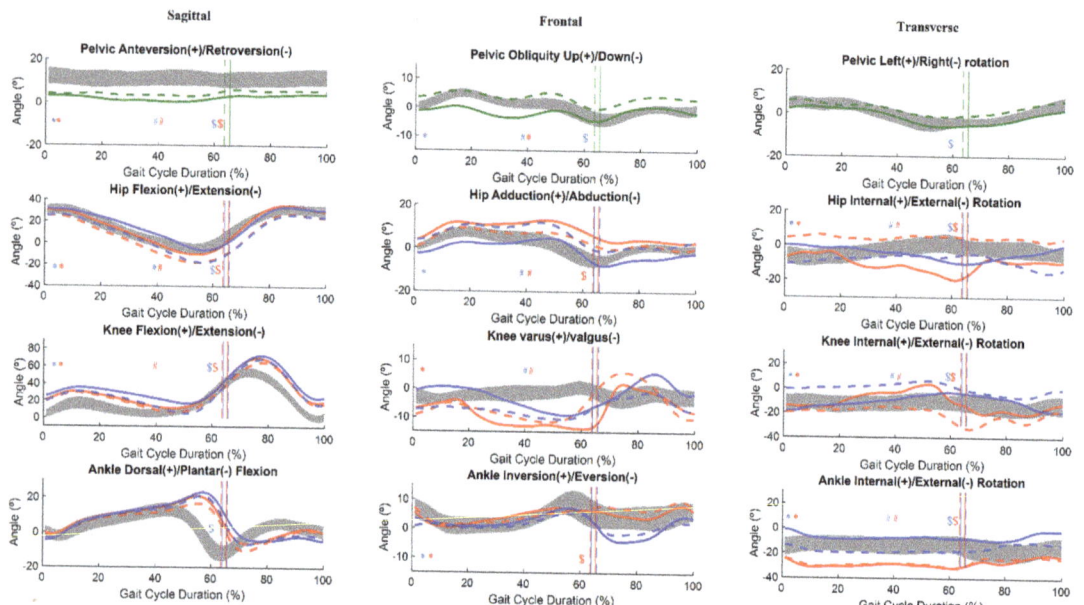

Figure A4. Average pelvis and lower limbs joint angles (in degrees) in the three anatomical planes during a gait cycle of the right (blue), left (red) lower limb and irrespective of the side (green). The joint angles at T0 are denoted by a solid line, while T1 is represented by a dashed line. The reference interval from the healthy gait dataset is shaded grey. A set of symbols are used to denote statistically significant differences, associated with large effect size, between T0 and T1 at the heel strike (*), midstance (#) and toe-off ($), with their color indicating the limb presenting such differences.

Appendix C.5. Participant 5

Table A23. Sagittal plane mean and standard deviation angles of different joints (hip, pelvis, knee and ankle), at T0 and T1, at the heel strike (HS), mid stance (MD), and toe off (TO), for both lower limbs, along with the *p*-value between both assessment periods. The effect size is presented as large ([a]), moderate ([b]) or small ([c]).

Joint Angle (Degrees)	Time of Assessment	Left Lower Limb			Right Lower Limb		
		HS	MD	LTO	HS	MD	TO
Pelvis	T0	−1.73 ± 1.63	−1.81 ± 1.10	5.74 ± 22.57	−3.85 ± 2.80	−2.01 ± 0.69	−4.50 ± 1.08
	T1	1.58 ± 0.79	1.10 ± 0.88	5.30 ± 0.91	1.03 ± 1.41	0.19 ± 0.94	−2.14 ± 0.82
	p-value	0.000 [a]	0.000 [a]	0.000 [a]	0.000 [a]	0.000 [a]	0.000 [a]
Left Hip	T0	21.24 ± 1.69	−4.48 ± 1.33	−7.81 ± 24.89	−19.64 ± 2.11	23.59 ± 1.53	17.83 ± 1.39
	T1	27.16 ± 2.50	1.66 ± 1.93	−4.68 ± 3.14	−13.89 ± 1.74	29.02 ± 1.57	22.93 ± 4.11
	p-value	0.000 [a]	0.000 [a]	0.000 [a]	0.000 [a]	0.000 [a]	0.000 [a]
Right Hip	T0	−20.86 ± 1.49	17.43 ± 1.40	23.55 ± 19.51	22.63 ± 1.63	−4.68 ± 1.70	−17.47 ± 1.40
	T1	−15.33 ± 2.55	24.06 ± 1.45	26.08 ± 3.16	30.13 ± 2.93	2.31 ± 2.74	−10.57 ± 4.49
	p-value	0.000 [a]	0.000 [a]	0.000 [a]	0.000 [a]	0.000 [a]	0.000 [a]

Table A23. Cont.

Joint Angle (Degrees)	Time of Assessment	Left Lower Limb			Right Lower Limb		
		HS	MD	LTO	HS	MD	TO
Left Knee	T0	13.69 ± 2.13	12.97 ± 2.01	39.18 ± 2.21	12.96 ± 1.74	66.3 ± 1.79	24.01 ± 2.15
	T1	14.71 ± 4.16	16.05 ± 4.04	47.93 ± 5.89	15.14 ± 3.6	29.02 ± 1.57	30.21 ± 3.78
	p-value	0.257 [c]	0.001 [b]	0.000 [a]	0.006 [b]	0.000 [a]	0.000 [a]
Right Knee	T0	4.87 ± 1.71	59.10 ± 2.13	26.25 ± 2.79	16.51 ± 1.85	11.39 ± 2.58	33.90 ± 2.19
	T1	11.93 ± 1.89	60.38 ± 2.31	29.79 ± 2.83	17.95 ± 3.05	13.87 ± 2.49	39.85 ± 5.87
	p-value	0.013 [b]	0.015 [a]	0.000 [a]	0.004 [b]	0.002 [a]	0.000 [a]
Left Ankle	T0	1.11 ± 1.10	9.15 ± 1.20	7.23 ± 2.81	25.02 ± 1.14	−6.15 ± 1.07	−1.54 ± 2.09
	T1	−3.11 ± 0.81	12.06 ± 1.78	2.45 ± 4.81	27.33 ± 1.98	−2.65 ± 1.33	4.15 ± 2.28
	p-value	0.000 [a]	0.000 [a]	0.000 [a]	0.000 [a]	0.000 [a]	0.000 [a]
Right Ankle	T0	20.25 ± 1.30	2.21 ± 0.81	2.98 ± 1.55	−0.01 ± 1.02	10.82 ± 1.22	6.89 ± 2.27
	T1	21.24 ± 1.34	−1.37 ± 1.33	4.44 ± 1.94	−2.68 ± 0.85	11.05 ± 1.28	3.53 ± 3.93
	p-value	0.005 [a]	0.000 [a]	0.002 [a]	0.000 [a]	0.371 [c]	0.000 [a]

Table A24. Frontal plane mean and standard deviation angles of different joints (hip, pelvis, knee and ankle), at T0 and T1, at the heel strike (HS), mid stance (MD), and toe off (TO), for both lower limbs, along with the p-value between both assessment periods. The effect size is presented as large ([a]), moderate ([b]) or small ([c]).

Joint Angle (Degrees)	Time of Assessment	Left Lower Limb			Right Lower Limb		
		HS	MD	TO	HS	MD	TO
Pelvis	T0	−6.20 ± 1.40	−8.65 ± 1.68	−6.35 ± 1.25	−5.75 ± 1.27	−7.31 ± 1.09	−8.14 ± 1.43
	T1	−1.15 ± 1.07	−3.34 ± 1.92	−1.67 ± 3.12	−0.68 ± 2.47	−1.87 ± 2.22	−4.33 ± 1.33
	p-value	0.000 [a]	0.000 [a]	0.000 [a]	0.000 [a]	0.000 [a]	0.000 [a]
Left Hip	T0	1.58 ± 1.93	5.28 ± 1.13	−3.48 ± 1.31	3.87 ± 2.51	2.09 ± 0.81	5.56 ± 1.84
	T1	−3.01 ± 1.44	2.41 ± 1.62	−6.22 ± 1.67	0.50 ± 2.59	−1.10 ± 1.03	1.71 ± 1.84
	p-value	0.000 [a]	0.000 [a]	0.000 [a]	0.000 [a]	0.000 [a]	0.434 [b]
Right Hip	T0	4.11 ± 2.17	0.14 ± 1.16	3.56 ± 4.56	−3.23 ± 3.13	5.46 ± 0.88	−0.86 ± 1.50
	T1	5.42 ± 1.64	1.87 ± 1.78	6.39 ± 2.13	−0.51 ± 2.72	5.46 ± 2.14	−1.83 ± 1.53
	p-value	0.001 [b]	0.001 [b]	0.000 [b]	0.001 [b]	0.829 [c]	0.000 [b]
Left Knee	T0	−0.89 ± 0.57	−0.97 ± 0.46	−7.42 ± 1.45	−1.56 ± 0.52	−4.24 ± 1.51	−1.26 ± 0.96
	T1	−0.59 ± 0.67	−0.27 ± 0.61	−2.45 ± 4.06	−0.96 ± 0.66	−1.10 ± 1.03	0.91 ± 1.26
	p-value	0.097 [b]	0.000 [b]	0.000 [b]	0.000 [a]	0.000 [a]	0.000 [a]
Right Knee	T0	−6.31 ± 3.82	7.91 ± 1.79	3.23 ± 2.14	0.86 ± 0.58	−0.32 ± 0.37	0.67 ± 0.66
	T1	−2.17 ± 0.64	2.31 ± 1.01	−0.70 ± 1.16	−1.48 ± 0.86	−1.48 ± 0.69	−1.18 ± 1.40
	p-value	0.000 [a]	0.000 [a]	0.000 [a]	0.000 [a]	0.000 [a]	0.000 [a]
Left Ankle	T0	0.97 ± 0.96	−4.53 ± 1.00	−4.10 ± 1.35	−5.00 ± 0.91	−5.30 ± 1.06	−3.57 ± 1.24
	T1	2.74 ± 1.00	0.06 ± 1.23	0.46 ± 1.11	0.50 ± 1.49	−2.62 ± 0.80	−1.26 ± 1.16
	p-value	0.000 [a]	0.000 [a]	0.000 [a]	0.000 [a]	0.000 [a]	0.000 [a]
Right Ankle	T0	3.76 ± 1.11	−4.05 ± 0.53	−2.72 ± 1.27	1.71 ± 0.78	−1.47 ± 1.18	3.40 ± 1.58
	T1	0.90 ± 1.32	−3.73 ± 2.05	−2.71 ± 1.84	2.84 ± 1.70	−1.76 ± 1.20	1.49 ± 2.14
	p-value	0.000 [a]	0.014 [b]	0.857 [c]	0.001 [a]	0.475 [c]	0.005 [a]

Table A25. Transverse plane mean and standard deviation angles of different joints (hip, pelvis, knee and ankle), at T0 and T1, at the heel strike (HS), mid stance (MD), and toe off (TO), for both lower limbs, along with the p-value between both assessment periods. The effect size is presented as large ([a]) or moderate ([b]).

Joint Angle (Degrees)	Time of Assessment	Left Lower Limb			Right Lower Limb		
		HS	MD	TO	HS	MD	TO
Pelvis	T0	89.55 ± 1.64	92.86 ± 1.72	101.39 ± 8.13	99.45 ± 1.62	94.12 ± 1.34	89.76 ± 1.72
	T1	87.40 ± 1.72	90.58 ± 1.68	97.02 ± 1.50	96.73 ± 1.84	92.25 ± 1.52	87.21 ± 1.90
	p-value	0.000 [b]	0.000 [a]	0.000 [a]	0.000 [a]	0.000 [a]	0.000 [a]
Left Hip	T0	−18.62 ± 3.40	−11.72 ± 1.90	−8.22 ± 13.92	−9.09 ± 1.78	−4.08 ± 2.11	−14.53 ± 2.78
	T1	−12.83 ± 2.52	−5.93 ± 3.84	−1.01 ± 4.84	−4.63 ± 3.56	6.23 ± 3.15	−9.73 ± 2.15
	p-value	0.000 [a]	0.000 [a]	0.000 [a]	0.000 [a]	0.000 [a]	0.000 [a]

Table A25. Cont.

Joint Angle (Degrees)	Time of Assessment	Left Lower Limb			Right Lower Limb		
		HS	MD	TO	HS	MD	TO
Right Hip	T0	−0.65 ± 1.89	4.60 ± 2.77	−5.24 ± 15.06	−5.13 ± 2.38	−0.43 ± 1.97	−1.67 ± 1.75
	T1	−3.22 ± 2.36	−0.55 ± 2.91	−10.39 ± 2.25	−13.44 ± 2.00	−4.66 ± 2.86	−4.18 ± 2.01
	p-value	0.000 a	0.000 a	0.000 a	0.000 a	0.000 a	0.000 a
Left Knee	T0	8.93 ± 2.54	13.96 ± 1.13	17.25 ± 1.62	18.06 ± 1.45	13.81 ± 1.43	10.67 ± 2.37
	T1	−8.55 ± 2.36	−4.18 ± 2.24	−0.76 ± 2.50	−0.60 ± 1.31	6.23 ± 3.15	−5.94 ± 1.92
	p-value	0.000 a	0.000 a	0.000 a	0.000 a	0.000 a	0.000 a
Right Knee	T0	13.57 ± 2.83	−18.78 ± 1.95	−25.08 ± 3.46	−27.53 ± 1.90	−21.18 ± 1.41	−20.37 ± 1.50
	T1	−2.96 ± 1.42	−6.50 ± 2.28	−7.25 ± 2.93	−11.38 ± 3.11	−6.39 ± 2.17	−7.66 ± 2.59
	p-value	0.000 a	0.000 a	0.000 a	0.000 a	0.000 a	0.000 a
Left Ankle	T0	1.32 ± 1.30	−8.29 ± 1.80	−7.80 ± 2.33	−6.99 ± 1.65	−11.44 ± 1.12	−8.59 ± 2.03
	T1	10.12 ± 2.47	3.32 ± 2.68	3.44 ± 2.14	2.33 ± 1.55	2.02 ± 1.24	4.19 ± 2.29
	p-value	0.000 a	0.000 a	0.000 a	0.000 a	0.000 a	0.000 a
Right Ankle	T0	−1.42 ± 1.27	−3.86 ± 1.59	−1.92 ± 1.64	4.41 ± 0.87	−1.89 ± 1.46	1.09 ± 2.37
	T1	−15.64 ± 1.20	−15.86 ± 1.94	−16.46 ± 2.54	−6.61 ± 1.57	−15.76 ± 1.43	−12.62 ± 2.30
	p-value	0.000 a	0.000 a	0.000 a	0.000 a	0.000 a	0.000 a

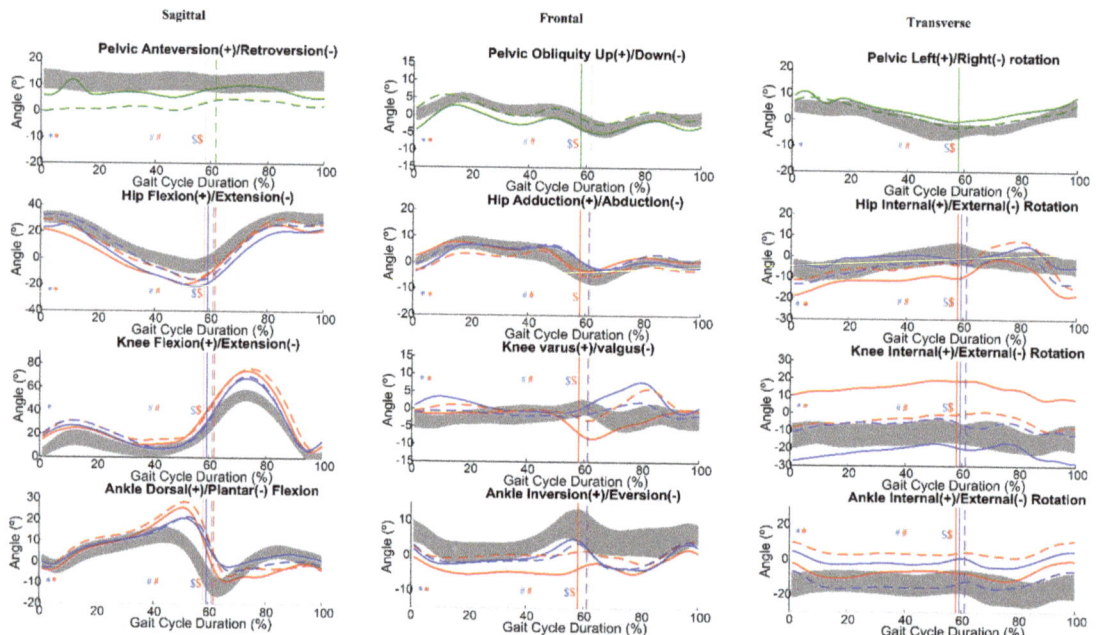

Figure A5. Average pelvis and lower limbs joint angles (in degrees) in the three anatomical planes during a gait cycle of the right (blue), left (red) lower limb and irrespective of the side (green). The joint angles at T0 are denoted by a solid line, while T1 is represented by a dashed line. The reference interval from the healthy gait dataset is shaded grey. A set of symbols are used to denote statistically significant differences, associated with large effect size, between T0 and T1 at the heel strike (*), midstance (#) and toe-off ($), with their color indicating the limb presenting such differences.

P5 has a delayed toe-off at T1 and a peak pelvic anteversion during loading response at T0. This peak disappeared at T1 which showed a more retroverted pelvic angle in general. However, this angle is generally within the reference values (at T0) and has a 5 degrees variation, in the sagittal plane. In the transverse plane, right rotations are more prominent than those in the reference gait data, and left rotation is within reference values. Variation is around −5 to 10 degrees. Hip extension is more prominent than the used reference population, although hip flexion is lower than reference values. Excessive transverse rotation (more than 10 degrees total displacement) is also observed in this patient. The stance phase knee flexion is higher at T1 than T0 and also than the reference population, and the following extension is lower. Swing phase knee flexion is also higher than reference data and higher at T1 than T0. The transverse plane analysis shows a very smooth rotation and more external than the used reference gait data in the case of the right lower limb cycles at T0 as well as a more internal rotation in the case of left lower limb cycles, also at T0. The ankle angle shows a higher plantar-flexion than the reference population on the swing phase, and a higher dorsiflexion (up to 30°) before the toe-off. In the frontal plane, the eversion is more prominent than the correspondent for the reference values, and the swing phase were different for all the assessments.

References

1. Planté-Bordeneuve, V.; Said, G. Familial amyloid polyneuropathy. *Lancet Neurol.* **2011**, *10*, 1086–1097. [CrossRef]
2. Schmidt, H.H.; Waddington-Cruz, M.; Botteman, M.F.; Carter, J.A.; Chopra, A.S.; Hopps, M.; Stewart, M.; Fallet, S.; Amass, L. Estimating the global prevalence of transthyretin familial amyloid polyneuropathy. *Muscle Nerve* **2018**, *57*, 829–837. [CrossRef] [PubMed]
3. Ines, M.; Coelho, T.; Conceicao, I.; Duarte-Ramos, F.; de Carvalho, M.; Costa, J. Epidemiology of Transthyretin Familial Amyloid Polyneuropathy in Portugal: A Nationwide Study. *Neuroepidemiology* **2018**, *51*, 177–182. [CrossRef]
4. Kato-Motozaki, Y.; Ono, K.; Shima, K.; Morinaga, A.; Machiya, T.; Nozaki, I.; Shibata-Hamaguchi, A.; Furukawa, Y.; Yanase, D.; Ishida, C.; et al. Epidemiology of familial amyloid polyneuropathy in Japan: Identification of a novel endemic focus. *J. Neurol. Sci.* **2008**, *270*, 133–140. [CrossRef]
5. Dardiotis, E.; Koutsou, P.; Papanicolaou, E.Z.; Vonta, I.; Kladi, A.; Vassilopoulos, D.; Hadjigeorgiou, G.; Christodoulou, K.; Kyriakides, T. Epidemiological, clinical and genetic study of familial amyloidotic polyneuropathy in Cyprus. *Amyloid* **2009**, *16*, 32–37. [CrossRef]
6. Parman, Y.; Adams, D.; Obici, L.; Galan, L.; Guergueltcheva, V.; Suhr, O.B.; Coelho, T. Sixty years of transthyretin familial amyloid polyneuropathy (TTR-FAP) in Europe: Where are we now? A European network approach to defining the epidemiology and management patterns for TTR-FAP. *Curr. Opin. Neurol.* **2016**, *29* (Suppl. S1), S3–S13. [CrossRef]
7. Coutinho, P.; Martins da Silva, A.; Lopes Lima, J.; Resende-Barbosa, A. Forty Years of Experience with Type I Amyloid Neuropathy. In *Amyloid and Amyloidosis*; Review of 483 cases; Glenner, G.G., Pinho e Costa, P., Falcão de Freitas, A., Eds.; Excerpta Medica: Amsterdam, The Netherlands, 1980; pp. 88–98.
8. Zhao, Y.; Xin, Y.; Song, Z.; He, Z.; Hu, W. Tafamidis, a Noninvasive Therapy for Delaying Transthyretin Familial Amyloid Polyneuropathy: Systematic Review and Meta-Analysis. *J. Clin. Neurol.* **2019**, *15*, 108–115. [CrossRef]
9. Adams, D.; Gonzalez-Duarte, A.; O'Riordan, W.D.; Yang, C.-C.; Ueda, M.; Kristen, A.V.; Tournev, I.; Schmidt, H.H.; Coelho, T.; Berk, J.L.; et al. Patisiran, an RNAi Therapeutic, for Hereditary Transthyretin Amyloidosis. *N. Engl. J. Med.* **2018**, *379*, 11–21. [CrossRef]
10. Benson, M.D.; Waddington-Cruz, M.; Berk, J.L.; Polydefkis, M.; Dyck, P.J.; Wang, A.K.; Planté-Bordeneuve, V.; Barroso, F.A.; Merlini, G.; Obici, L.; et al. Inotersen Treatment for Patients with Hereditary Transthyretin Amyloidosis. *N. Engl. J. Med.* **2018**, *379*, 22–31. [CrossRef]
11. Plante-Bordeneuve, V. Transthyretin familial amyloid polyneuropathy: An update. *J. Neurol.* **2018**, *265*, 976–983. [CrossRef]
12. Escolano Lozano, F.; Barreiros, A.P.; Birklein, F.; Geber, C. Transthyretin familial amyloid polyneuropathy (TTR-FAP): Parameters for early diagnosis. *Brain Behav.* **2018**, *8*, e00889. [CrossRef] [PubMed]
13. Vinik, E.J.; Hayes, R.P.; Oglesby, A.; Bastyr, E.; Barlow, P.; Ford-Molvik, S.L.; Vinik, A.I. The Development and Validation of the Norfolk QOL-DN, a New Measure of Patients' Perception of the Effects of Diabetes and Diabetic Neuropathy. *Diabetes Technol. Ther.* **2005**, *7*, 497–508. [CrossRef] [PubMed]
14. Vilas-Boas, M.d.C.; Cunha, J.P.S. Movement Quantification in Neurological Diseases: Methods and Applications. *IEEE Rev. Biomed. Eng.* **2016**, *9*, 15–31. [CrossRef]
15. Adams, D.; Koike, H.; Slama, M.; Coelho, T. Hereditary transthyretin amyloidosis: A model of medical progress for a fatal disease. *Nat. Rev. Neurol.* **2019**, *15*, 387–404. [CrossRef] [PubMed]
16. Adams, D. Recent advances in the treatment of familial amyloid polyneuropathy. *Ther. Adv. Neurol. Disord.* **2013**, *6*, 129–139. [CrossRef] [PubMed]
17. Whittle, M.W. *Gait Analysis An Introduction*, 4th ed.; Elsevier Ltd.: Amsterdam, The Netherlands, 2007.
18. Roetenberg, D. Inertial and Magnetic Sensing of Human Motion. Ph.D. Thesis, University of Twente, Enschede, The Netherlands, 2006.
19. Vilas-Boas, M.C.; Rocha, A.P.; Choupina, H.M.P.; Fernandes, J.M.; Coelho, T.; Cunha, J.P.S. The First Transthyretin Familial Amyloid Polyneuropathy Gait Quantification Study—Preliminary Results. In Proceedings of the 2017 39th Annual International Conference of the IEEE Engineering in Medicine and Biology Society (EMBC), Jeju, Korea, 11–15 July 2017.
20. Vilas-Boas, M.D.C.; Rocha, A.P.; Cardoso, M.N.; Fernandes, J.M.; Coelho, T.; Cunha, J.P.S. Clinical 3-D Gait Assessment of Patients With Polyneuropathy Associated With Hereditary Transthyretin Amyloidosis. *Front. Neurol.* **2020**, *11*, 605282. [CrossRef]

21. Vilas-Boas, M.d.C.; Rocha, A.P.; Cardoso, M.N.; Fernandes, J.M.; Coelho, T.; Cunha, J.P.S. Supporting the Assessment of Hereditary Transthyretin Amyloidosis Patients Based On 3-D Gait Analysis and Machine Learning. *IEEE Trans. Neural Syst. Rehabil. Eng.* **2021**, *29*, 1350–1362. [CrossRef] [PubMed]
22. Compston, A. Aids to the Investigation of Peripheral Nerve Injuries. Medical Research Council: Nerve Injuries Research Committee. His Majesty's Stationery Office: 1942; pp. 48 (iii) and 74 figures and 7 diagrams; with Aids to the Examination of the Peripheral Nervous System. By Michael O'Brien for the Guarantors of Brain. Saunders Elsevier: 2010; pp. [8] 64 and 94 Figures. *Brain* **2010**, *133*, 2838–2844. [CrossRef]
23. Adams, D.; Suhr, O.B.; Hund, E.; Obici, L.; Tournev, I.; Campistol, J.M.; Slama, M.S.; Hazenberg, B.P.; Coelho, T. First European consensus for diagnosis, management, and treatment of transthyretin familial amyloid polyneuropathy. *Curr. Opin. Neurol.* **2016**, *29* (Suppl. S1), S14–S26. [CrossRef]
24. Cappozzo, A.; Catan, F.; Croce, U.D.; Leardini, A. Position and orientation in space of bones during movement: Experimental artefacts. *Clin. Biomech.* **1995**, *10*, 171–178. [CrossRef]
25. Benedetti, M.G.; Catani, F.; Leardini, A.; Pignotti, E.; Giannini, S. Data management in gait analysis for clinical applications. *Clin. Biomech.* **1998**, *13*, 204–215. [CrossRef]
26. Kim, K.; Song, W.K.; Lee, J.; Lee, H.Y.; Park, D.S.; Ko, B.W.; Kim, J. Kinematic analysis of upper extremity movement during drinking in hemiplegic subjects. *Clin. Biomech.* **2014**, *29*, 248–256. [CrossRef] [PubMed]
27. Cohen, J.W. *Statistical Power Analysis for the Behavioral Sciences*, 2nd ed.; Lawrence Erlbaum Associates: Hillsdale, NJ, USA, 1988.
28. Richards, J. *Biomechanics in Clinic and Research*; Churchill Livingstone Elsevier: London, UK, 2009.
29. Martinelli, A.R.; Mantovani, A.M.; Nozabieli, A.J.L.; Ferreira, D.M.A.; Barela, J.A.; Camargo, M.R.d.; Fregonesi, C.E.P.T. Muscle strength and ankle mobility for the gait parameters in diabetic neuropathies. *Foot* **2013**, *23*, 17–21. [CrossRef] [PubMed]
30. Perry, J. *Gait Analysis—Normal and Pathological Function*; SLACK Incorporated: Thorofare, NJ, USA, 1992.
31. Abu-Zidan, F.M.; Abbas, A.K.; Hefny, A.I. Clinical "case series": A concept analysis. *Afr. Health Sci.* **2013**, *12*, 557–562. [CrossRef]
32. Katoulis, E.C.; Ebdon-Parry, M.; Lanshammar, H.; Vlleikyte, L.; Kulkarni, J.; Boulton, A.J.M. Gait Abnormalities in Diabetic Neuropathy. *Diabetes Care* **1997**, *20*, 1904–1907. [CrossRef]
33. Brown, S.J.; Handsaker, J.C.; Bowling, F.L.; Maganaris, C.N.; Boulton, A.J.; Reeves, N.D. Do patients with diabetic neuropathy use a higher proportion of their maximum strength when walking? *J. Biomech.* **2014**, *47*, 3639–3644. [CrossRef]
34. Karmakar, M.K.; Samy, W.; Li, J.W.; Lee, A.; Chan, W.C.; Chen, P.P.; Ho, A.M.-H. Thoracic paravertebral block and its effects on chronic pain and health-related quality of life after modified radical mastectomy. *Reg. Anesth. Pain Med.* **2014**, *39*, 289–298. [CrossRef]
35. Adams, D.; Samuel, D.; Goulon-Goeau, C.; Nakazato, M.; Costa, P.M.; Feray, C.; Planté, V.; Ducot, B.; Ichai, P.; Lacroix, C.; et al. The course and prognostic factors of familial amyloid polyneuropathy after liver transplantation. *Brain* **2000**, *123*, 1495–1504. [CrossRef]
36. Yamamoto, S.; Wilczek, H.E.; Nowak, G.; Larsson, M.; Oksanen, A.; Iwata, T.; Gjertsen, H.; Soderdahl, G.; Wikstrom, L.; Ando, Y.; et al. Liver transplantation for familial amyloidotic polyneuropathy (FAP): A single-center experience over 16 years. *Am. J. Transpl.* **2007**, *7*, 2597–2604. [CrossRef]
37. Coelho, T. Familial amyloid polyneuropathy: New develpments in genetics and treatment. *Curr. Opin. Neurol.* **1996**, *9*, 355–359. [CrossRef]
38. Fabio, A.B.; Daniel, P.J.; Ben, E.; Huihua, L.; Michelle, S.; Amass, L.; Sultan, M.B. Long-term safety and efficacy of *tafamidis* for the treatment of hereditary transthyretin amyloid polyneuropathy: Results up to 6 years. *Amyloid* **2017**, *24*, 194–204. [CrossRef]
39. Monteiro, C.; Mesgazardeh, J.S.; Anselmo, J.; Fernandes, J.; Novais, M.; Rodrigues, C.; Brighty, G.J.; Powers, D.L.; Powers, E.T.; Coelho, T.; et al. Predictive model of response to tafamidis in hereditary ATTR polyneuropathy. *JCI Insight* **2019**, *4*, e126526. [CrossRef] [PubMed]

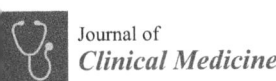

Article

Differences in the Time Course of Recovery from Brain and Liver Dysfunction in Conventional Long-Term Treatment of Wilson Disease

Harald Hefter [1,*], Theodor S. Kruschel [1], Max Novak [1], Dietmar Rosenthal [1], Tom Luedde [2], Sven G. Meuth [1], Philipp Albrecht [1,3], Christian J. Hartmann [1] and Sara Samadzadeh [1,4,5,6]

[1] Departments of Neurology, University of Düsseldorf, Moorenstrasse 5, D-40225 Düsseldorf, Germany; theo.kruschel@gmx.de (T.S.K.); max.novak@uni-duesseldorf.de (M.N.); dietmar.rosenthal@med.uni-duesseldorf.de (D.R.); svenguenther.meuth@med.uni-duesseldorf.de (S.G.M.); philipp.albrecht@med.uni-duesseldorf.de (P.A.); christian.hartmann@med.uni-duesseldorf.de (C.J.H.); sara.samadzadeh@yahoo.com (S.S.)
[2] Departments of Gastroenterology, University of Düsseldorf, Moorenstrasse 5, D-40225 Düsseldorf, Germany; tom.luedde@med.uni-duesseldorf.de
[3] Department of Neurology, Kliniken Maria Hilf GmbH Mönchengladbach, 41063 Mönchengladbach, Germany
[4] Charité–Universitätsmedizin Berlin, Corporate Member of Freie Universität Berlin and Humboldt-Unverstät zu Berlin, Experimental and Clinical Research Center, 13125 Berlin, Germany
[5] Department of Regional Health Research and Molecular Medicine, University of Southern Denmark, 5230 Odense, Denmark
[6] Department of Neurology, Slagelse Hospital, 4200 Slagelse, Denmark
* Correspondence: harald.hefter@online.de; Tel.: +49-211-811-7025; Fax: +49-211-810-4903

Abstract: Background: The aim of this study was to demonstrate that both neurological and hepatic symptoms respond to copper chelation therapy in Wilson disease (WD). However, the time course of their recovery is different. Methods: Eighteen patients with neurological WD from a single specialized center who had been listed for liver transplantation during the last ten years and two newly diagnosed homozygous twins were recruited for this retrospective study. The mean duration of conventional treatment was 7.3 years (range: 0.25 to 36.2 years). A custom Wilson disease score with seven motor items, three non-motor items, and 33 biochemical parameters of the blood and urine, as well as the MELD score, was determined at various checkup visits during treatment. These data were extracted from the charts of the patients. Results: Treatment was initiated with severity-dependent doses ($\geq$900 mg) of D-penicillamine (DPA) or triethylene-tetramin-dihydrochloride (TRIEN). The motor score improved in 10 and remained constant in 8 patients. Worsening of neurological symptoms was observed only in two patients who developed comorbidities (myasthenia gravis or hemispheric stroke). The neurological symptoms continuously improved over the years until the majority of patients became only mildly affected. In contrast to this slow recovery of the neurological symptoms, the MELD score and liver enzymes had already started to improve after 1 month and rapidly improved over the next 6 months in 19 patients. The cholinesterase levels continued to increase significantly ($p < 0.0074$) even further. One patient whose MELD score indicated further progression of liver disease received an orthotopic liver transplantation 3 months after the diagnosis of WD and the onset of DPA treatment. Conclusions: Neurological and hepatic symptoms both respond to copper chelation therapy. For patients with acute liver failure, the first 4 months are critical. This is the time span in which patients have to wait either for a donor organ or until significant improvement has occurred under conventional therapy. For patients with severe neurological symptoms, it is important that they are treated with fairly high doses over several years.

Keywords: Wilson disease; spectrum of symptoms; recovery; cholinesterase; biomarker; orthotopic liver transplantation

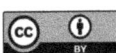

1. Introduction

Wilson disease (WD) is a recessively inherited disorder of copper metabolism predominantly affecting the liver and brain that was named after S.A.K. Wilson [1]. Inspecting post-mortem WD brains, he was impressed by the damage to the brain, especially to the putamen (the lenticular nucleus), in addition to liver cirrhosis. Therefore, he called this disease entity progressive hepatolenticular degeneration [1].

About 110 years later, knowledge about the pathophysiology of WD has considerably improved [2,3]. The essential trace element copper, which is necessary for iron oxidation in the mitochondria and a variety of other enzymatic intracellular reactions, turned out to play a crucial role in this disease [3–5]. Copper is taken up from the gut and the portal veins by the human copper transporter (CTR1/hCTR1 [6]) into hepatocytes and transported to the trans-Golgi network. Here, the P-adenotriphosphate protease ATP7B (ATP7B) modifies apo-ceruloplasmin to ceruloplasmin (CER) by incorporating copper [7]. Intact ceruloplasmin regulates iron metabolism and the transport of copper to non-hepatic cells [7,8]. Furthermore, ATP7B is necessary for the excretion of excessive copper into the bile [9,10].

In 1993, causal mutations in the *ATP7B* gene (locus 13q14.3-q21.1) that are responsible for the development of WD were identified [11]. During the last 30 years, more than 1000 mutations have been reported [12,13]. However, there seems to be no genotype–phenotype correlation [14]. Even in homozygotic WD twins, the phenotype may be considerably discordant [15–17].

The spectrum of both hepatic and neurological symptoms is broad. On the one hand, WD may become manifest as fulminant liver failure [18]; on the other hand, it may be diagnosed in elderly people without or with mild hepatic symptoms by chance [19]. Neurologic WD may become manifest as a severe generalized movement disorder [2,3,15] or a mild tremor of the hands, voice, and tongue only [20]. These differences in its clinical manifestation are still poorly understood. Since neurological manifestations usually occur later than hepatic manifestations, the blood–brain barrier (BBB) is thought to protect against brain damage due to the influx of copper [21]. However, even that is doubted since free copper can penetrate and damage the BBB [22,23].

The response to treatment is similarly as broad as the clinical manifestations. Different symptoms respond differently to therapy [24]. Tremors seem to improve faster and better than dystonia in WD [24]. Even in homozygotic twins, the response to therapy, including liver transplantation, and the spectrum of the side effects of WD-specific therapy may be different [15,25]. However, the response to long-term treatment was not the only difference for different symptoms; additionally, the speed of improvement is different for different symptoms in WD.

To demonstrate this clearly and provide a solid base of information for advising newly diagnosed patients on what can be expected realistically during continuous WD-specific treatment, the time course of improvement in neurological and hepatic symptoms was compared in 20 WD patients who had been listed for orthotopic liver transplantation (LTX) but underwent conventional treatment.

2. Materials and Methods

This retrospective study was performed according to the Declaration of Helsinki and approved by the local ethics committee of the University of Düsseldorf (Germany).

2.1. Patient Recruitment

In the Clinic of Neurology of the University Hospital in Düsseldorf (Germany), a special outpatient department ward for rare metabolic diseases was implemented in 1985. About 1 to 3 new WD patients per year have been diagnosed in this institution since then. For the present retrospective study, 20 new WD patients were recruited. Seventeen fulfilled the following criteria: (i) their WD had been diagnosed in our department, (ii) the patient had been listed for liver transplantation (LTX) by colleagues from the regional departments of gastroenterology, and (iii) the patient had a well-documented course of conservative treatment since the onset of therapy in our institution. In addition, the data included one girl who (i) was diagnosed in a nearby city, (ii) was listed for liver transplantation, and (iii) whose mother had documented the course of treatment from the very beginning. Furthermore, two newly diagnosed homozygous twins with different disease severity and symptoms were included; their clinical data have already been presented elsewhere [15]. Although there was an indication for LTX in one of the twins, both had not been listed for LTX since both patients did not want to be transplanted. In summary, apart from the twins, all other patients had been listed for LTX.

The diagnosis of WD was based on an analysis of the Kayser–Fleischer rings, anterior segmental optical coherence tomography [26], cranial magnetic resonance imaging, acoustic radiation force impulse investigation [27,28], and typical biochemical findings.

2.2. Scoring of the Neurological Findings

At each therapeutic checkup visit in our outpatient department, the WD patients underwent a detailed neurological examination and were asked for their actual body weight. Then, the customized Düsseldorf Wilson Disease score (DWDS) was determined. This scale scores whether 10 specific symptoms are mildly (1 point), moderately (2 points), or severely (3 points) present or absent (0 points). The seven motor items of the DWDS (dysarthria/dysphagia, dystonia, bradykinesia, tremor, gait, cerebellar symptoms, and ophthalmological/brain stem symptoms) were summed up to yield the motor score (MotS; range: 0–21 points), and the three non-motor items of the DWDS (reflexes, sensory symptoms, and neuropsychiatric symptoms) were summed to yield the non-motor score (N-MotS; range: 0–9 points). MotS and N-MotS were summed to yield a total score (TS; range: 0–30 points). This scoring system can be completed by a treating physician within 1 min after a neurological examination and has been used in our institution since 1985 [29]; it is similar to a score used by the Italian OLT study group [30] and covers most of the neurological findings described by Shribman et al. [31].

2.3. Analysis of the Biochemical Parameters

After the neurological examination, a blood sample was taken. Furthermore, the WD patients in our department have been trained to collect their urine over 24 h without medication after previous cessation of WD-specific medication for 2 days and to bring a sample of the 24 h urine collection with them. For monitoring the therapy, 33 biochemical parameters were determined from the blood or the urine sample. These 33 biochemical parameters included: (i) four parameters of copper metabolism (ceruloplasmin (CER), serum copper (CUS), copper concentration in the 24 h urine collection (24 h-UCU/L), copper excreted in the urine over 24 h (24 h-UCU/d); (ii) four liver enzymes (AP, AST, ALT, and GGT) and pseudocholinesterase (CHE); (iii) four parameters testing kidney function (serum level of creatinine (CREA), clearance of creatinine in the 24 h urine collection (24 h-CREAC), concentration of protein excreted over 24 h (24 h-PROT/L), total amount of protein excreted over 24 h (24 h-PROT/d)); (iv) five parameters of the coagulation system (thrombocyte count (THROM), thromboplastin time (PTT), Quick´s test (Quick), international normalized ratio (INR), serum level of fibrinogen (FIBR)); and (v) four parameters of the iron metabolism (serum levels of iron (FE), transferrin (TRANS), ferritin (FERR), and hemoglobin (Hb), and erythrocyte count (ERY)). The other parameters were albumin (ALB), the serum level of bilirubin (BILI), leucocyte counts (LEUCC), and nine more parameters. As a further parameter, the MELD score was determined (MELD score = $10 \times (0.957 \times \ln(CREA) + 0.378 \times \ln(BILI) + 1.12 \times \ln(INR) + 0.643)$). These 34 parameters were determined at each checkup visit by the central laboratory of the University Hospital of Düsseldorf (Germany).

Demographic- and treatment-related data, body weight, the DWDS score, and biochemical findings were extracted from the charts of the patients.

2.4. Statistics

Patients were subdivided into patients with a MELD score of ≤10 and patients with a MELD score of >10. The parameters determined at the first visit to our department (initial data) were compared with the parameters determined at enrollment in this study (final data). The significance level was set to $p = 0.05$. Bonferroni's alpha adjustments were applied for multiple comparisons. A two-group repeated measurement ANOVA was calculated to detect significant differences between groups and among repeated measurements for all 34 parameters of the blood and urine. For the correlation analysis, the rank correlation coefficient was determined. When a regression line was calculated, Pearson's correlation coefficient (PCC = r) was also determined. ANOVA, rank correlation, and PCC were conducted/calculated using the commercially available SPSS statistics package (version 25: IBM Analytics, Armonk, NY, USA).

3. Results

3.1. Demographic and Treatment-Related Data and Spectrum of Initial Clinical Symptoms

The age at recruitment varied between 23.3 and 54.7 years (median: 38.2 years; interquartile range (Q25–Q75): 21 years). The age at the manifestation of WD varied between 7.5 and 50.4 years (median: 19.5 years; interquartile range: 12.1 years). Twelve patients were females; eight were males.

In Table 1, the clinical type of WD (asymptomatic, hepatic, etc.) is presented, as well as the result of the initial neurological investigation. Four patients did not have any neurological symptoms (TS = 0). Seven (35%) patients were classified as being mildly affected (total score: TS < 3), seven patients were moderately affected (2 < TS < 7), and six (30%) were severely affected (TS > 6). The initial TS did not correlate with age at manifestation of WD.

For the initial copper elimination treatment (CET), D-penicillamine (DPA) was used in 13 (65%) patients, and trientine dihydrochloride (TRIEN) was used in 6 (30%) patients. One asymptomatic patient remained on zinc monotherapy until he developed a hand tremor. He then agreed to be treated with TRIEN (for details, see [25]). The mean dose of DPA was 1131 mg (SD = 427), and the mean TRIEN dose was 1050 mg (SD = 266).

Retrospective analysis showed that, apart from two exceptions (the open circles in Figure 1), the dose of DPA chosen for the initial treatment was significantly correlated ($r = 0.7545$, $p < 0.01$) with the severity of WD (TS; full circles). Apart from two further cases (the open triangles in Figure 1), the dose of TRIEN was also correlated with TS, but because of the lower number of patients, this correlation was not significant ($r = 0.833$, n.s.) (Figure 1; full triangles). Body weight did not correlate with either the dose of DPA ($r = 0.440$, n.s.) or of TRIEN ($r = 0.297$, n.s.).

Table 1. General clinical classification and results of the initial neurological investigation.

No. of Patients	Type	General Clinical Classification
1	Asymptomatic	No symptoms at all
3	Hepatic	1 patient with acute liver failure 2 patients with reduced daily activities and fatigue
1	Neuropsychiatric	Intellectual decline and moderate depression
15	Neurologic	7 patients with tremor of the extremities, head, and/or trunk 5 patients with Parkinsonian symptoms 3 patients with other movement disorders (cerebellar ataxia, chorea, generalized dystonia)

Table 1. *Cont.*

No. of Patients	Symptom	Initial Neurological Investigation
		Motor Symptoms
14	Bradykinesia	Slowness in fast alternating movements of the fingers or tongue
9	Tremor	Clinically manifest tremors of the extremities, head, and/or trunk
8	Dysarthria	Dysarthria and/or dysphagia
7	Gait disorder	Spastic, cerebellar, or Parkinsonian gait disorder
7	Dystonia	Focal and/or generalized dystonia
6	Cerebellar	Ataxia of extremities
5	Oculomotor deficits	Oculomotor impairment or oculogyric crisis
		Non-Motor Symptoms
0	Sensory abnormalities	Sensory deficits of the legs, arms, hands, or fingers
3	Reflexes abnormalities	Reflex abnormalities (either enhanced reflexes with positive pyramidal tract signs or reduced or missing reflexes)
4	Neuropsychiatric symptoms	Neuropsychiatric symptoms; only 1 patient needed specific treatment

In column 2 the 7 motor subscores (Bradykinesia, Tremor, Dysarthria, Gait disorder, Dystonia, Cerebellar disorders, Oculomotor deficits) and the 3 non-motor subscores (Sensory abnormalities, Reflex abnormalities, Neuropsychiatric symptoms) of the Düsseldorf Wilson´s disease Score (DWDS) are listed.

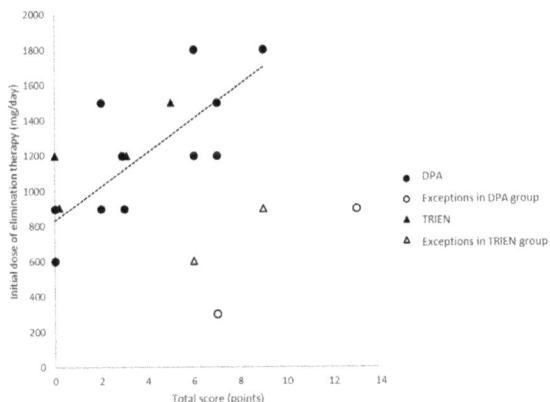

Figure 1. Relationship between the total score (TS; *x*-axis) and the dose of copper elimination therapy (DPA, circles; TRIEN, triangles; *y*-axis). Apart from two exceptions for DPA (open circles) and two exceptions for TRIEN (open triangles), there was a significant correlation between TS and the dose, which was significant ($p < 0.01$) only for DPA (full circles). The regression line was calculated for the relationship between TS and the dose of DPA.

3.2. Course of Treatment and Improvement in Neurological Symptoms

During the course of treatment, the dose of DPA was further increased in three patients, remained constant in five patients, and reduced from 900 to 600 mg in one patient. In one patient, the treatment was switched from 900 mg TRIEN to 900 mg DPA. After a duration of 10.6 years (SD: 13.3), the mean dose of DPA was 1309 mg (SD: 345). One patient received DPA until he underwent LTX. The other 10 patients received TRIEN. After a duration of 17.4 years (SD: 10.4), the mean dose of TRIEN was increased to 1325 mg (SD: 381). Neither the increase in the dose of DPA nor the increase in the dose of TRIEN was significant. At recruitment, neither the dose of DPA nor the dose of TRIEN was significantly correlated with TS or body weight.

In 10 patients, MotS improved, whereas in 8 other patients, MotS remained constant. In only two patients, MotS worsened. These two patients developed comorbidities: one female patient (Patient 8) developed myasthenia gravis, and one male patient (Patient 19) had a left-hemispheric stroke (hatched arrow in Figure 2A,B). When TS was plotted against time since the onset of therapy, the severity of WD (TS) approached a mildly affected level (TS < 3) in the majority of patients (Figure 2A: dark grey area). In some patients, however, TS remained in the moderately affected range (2 < TS < 6; light grey area in Figure 2A). When TS was plotted against age at investigation, it was obvious that all patients aged below 37 years showed an improvement (Figure 2B). Some patients above the age of 37 (indicated by the vertical hatched line in Figure 2B) experienced a worsening of their condition, which was either due to comorbidities or due to a worsening of N-MotS. TS did not correlate with age at recruitment.

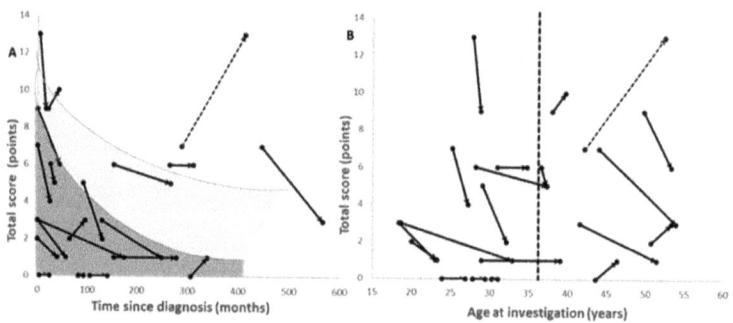

Figure 2. Temporal change in the total score (TS) depending on the time since diagnosis (**A**) and on age at investigation (**B**). The neurological symptoms responded well to therapy, and the total score was reduced to values below 3, indicating that the patients were only mildly affected (dark grey area in (**A**)). However, some patients remained moderately (2 < TS < 7) affected (light grey area in (**A**)). All patients below the age of 37 years (vertical line) improved (**B**). For patients above the age of 37 years (vertical hatched line), secondary worsening may occur (**B**). The hatched arrow indicates an exceptional case with a left-hemispheric stroke.

3.3. Improvement in the MELD Score and Biochemical Parameters

At the first presentation, 10 patients had a MELD score of >10. Within fewer than 240 days of treatment, the MELD score was less than 12 in all patients (Figure 3A), except in Patient 3, who received a transplant after 3 months of conservative treatment and whose data are presented in more detail below. The copper concentration in the 24 h urine collection showed high variability and decreased down to values below 0.030 mg/L in most of the patients during the first 700 days of treatment (Figure 3B). Apart from one exception, pseudocholinesterase (CHE) showed a continuous increase during a period of treatment of 700 days (Figure 4A). The serum levels of liver enzymes rapidly improved during the first 200 days of treatment and approached normal levels. This was also demonstrated for the levels of AST in Figure 4B.

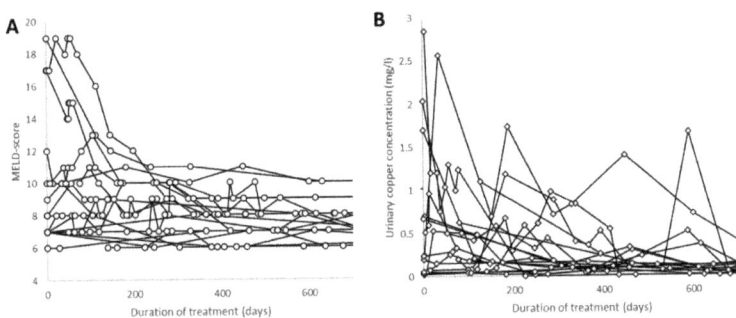

Figure 3. In all patients (except the patient who received a transplant), the model of end-stage liver disease (MELD) score declined to values below 12 after a treatment period of more than 200 days (**A**). The 24 h concentration of copper in the urine (**B**) showed high variability and declined to close to normal values (<0.03 mg/L) with increasing duration of therapy. The exceptionally high values are from patients with low compliance.

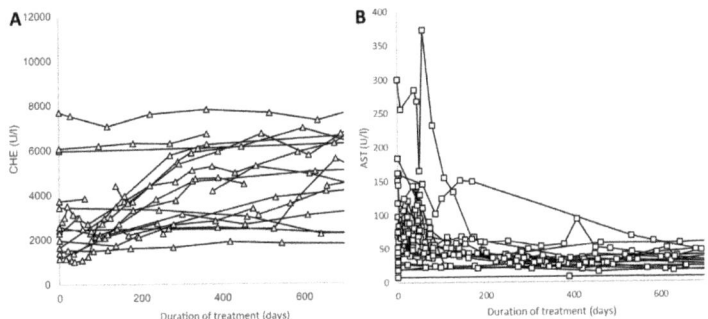

Figure 4. In most patients, pseudocholinesterase (CHE) continuously increased during therapy over a time period of up to 700 days (**A**). In one non-compliant patient, a further deterioration of CHE was observed despite treatment. In most patients, the liver enzyme aspartate transaminase (AST)-levels declined to close to normal values (around 50 U/L) within a treatment period of 200 days (**B**).

In Table 2 (upper part), seven parameters for which a significant change could be detected under CET by rm-ANOVA are presented in detail. The two parameters with the most significant change after the onset of CET were the concentration of protein excreted (24 h-PROT/L) and the total amount of protein excreted daily (24 h-PROT/d). This implies that kidney function has to be carefully controlled during copper chelation therapy. Improvements in cirrhosis of the liver were demonstrated by the significant increase in CHE and the significant decrease in AP and AST levels. The significant increase in albumin (ALB) indicated significant improvements in protein synthesis. A variety of parameters did not show significant changes under CET because of the large initial interindividual variability.

When patients were split into 10 patients with an initial MELD score of >10 and 10 patients with an initial MELD score of ≤10, nine parameters showed a highly significant ($p < 0.01$) difference between these two groups (Table 2 (middle part)) and seven other parameters had a significant ($p < 0.05$) difference (not presented). Only three parameters (PTT, ceruloplasmin, and transferrin) remained significantly ($p < 0.05$) different under CET (Table 2 (lower part)). This underlines the excellent recovery of the biochemical parameters, especially in the patients who were initially more affected.

Table 2. Improvement in the laboratory findings for the entire cohort and in two subgroups.

Parameter	Units	Initial Values		Final Values		Significance
		Initial MV	Initial SD	Final MV	Final SD	$p<$
24 h-PROT/L	mg/L	107.9	107.9	142.0	329.4	0.00049
24 h-PROT/d	mg/d	173.5	152.2	195.5	354.5	0.00604
CHE	U/L	3028	1886	5220	1379	0.00740
AP	U/L	131.0	71.6	87.3	25.7	0.01010
ALB (%)	%	54.5	6.6	60.2	2.7	0.02095
AST	U/L	78.8	76.2	31.6	17.3	0.04024
ALB (g/dL)	g/dL	6.1	7.6	4.4	1.0	0.04813
Parameter	Units	MELD ≤ 10 MV: Initial MELD ≤ 10	Initial SD: Initial MELD ≤ 10	MELD > 10 MV: Initial MELD > 10	SD: Initial MELD > 10	Significance $p<$
Quick	%	91.1	5.93	54.5	16.07	0.00004
HB	g/L	14.73	0.69	12.66	1.14	0.00069
CHE	U/L	4502	1939	1849	567	0.00077
PTT	Sec	29.0	2.65	41.28	7.50	0.00106
ERY	$10^6/\mu L$	4.97	0.31	4.14	0.54	0.00252
24 h-UCU/L	mg/L	0.16	0.20	1.31	0.98	0.00740
ALB (%)	%	58.9	3.56	50.5	6.2	0.00763
24 h-UCU/d	mg/d	0.26	0.36	2.41	1.89	0.00846
INR		1.04	0.05	1.55	0.44	0.00865
Parameter	Units	MELD ≤ 10 MV: Final MELD ≤ 10	Final SD: Final MELD ≤ 10	MELD > 10 MV: Final MELD > 10	SD: Final MELD > 10	Significance $p<$
PTT	s	25.67	2.00	29.86	4.59	0.02172
CER	mg/dL	7.22	3.31	12.40	5.64	0.02910
TRANS	mg/dL	254.6	31.8	285.7	24.5	0.03343

MELD—model for end-stage liver disease; MV—mean value; SD—standard deviation; 24 h-PROT/L—concentration of protein in the 24 h urine collection; 24 h-PROT/d—urinary protein excretion over 24 h; CHE—pseudocholinesterase; AP—alkaline phosphatase; ALB (%)—percentage of albumin; AST—aspartate transaminase; ALB (g/dL)—albumin in g/dL; Quick—Quick´s test; HB—serum level of hemoglobin; ERY—erythrocyte count; 24 h-UCU/L—concentration of copper in the 24 h urine collection; 24 h-UCU/d—copper excreted in the urine over 24 h; INR—international normalized ratio; PTT—thromboplastin time; CER—ceruloplasmin; TRANS—transferrin.

3.4. Liver Transplantation in a Wilson Disease Patient with Acute Liver Failure

A 19-year-old male patient (Patient 3) noticed fatigue and reduced mental drive and capacity in school. Laboratory testing detected elevated liver enzymes, increased serum levels of bilirubin, and an elevated INR, resulting in a MELD score of 22. Acute liver failure was diagnosed. Extensive testing for liver infection or autoimmune hepatitis was negative. He was admitted to our institution for further examination. Detailed laboratory testing revealed highly elevated copper excretion in the urine over 24 h and a decreased serum level of ceruloplasmin. Therefore, WD was diagnosed. The neurological examination and a slit-lamp investigation of the cornea were normal, as was the cranial MRI scan.

The patient was taken to a gastrointestinal ward, and DPA therapy was initiated. From the very beginning, a debate arose among the treating physicians about whether this patient should undergo LTX or whether he could be kept on conservative therapy. On the one hand, it was argued that the patient had a progressive increase in his MELD score, indicating a higher risk for mortality [32]. On the other hand, the patient was positively genetically tested for the presence of Gilbert syndrome (Morbus Meulengracht). This implied that the MELD score overestimated the degree of liver disease. In Figure 5A, the MELD score of the patient (full circles) is presented in comparison with a corrected MELD score (MELD score (corr), full diamonds) calculated under the assumption of a normal serum level of bilirubin. Furthermore, the cholinesterase started to increase (Figure 5B), and the liver enzymes (Figure 5C: AST (full circles) and ALT (full diamonds)) decreased 40 days after the onset of CET. Intermittently, the patient received antibiotic treatment several times, which led to transient increases in his liver enzymes (Figure 5C).

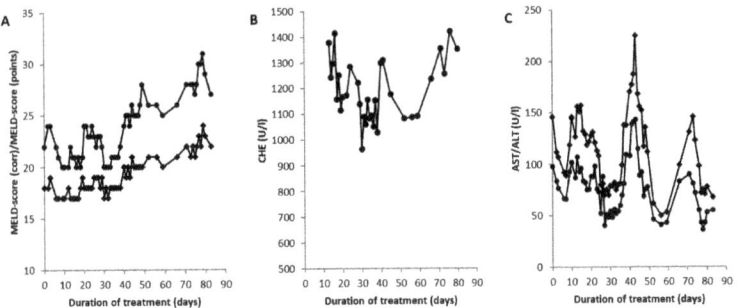

Figure 5. Temporal changes in the model of end-stage liver disease (MELD) score and the corrected MELD score (MELD score (corr)) (**A**) of serum levels of pseudocholinesterase (CHE) (**B**) and serum levels of aspartate transaminase (AST) and alanine transaminase (ALT) (**C**) in the patient receiving the transplant since the onset of copper elimination therapy (CET). CHE, AST, and ALT levels (**B**,**C**) started to improve 30 to 40 days after the onset of CET. The MELD score progressively worsened despite his liver function beginning to recover (**A**).

When a suitable young donor organ was allocated to the center, the patient successfully received a transplant without any perioperative complications about 4 months after onset of CET. His fatigue and mood disturbances rapidly improved, and his parameters of copper metabolism normalized within 3 months, and the patient went back to school again. Another extensive test for the presence of viral infections demonstrated that the patient had become EBV-positive after the transplantation.

3.5. Recovery of Pseudocholinesterase in 10 Selected Patients

In this section, the patient receiving the transplant (full circles in Figure 6B–D) is compared with seven new WD patients with subacute liver failure (open circles in Figure 6B–D) who had been listed as candidates for LTX but had conservatively been treated with copper chelation therapy, and two new conservatively treated WD patients who were homozygous twins (open squares in Figure 6B–D).

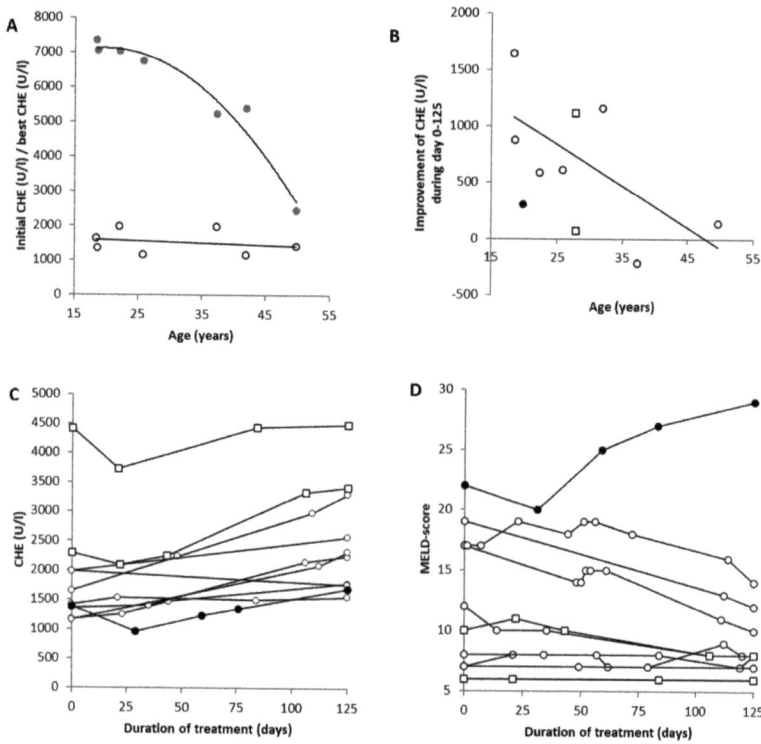

Figure 6. Comparison of the initial (open circles) and best (grey dots) serum levels of pseudo-cholinesterase (CHE) after the onset of copper elimination therapy (CET), revealing an age-dependent recovery of liver dysfunction (**A**). The recovery of CHE serum levels during the first 125 days of treatment was also age-dependent (**B**). Open circles in (**B**) indicate the values of the seven conservatively treated patients, the full circles indicate the data of the 19-year-old patient before transplantation, and the open squares are the values of the homozygotic twins. CHE significantly ($p < 0.043$) improved during the first 125 days of CET (**C**). With only one exception (the eldest patient), an improvement in CHE was observed in all patients, including the patient receiving the transplant (full circle) and the twins (open squares). Moreover, the model-end-stage-liver disease (MELD)scores of all patients improved or remained constant during the first 125 days of CET (**D**), except in the patient who had received the transplant (full circle in D) about 4 months after onset of CET.

In the seven conservatively treated WD patients, excellent recovery of liver function was observed. This is demonstrated in Figure 6A, where the initial values of CHE (open circles) are plotted against the age at the onset of WD, as well as the best values of CHE (grey dots) under CET. The non-linear regression analysis between the best value of CHE and age revealed a highly significant ($r = 0.9776$; $p < 0.001$) age-dependent recovery from liver disease.

In Figure 6B, the temporal development of CHE during the first 125 days of treatment is presented for all 10 patients. The value on Day 125 was interpolated for all seven conservatively treated patients (open circles), the homozygous twins (open squares), and then extrapolated in the patient receiving the (full dots) since he underwent transplantation before Day 125. In the patient with the transplant and in the twins, a further small initial decline in CHE after initiation of CET can be seen (Figure 6B). After about 40 days, CHE started to improve. The mean initial CHE of the seven conservatively treated patients was 1541 U/L (SD: 349); after 125 days of treatment, CHE significantly ($p < 0.043$) increased to a mean of 2218 U/L (SD: 598). The increase in CHE during the first 125 days was age-dependent (r = −0.549; $p < 0.05$ (one-sided testing)). In Figure 6D, the temporal development of the MELD score is presented for all 10 patients during the first 125 days of CET. In four patients, a clear improvement (>2 score points) was seen in the MELD score, but in five patients, only a small change (−1 to +2) could be observed. Later on, in the patient who received the transplant, the MELD score clearly worsened during conservative treatment.

4. Discussion

4.1. The Broad Spectrum of Neurological Symptoms in Wilson´s Disease before and after Therapy

The spectrum of clinical neurological symptoms is broad in Wilson disease [2,3,21]. A variety of factors influence the phenotype [15]. Differences in copper exposure, differences in hormonal status including pregnancy, possible modifier genes, and differences in genotype and in the function of the blood–brain barrier may lead to differences in the clinical manifestation of WD [15]. To score the main neurological symptoms, we used a simple score (DWDS; see the Methods), which can be easily completed within 1 min after a clinical neurological investigation. It covers most of the symptoms mentioned in previous reports on the neurological symptoms of WD [3,31,33]. In the present cohort, only one patient had involuntary choreatic movements (Patient 10), which were not scored by the DWDS. In a much larger sample of 115 WD patients, only two patients had chorea and had not been tested for additional comorbidity with benign hereditary chorea or Huntington´s disease [33].

In general, the neurological symptoms manifest after the hepatic symptoms [21], but in the present cohort, no significant positive correlation between age and the severity of neurological symptoms could be detected. Retrospective analysis revealed that apart from four exceptions, the dose of CET was significantly correlated with the severity of the initial symptoms (Figure 1). This correlation disappeared during the course of treatment simply because the dose was kept constant or slightly increased, whereas the symptoms improved, especially in the more affected patients.

The spectrum of symptoms remained broad, but the frequency of individual symptoms changed since the sensitivity to CET is different for different symptoms, as described previously [24]. Motor symptoms improved in 50% of the patients and remained constant in a further 40% of the patients. Tremors and cerebellar symptoms responded best to CET, as reported previously, whereas bradykinesia or dystonia did not show many changes during therapy [24,29].

The present study shows clearly that the neurological symptoms improved over time. However, continuous treatment with fairly high doses (≥900 mg DPA or TRIEN) over several years seemed to be necessary for the majority of WD patients until they became only mildly affected.

In a cross sectional study, the motor symptoms of WD patients under long-term treatment did not significantly change with age, in contrast to the non-motor symptoms [34]. This is in line with the present longitudinal observations (Figure 2), which showed an improvement in all patients aged <37 years and a mild worsening in some patients older than 37 years. Initial improvements and a secondary worsening for various reasons beyond the age of 40 have also been observed in a much larger cohort of 115 WD patients under long-term treatment [33].

4.2. Improvement in Biochemical Parameters during the Course of Therapy in Wilson´s Disease

The two-group rm-ANOVA revealed a significant time × group interaction: many more parameters improved during CET in the patients with a MELD score of >10 than in the patients with a MELD score of ≤10. Impaired coagulation and bleeding are critical complications of acute liver failure [18,35]. INR and PTT increased significantly, and thrombocyte counts were significantly reduced, indicating that, initially, different components of the coagulation system were affected in the patients with a MELD score of >10. Impaired coagulation was the main reason why Patient 3 received a transplant (see Section 3.4).

Significantly elevated levels of liver enzymes (AP, AST, ALT, GGT) and decreased levels of CHE indicated liver impairment and the beginning of cirrhosis, whereas elevated levels of ferritin and decreased levels of transferrin and hemoglobin indicated an impairment in iron metabolism in the untreated WD patients with a MELD score of >10. However, all these parameters responded excellently to CET. Only PTT and transferrin levels remained different between the two groups of patients under CET. We believe that the use of rather high doses of DPA or TRIEN to reduce neurological symptoms was the reason why many biochemical parameters responded so well and quickly.

4.3. Difference in Time Course of the Improvement in Neurological and Hepatic Symptoms

In the brains of WD patients post-mortem, the copper content is elevated [36]. Over the course of therapy, the brain's copper content decreases [34]. In WD patients, the brain's metabolism recovers over the duration of therapy [37]. However, doses of copper chelators below 900 mg do not seem to be high enough to maintain the initial level of improvement in neurological symptoms reached during continuous treatment during the first years after the diagnosis of WD [37]. A low serum level of free copper seems to be necessary to guarantee the continuous efflux of copper from the brain of a WD patient, especially from structures with a high affinity to copper, such as the basal ganglia [38]. Therefore, continuous treatment with rather high doses seems to be necessary to reduce the neurological symptoms slowly over the years (Figure 2A).

The blood–brain barrier (BBB) probably plays a crucial role in the influx and efflux of copper to and from the brain [23,39]. Copper is an ion that has to be actively transported across the BBB. Thus, the BBB also reduces the efflux of copper from the brain into the blood under CET. The initial worsening of neurological symptoms after the onset of DPA therapy has been explained by the mobilization of free copper in combination with DPA-induced damage to the BBB and a subsequent increase in the influx of copper to the brain [23,39]. With a fast initial increase in the dose of DPA or TRIEN over 3 weeks, we did not observe this initial worsening and therefore think that the efflux of copper from different structures of the brain with different levels of affinity to copper is also a plausible explanation for the initial worsening. Whether neurological symptoms respond better to tetramolybdate (which does not damage the BBB [23]) than to DPA has yet to be analyzed in long-term cross-over studies.

It has been observed previously that the neurological symptoms in WD may recover greatly within months after LTX [40,41]. This has recently been confirmed again [42]. Nevertheless, it seems to be a challenging task to convince transplantation centers to operate on WD patients because of the neurological indications.

In contrast to the slow improvement in neurological symptoms over years under conventional treatment, the biochemical parameters of the blood and urine responded rapidly within weeks after the onset of CET. A decline in the copper concentration in the 24 h urine collection looked like a wash-out curve (see Figure 3B). In parallel, the liver enzymes improved, and the CHE recovered continuously (Figure 4A,B). In most of the patients, the serum levels of liver enzymes approached the normal range within 200 days. This recovery seemed to depend on the age of the patient (see Figure 6). However, this recovery also depends heavily on the compliance of the patient and the velocity of the increase in the initial dose.

4.4. Is There a Time Window for Conservative Therapy in Patients with Acute Liver Failure?

The present study, on the one hand, confirmed that the CHE level is a sensitive biomarker for detecting untreated WD [43]. On the other hand, it indicated that CHE measurements may also be an appropriate tool for monitoring the conventional treatment of WD. The analysis of the levels of liver enzymes and CHE in patients with an initial CHE of <2000 U/L revealed that an improvement in liver function can be expected from Days 30 to 40 after the initiation of CET (Figure 6). After 125 days of therapy, the recovery from liver dysfunction had clearly progressed, and after 200 days of continuous CET, the danger arising from liver failure [18,35] seemed to be over. Since the time from listing for LTX to the availability of a suitable donor organ usually lasts several months in an industrialized country [44,45], there is a realistic chance that LTX may not be necessary after 200 days as long as conservative therapy has been performed consequentially for several months (see also [46]).

Nevertheless, the example of Patient 3, who received a transplant, clearly demonstrated that the MELD score may continue to increase although the liver enzymes have started to improve (see Figure 5). This is a clear sign of a life-threatening situation [32] and a clear indication of LTX.

There is hope that, in the future, even more rapidly acting copper-eliminating substances than DPA or TRIEN will become available. Methanobactin, a yeast product, has an extremely high affinity for copper [47,48]. In a rat model of WD (LEG-rat), methanobactin improved mitochondrial dysfunction within days after the onset of treatment and reversed acute liver failure [49,50]. There is good reason to assume that this will also happen in humans; however, applications of methanobactin in humans are lacking so far.

5. Conclusions

In WD, both the neurological and hepatic symptoms respond to copper elimination therapy (CET) quite well. However, the hepatic symptoms respond much faster than the neurological symptoms. Within 200 days of treatment, the MELD score declined to values around 10, and liver enzyme levels returned to normal values, whereas some neurological symptoms may persist over several years despite continuous treatment. CET should be initiated with sufficiently high doses of DPA or TRIEN to reduce the neurological impairment to a mild level, which would allow a fairly normal life. The patients in the present study were treated with rather high doses. A subsequent study is recommended to prospectively analyze whether patients with mild or no neurological symptoms should be treated with doses as high as those given to patients with moderate or severe neurological findings. In the case of acute liver failure, conservative treatment with doses above 900 mg of DPA or 1200 mg of TRIEN during the first 4 months after the diagnosis of WD may be sufficient to improve liver function to such an extent that LTX is not required.

6. Strengths and Limits of the Study

The temporal development of biochemical parameters was well documented over a long period of therapy in most of the 20 new WD patients. The number of patients (n = 20) seems small; however, the primary selection criterion was "listed for liver transplantation". Such patients are rare in a neurological department. They had been frequently monitored, which allowed us to analyze the improvements in their liver function during the first 4 months and their neurological outcomes over several years. The present study was retrospective and was performed on selected patients from a single specialized center. Therefore, a multi-center prospective study is recommended to confirm the differences in the recovery of the brain and liver under CET.

Author Contributions: Conceptualization, H.H. and S.S.; methodology, S.S.; software, S.S. and D.R.; validation, H.H. and S.S.; formal analysis, S.S.; investigation, H.H., T.S.K. and M.N.; resources, S.S., M.N. and T.S.K.; data curation, M.N.; writing—original draft preparation, H.H. and S.S.; writing—review and editing, H.H., T.L., S.G.M. and S.S.; visualization, S.S.; supervision, H.H., C.J.H. and P.A.; project administration, H.H.; funding acquisition, H.H. All authors have read and agreed to the published version of the manuscript.

Funding: This research received no external funding.

Institutional Review Board Statement: The study was conducted according to the guidelines of the Declaration of Helsinki and approved by the ethics committee of Heinrich Heine University of Düsseldorf (No. 2018-20, 8 May 2018).

Informed Consent Statement: Informed consent forms were obtained from all patients or the patients' guardians for all retrospective studies on the topic of Wilson disease in the outpatient clinic of the University Hospital of Düsseldorf.

Data Availability Statement: The datasets generated and/or analyzed during the current study are not publicly available because the datasets are part of a dissertation for a Doctor of Medicine but are available from the corresponding author upon reasonable request.

Conflicts of Interest: The authors declare no conflict of interest.

Abbreviations

ALB, albumin; ALB%, percentage of albumin; ALT, alanine transaminase; ANOVA, analysis of variance; AP, alkaline phosphatase; AST, aspartate transaminase; ATP7B, P-adenotriphosphate protease; BBB, blood–brain barrier; BILI, serum level of bilirubin; CER, ceruloplasmin; CET, copper elimination therapy; CHE, pseudocholinesterase; CREA, creatinine; 24 h-CREAC, clearance of creatinine over 24 h; CTR/hCTR, human copper transporter 1; DPA, D-penicillamine; CUS, serum level of copper; DWDS, Düsseldorf Wilson disease score; ERY, erythrocyte count; FE, serum level of iron; FERR, ferritin; FIBR, serum level of fibrinogen; GGT = gamma-glutamyl transferase; HB, serum level of hemoglobin; INR, international normalized ratio; LEUCC, white blood cell count; LTX, orthotopic liver transplantation; MELD, model for end-stage liver disease; MotS, motor score; MV, mean value; N-MotS, non-motor score; Quick, Quick's test; PCC, prothrombin complex concentrates; PTT, thromboplastin time; SD, standard deviation; TRIEN, trientine dihydrochloride; THROM, thrombocyte counts; TRANS, transferrin; TS, total score; WD, Wilson disease; 24 h-PROT/d, urinary protein excretion over 24 h; 24 h-PROT/L, concentration of protein in the 24 h urine collection; 24 h-UCU/d, copper excreted in the urine over 24 h; 24h-UCU/L, concentration of copper in the 24 h urine collection.

References

1. Wilson, S.A.K. Progressive lenticular degeneration: A familial nervous disease associated with cirrhosis of the liver. *Brain* **1912**, *34*, 295–507. [CrossRef]
2. Bandmann, O.; Weiss, K.H.; Kaler, S.G. Wilson's disease and other neurological copper disorders. *Lancet Neurol.* **2015**, *15*, 103–113. [CrossRef] [PubMed]
3. Członkowska, A.; Litwin, T.; Dusek, P.; Ferenci, P.; Lutsenko, S.; Medici, V.; Rybakowski, J.K.; Weiss, K.H.; Schilsky, M.L. Wilson disease. *Nat. Rev. Dis. Prim.* **2018**, *4*, 21. [CrossRef] [PubMed]
4. Cumings, J.N. The copper and iron content of brain and liver in the normal and in hepato-lenticular degeneration. *Brain* **1948**, *71*, 410–415. [CrossRef]
5. Madsen, E.; Gitlin, J.D. Copper and iron disorders of the brain. *Annu. Rev. Neurosci.* **2007**, *30*, 317–337. [CrossRef]
6. Nose, Y.; Kim, B.E.; Thiele, D.J. Ctr1 drives intestinal copper absorption and is essential for growth, iron metabolism, and neonatal cardiac function. *Cell Metab.* **2006**, *4*, 235–244. [CrossRef]
7. Hellman, N.E.; Gitlin, J.D. Ceruloplasmin metabolism and function. *Ann. Rev. Nut* **2002**, *22*, 439–458. [CrossRef]
8. Mukhopadhyay, C.K.; Attieh, Z.K.; Fox, P.L. Role of ceruloplasmin in cellular iron uptake. *Science* **1998**, *279*, 714. [CrossRef]
9. Stremmel, W.; Merle, U.; Weiskirchen, R. Clinical features of Wilson disease. *Ann. Transl. Med.* **2019**, *7* (Suppl. S2), S61. [CrossRef]
10. Ferenci, P. Wilson's disease. *Clin. Gastroenterol. Hepatol.* **2005**, *3*, 726–733. [CrossRef]
11. Bull, P.C.; Thomas, G.R.; Rommens, J.M.; Forbes, J.R.; Cox, D.W. The Wilson disease gene is a putative copper transporting P-type ATPase similar to the Menkes gene. *Nat. Genet.* **1993**, *5*, 327–337. [CrossRef] [PubMed]
12. Cooper, D.N.; Ball, E.V.; Stenson, P.D.; Phillips, A.D.; Evans, K.; Heywood, S.; Hayden, M.J.; Chapman, M.M.; Mort, M.E.; Azevedo, L.; et al. The Human Gene Mutation Database. QIAGEN. 2018. Available online: http://www.hgmd.cf.ac.uk/ac/index.php (accessed on 2 May 2023).
13. Stenson, P.D.; Mort, M.; Ball, E.V.; Evans, K.; Hayden, M.; Heywood, S.; Hussain, M.; Phillips, A.D.; Cooper, D.N. The Human Gene Mutation Database: Towards a comprehensive repository of inherited mutation data for medical research, genetic diagnosis, and next-generation sequencing studies. *Hum. Genet.* **2017**, *136*, 665–677. [CrossRef] [PubMed]
14. Ferenci, P.; Stremmel, W.; Czlonkowska, A.; Szalay, F.; Viveiros, A.; Stättermayer, A.F.; Bruha, R.; Houwen, R.; Pop, T.L.; Stauber, R.; et al. Age and sex but not ATP7B genotype effectively influence the clinical phenotype of Wilson disease. *Hepatology* **2018**, *69*, 1464–1476. [CrossRef]
15. Samadzadeh, S.; Kruschel, T.; Novak, M.; Kallenbach, M.; Hefter, H. Different Response Behavior to Therapeutic Approaches in Homozygotic Wilson's Disease Twins with Clinical Phenotypic Variability: Case Report and Literature Review. *Genes* **2022**, *13*, 1217. [CrossRef]

16. Castillo-Fernandez, J.E.; Spector, T.D.; Bell, J.T. Epigenetics of discordant monozygotic twins: Implications for disease. *Genome Med.* **2014**, *6*, 60. [CrossRef]
17. Członkowska, A.; Gromadzka, G.; Chabik, G. Monozygotic female twins discordant for phenotype of Wilson's disease. *Mov. Disord.* **2009**, *24*, 1066–1069. [CrossRef]
18. Eisenbach, C.; Sieg, O.; Stremmel, W.; Encke, J.; Merle, U. Diagnostic criteria for acute liver failure due to Wilson disease. *World J. Gastroenterol.* **2007**, *13*, 1711–1714. [CrossRef]
19. Reyes, C.V. Hepatocellular carcinoma in Wilson disease-related liver cirrhosis. *Gastroenterol. Hepatol.* **2008**, *4*, 435–437.
20. Hartmann, C.J.; Hefter, H. Manifestation of Wilson disease despite ongoing zinc-monotherapy and improvement after adding trientine: A case report. *Basal Ganglia* **2014**, *4*, 81–83. [CrossRef]
21. Ghika, J.; Vingerhoets, F.; Maeder, P.; Borruat, F.-X.; Bogousslavsky, J. Maladie de Wilson. *EMC Neurol.* **2004**, *1*, 481–511. [CrossRef]
22. Rajan, A.; Kalita, J.; Kumar, V.; Misra, U.K. MRI and oxidative stress markers in neurological worsening of Wilson disease following penicillamine. *Neurotoxicology* **2015**, *49*, 45–49. [CrossRef] [PubMed]
23. Borchard, S.; Raschke, S.; Zak, K.M.; Eberhagen, C.; Einer, C.; Weber, E.; Müller, S.M.; Michalke, B.; Lichtmannegger, J.; Wieser, A.; et al. Bis-choline tetrathiomolybdate prevents copper-induced blood-brain barrier damage. *Life Sci. Alliance* **2021**, *4*, e202101164. [CrossRef]
24. Burke, J.F.; Dayalu, P.; Nan, B.; Askari, F.; Brewer, G.J.; Lorincz, M.T. Prognostic significance of neurologic examination findings in Wilson disease. *Park. Relat. Disord.* **2011**, *17*, 551–556. [CrossRef]
25. Senzolo, M.; Loreno, M.; Fagiuoli, S.; Zanus, G.; Canova, D.; Masier, A.; Russo, F.P.; Sturniolo, G.C.; Burra, P. Different neurological outcome of liver transplantation for Wilson's disease in two homozygotic twins. *Clin. Neurol. Neurosurg.* **2007**, *109*, 71–75. [CrossRef]
26. Broniek-Kowalik, K.; Dziezyc, K.; Litwin, T.; Członkowska, A.; Szaflik, J.P. Anterior segment optical coherence tomography (AS-OCT) as a new method of detecting copper deposits forming the Kayser-Fleischer ring in patients with Wilson disease. *Acta Ophthalmol.* **2019**, *97*, e757–e760. [CrossRef]
27. Yap, W.W.; Kirke, R.; Yoshida, E.M.; Owen, D.; Harris, A.C. Non-invsive assessment of liver fibrosis using ARFI with pathological correlation, a prospective study. *Ann. Hepatol.* **2013**, *12*, 440–447. [CrossRef]
28. Li, Y.; Ma, J.; Li, B.; Zhu, X.; Wang, J. Cirrhosis of Wilson's disease: High and low cutoff using acoustic radiation force pulse (ARFI)-comparison and combination of serum fibrosis index. *Clin. Hemorheol. Microcirc.* **2021**, *79*, 575–585. [CrossRef]
29. Hefter, H.; Tezayak, O.; Rosenthal, D. Long-term outcome of neurological Wilson's disease. *Park. Relat. Disord.* **2018**, *49*, 48–53. [CrossRef]
30. Medici, V.; Mirante, V.G.; Fassati, L.R.; Pompili, M.; Forti, D.; Del Gaudio, M.; Trevisan, C.P.; Cillo, U.; Sturniolo, G.C.; Fagiuoli, S. Liver transplantation for Wilson´s disease: The burden of neurological and psychiatric disorders. *Liver Transpl.* **2005**, *11*, 1056–1063. [CrossRef]
31. Shribman, S.; Warner, T.T.; Dooley, J.S. Clinical presentations of Wilson disease. *Ann. Transl. Med.* **2019**, *7* (Suppl. S2), S60. [CrossRef]
32. Londono, M.-C.; Cardenas, A.; Guevara, M.; Quintó, L.; Heras, D.D.L.; Navasa, M.; Rimola, A.; Garcia-Valdecasas, J.-C.; Arroyo, V.; Ginès, P. MELD score and serum sodium in the prediction of survival of patients with cirrhosis awaiting liver transplantation. *Gut* **2007**, *56*, 1283–1290. [CrossRef]
33. Samadzadeh, S. Long-Term Follow-Up of 115 Patients with Wilson's Disease. Ph.D. Thesis, University of Düsseldorf, Düsseldorf, Germany, 2022. Available online: https://docserv.uni-duesseldorf.de/servlets/DocumentServlet?id=59305 (accessed on 3 May 2023).
34. Horoupian, D.S.; Sternlieb, I.; Scheinberg, I.H. Neuropathological findings in penicillamine-treated patients with Wilson's disease. *Clin. Neuropathol.* **1988**, *7*, 62–67.
35. Stravitz, R.T.; Ellerbe, C.; Durkalski, V.; Schilsky, M.; Fontana, R.J.; Peterseim, C.; Lee, W.M.; The Acute Liver Failure Study Group. Bleeding complications in acute liver failure. *Hepatology* **2018**, *67*, 1931–1942. [CrossRef]
36. Walshe, J.M.; Gibbs, K.R. Brain copper in Wilson's disease. *Lancet* **1987**, *2*, 1030. [CrossRef]
37. Hefter, H.; Arendt, G.; Kuwert, T.; Herzog, H.; Feinendegen, L.E.; Stremmel, W. Relationship between striatal glucose consumption and copper excretion in patients with Wilson's disease treated with D-penicillamine. *J. Neurol.* **1993**, *241*, 49–53. [CrossRef]
38. Ijomone, O.M.; Ifenatuoha, C.W.; Aluko, O.M.; Ijomone, O.K.; Aschner, M. The aging brain: Impact of heavy metal neurotoxicity. *Crit. Rev. Toxicol.* **2020**, *50*, 801–814. [CrossRef]
39. Stuerenburg, H.J. CSF copper concentrations, blood barrier function, and coeruloplasmin synthesis during treatment of Wilson's disease. *J. Neural Transm.* **2000**, *107*, 321–329. [CrossRef]
40. Polson, R.J.; Rolles, K.; Calne, R.Y.; Williams, R.; Marsden, D. Reversal of severe neurological manifestations of Wilson's disease following liver transplantation. *Q. J. Med.* **1987**, *64*, 685–691.
41. Bax, R.T.; Hässler, A.; Luck, W.; Hefter, H.; Krägeloh-Mann, I.; Neuhaus, P.; Emmrich, P. Cerebral manifestation of Wilson´s disease successfully treated with liver transplantation. *Neurology* **1998**, *51*, 863–865. [CrossRef]
42. Poujois, A.; Sobesky, R.; Meissner, W.G.; Brunet, A.-S.; Broussolle, E.; Laurencin, C.; Lion-François, L.; Guillaud, O.; Lachaux, A.; Maillot, F.; et al. Liver transplantation as a rscue therapy for severe forms of Wilson disease. *Neurology* **2020**, *94*, e2189–e2202. [CrossRef]

43. Hefter, H.; Arslan, M.; Kruschel, T.; Novak, M.; Rosenthal, D.; Meuth, S.G.; Albrecht, P.; Hartmann, C.J.; Samadzadeh, S. Pseudocholinesterase as a biomarker for untreated Wilson´s disease. *Biomolecules* **2022**, *12*, 1791. [CrossRef]
44. Gheorge, L.; Popescu, I.; Iacob, R.; Gheorghe, C. Predictors of death on the waiting list for liver transplantation characterized by a long waiting time. *Transpl. Intern.* **2005**, *18*, 572–576. [CrossRef]
45. Ahmad, J.; Bryce, C.L.; Cacciarelli, T.; Roberts, M.S. Differences in access to liver transplantation: Disease severity, waiting time, and transplantation center volume. *Ann. Intern. Med.* **2007**, *146*, 735–741. [CrossRef]
46. Kido, J.; Matsumoto, S.; Sakamoto, R.; Mitsubuchi, H.; Inomata, Y.; Nakamura, K. Recovery of severe acute liver failure without transplantation in patients with Wilson disease. *Pediatr. Transplant.* **2018**, *22*, e13292. [CrossRef]
47. Summer, K.H.; Lichtmannegger, J.; Bandow, N.; Choi, D.W.; Di Spirito, A.A.; Michalke, B. The biogenic methanobactin is an effective chelator for copper in a rat model for Wilson disease. *J. Trace Elem. Med. Biol.* **2011**, *25*, 36–41. [CrossRef]
48. Dispirito, A.A.; Choi, D.W.; Semrau, J.D.; Keeney, D. Use of Methanobactin. U.S. Patent US 8,735,538 B1, 27 May 2014.
49. Lichtmannegger, J.; Leitzinger, C.; Wimmer, R.; Schmitt, S.; Schulz, S.; Kabiri, Y.; Eberhagen, C.; Rieder, T.; Janik, D.; Neff, F.; et al. Methanobactin reverses acute liver failure in a rat model of Wilson disease. *J. Clin. Investig.* **2016**, *126*, 2721–2735. [CrossRef]
50. Müller, J.C.; Lichtmannegger, J.; Zischka, H.; Sperling, M.; Karst, U. High spatial resolution LA-ICP-MS demonstrates massive liver copper depletion in Wilson disease rats upon Methanobactin treatment. *J. Trace Elem. Med. Biol.* **2018**, *49*, 119–127. [CrossRef]

Disclaimer/Publisher's Note: The statements, opinions and data contained in all publications are solely those of the individual author(s) and contributor(s) and not of MDPI and/or the editor(s). MDPI and/or the editor(s) disclaim responsibility for any injury to people or property resulting from any ideas, methods, instructions or products referred to in the content.

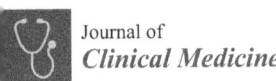

Article

Efficacy and Safety of Two Salts of Trientine in the Treatment of Wilson's Disease

France Woimant [1], Dominique Debray [2], Erwan Morvan [3], Mickael Alexandre Obadia [4,*,†] and Aurélia Poujois [4,†]

1. Department of Neurology, Lariboisière Hospital, AP-HP, 75010 Paris, France; france.woimant@live.fr
2. Department of Liver Pediatrics, Necker Hospital, AP-HP, 75015 Paris, France; dominique.debray@aphp.fr
3. Department of Neurology, Rothschild Foundation Hospital, 75019 Paris, France; emorvan@for.paris
4. National Reference Centre for Wilson's Disease, Rothschild Foundation Hospital, 75019 Paris, France; apoujois@for.paris
* Correspondence: mickael.alexandre.obadia@gmail.com
† These authors contributed equally to this work.

Abstract: Background: Wilson's disease (WD) is one of the few genetic disorders that can be successfully treated with pharmacological agents. Copper-chelating agents (D-penicillamine and Trientine salts) and zinc salts have been demonstrated to be effective. There are two salts of trientine. Trientine dihydrochloride salt (TETA 2HCL) is unstable at room temperature and requires storage at 2–8 °C. Trientine tetrahydrochloride (TETA 4HCL) is a more stable salt of trientine that can be stored at room temperature. No comparative study between both of the salts of trientine has been performed to date. As the two chemical forms were available in France between 1970 and 2009, we conducted a study to evaluate their efficacy and safety profiles. Methods: This retrospective cohort study was conducted by reviewing data from the national WD registry in France. Forty-three WD patients who received TETA 2HCL or TETA 4HCL monotherapy for at least one year until 2010 were included. The primary endpoints were hepatic and neurological outcomes. Secondary endpoints were the events leading to a discontinuation of medication. Results: Changes in medication were common, leading to the analysis of 57 treatment sequences of TETA 4HCL or TETA 2HCL. The mean duration of treatment sequence was significantly longer in the TETA 4 HCL group (12.6 years) than in the TETA 2HCL group (7.6 years) ($p = 0.011$). Ten patients experienced both trientine salts: eight stopped TETA 4 HCL (six had a hepatologic phenotype and two had a neurological phenotype) because this treatment was not available anymore (mean duration 7.4 years). Three of these patients already experienced TETA 2 HCL before the sequence. Two patients with a hepatologic phenotype (one had a previous sequence of TETA 4 HCL before) stopped TETA 2 HCL because of cold storage issues (mean duration 42.8 years). The total number of sequences was 57. All of the patients were clinically stable. No difference in efficacy was detected. Both treatments were well tolerated, except for a case of recurrence of lupus erythematosus-like syndrome in the TETA 2HCL group. The major reason for interruption of TETA 4HCL was due to a discontinuation in production of this salt. The reasons for stopping TETA 2HCL were mainly due to adherence issues largely attributed to the cold storage requirement. Conclusions: The two salts of trientine were effective in treating patients with WD. However, interruption of TETA 2HCL was frequent, linked to the cold storage requirement. As adherence to treatment is a key factor in the successful management of WD, physicians need to be even more vigilant in detecting adherence difficulties in patients receiving treatment with TETA 2HCL.

Keywords: Wilson's disease; medication adherence; chronic disease; trientine salts; D-penicillamine; zinc salts; efficacy; safety

Citation: Woimant, F.; Debray, D.; Morvan, E.; Obadia, M.A.; Poujois, A. Efficacy and Safety of Two Salts of Trientine in the Treatment of Wilson's Disease. *J. Clin. Med.* **2022**, *12*, 3975. https://doi.org/10.3390/jcm11143975

Academic Editor: Lazzaro di Biase

Received: 30 May 2022
Accepted: 6 July 2022
Published: 8 July 2022

Publisher's Note: MDPI stays neutral with regard to jurisdictional claims in published maps and institutional affiliations.

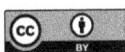

Copyright: © 2022 by the authors. Licensee MDPI, Basel, Switzerland. This article is an open access article distributed under the terms and conditions of the Creative Commons Attribution (CC BY) license (https://creativecommons.org/licenses/by/4.0/).

1. Introduction

Wilson's disease (WD) is an autosomal recessive disorder characterized by pathological copper accumulation in many organs, initially the liver, and then essentially the cornea and brain. It is caused by homozygous or compound heterozygous mutations in the ATP7B gene which encodes a transmembrane copper-transporting P-type ATPase [1]. WD is one of the few genetic disorders that can be successfully treated with pharmacological agents. The treatment is based on the generation of a negative copper balance. Copper-chelating agents and zinc salts have been demonstrated to be effective in the treatment of WD, associated with a low copper diet [2]. However, the best therapeutic approach remains controversial because no randomized controlled trials have compared these treatments and the use of drugs depends mainly on center experience and access to treatment in different countries or regions. Treatment is a lifelong necessity and should be started as early as possible. Whatever the chosen medical therapy, non-adherence to or discontinuation of therapy is associated with a high risk of very severe hepatic or neurologic deterioration [3]. The optimum goal for the patients requiring this lifelong medical therapy should therefore be to limit the side effects and difficulties associated with treatment dispensation and conservation.

Copper-chelating agents (D-penicillamine and Trientine salts) bind with excess copper, forming a stable complex which is excreted mainly in the urine. It has been suggested that trientine salts may also decrease intestinal copper absorption [2,4]. Zinc salts decrease the intestinal absorption of copper, inducing the synthesis of metallothioneins, proteins that sequester copper in the enterocytes [5]. Zinc salts are indicated in pre-symptomatic patients and during the maintenance phase of treatment [2], but some data indicate that zinc may also be considered in patients who exhibit neurological symptoms during the acute phase of the disease [6]. Zinc is generally well-tolerated in adults, although gastritis and nausea may lead to discontinuation of the treatment [7]. In pre-symptomatic children, gastrointestinal adverse effects are present in nearly 20% of the patients, associated with poor efficacy [8].

D-penicillamine is the reference treatment in many European countries, but severe adverse effects are frequent, leading to a discontinuation of this therapy in up to 30 % of patients [9]. The other copper chelators are trientine salts, currently indicated in WD patients who are intolerant to D-penicillamine. There are two currently available trientine salts. The trientine dihydrochloride salt (TETA 2HCL) is unstable at room temperature and requires storage between 2 and 8 °C. In Europe, TETA 2HCL was approved by the Medicines Health and Regulatory Agency (MHRA) in the United Kingdom (UK) for the treatment of WD in 1985, and was supplied to some other European Union (EU) countries. In France, TETA 2HCL (Trientine® from Univar, Downers Grove, IL, USA) was used through a compassionate use program for those patients intolerant to D-penicillamine and was only dispensed by hospital pharmacies. This salt is now marketed in the EU as Cufence®, following EU marketing authorization in 2019. Trientine tetrahydrochloride (TETA 4HCL) is a more stable salt of trientine that can be stored at room temperature. In France, TETA 4HCL was available from the mid-1970s until 2009, as a hospital preparation supplied by AGEPS (Agence Générale des Equipements des Produits de Santé) of the Assistance Publique—Hôpitaux de Paris. This salt was granted a European marketing authorization in 2018 and is currently marketed in Europe as Cuprior® (Orphalan, Paris, France).

No comparative study between both of the salts of trientine (dihydrochloride and tetrahydrochloride) has previously been performed. As the two chemical forms were available in France between 1970 and 2009, we conducted a study to evaluate the efficacy and safety profiles of both of the salts.

2. Materials and Methods

2.1. Ethics Approval and Consent to Participate

This study was approved by the Institutional Review Board of HUPNVS, Paris 7 University, AP-HP (n°1343579). An informed consent was obtained from all of the subjects and/or their legal guardian(s). All of the patients signed a written consent form. All of the methods were carried out in accordance with relevant guidelines and regulations, and in accordance with the Declaration of Helsinki.

2.2. Patients

This retrospective cohort study was conducted by reviewing data from the national WD registry. The WD patients who were followed in Lariboisière hospital—Paris (National Centre for Wilson's disease) and treated until 2010 were selected. This final date corresponded to the year after which the production of TETA 4HCL by AGEPS was discontinued. The diagnosis of WD was based on clinical symptoms, abnormal copper metabolism and genetic testing with a Leipzig score ≥ 4 [2]. Only the patients receiving TETA 2HCL or TETA 4 HCL monotherapy for at least one year were included. The specific duration of one year of trientine monotherapy was considered as the minimum time required to show a treatment effect. The patients were in the initial or maintenance phase of treatment and received trientine as a first, second or third line treatment. The patients who successively received both forms of trientine (TETA 4HCL and 2HCL) were included in the analysis. The patients who received either TETA 2HCL or TETA 4HCL in association with zinc salts were excluded.

2.3. Analysis of Treatments

The different courses of treatment with TETA 4HCL and 2HCL were identified and the treatment sequences of TETA 4HCL or 2 HCL with a follow-up period superior to one year of continuous treatment were analyzed. The events leading to a discontinuation of medication were recorded and classified.

2.4. Baseline Comparison of Treatments

The clinical and laboratory data were recorded at the beginning and at the end of each trientine treatment sequence; the duration of the sequence was noted. The patients included in the study were divided into two groups, according to the absence or presence of neurological symptoms. The hepatic assessment included clinical symptoms, measurement of serum transaminase levels, bilirubin and prothrombin time (PT). The presence of cirrhosis (typical findings on imaging and/or presence of clinical signs of portal hypertension) was recorded. The neurological evaluation was based on clinical symptoms. The presence of Kayser–Fleischer rings at slit-lamp examination was documented. The adherence to treatment was recorded by reports of compliance from the patients that were recorded in their medical records.

2.5. Study Endpoints

Primary endpoints were hepatic and neurological outcomes. The hepatic outcome was based on clinical symptoms and a course of liver enzymes and liver function tests. The neurological outcome was evaluated by neurological symptoms. Both hepatic and neurologic outcomes were scored as follows: unchanged, improved or deteriorated. The evolution of Kayser–Fleischer rings was also scored as unchanged, improved, disappeared or increased.

The secondary endpoints were the events leading to a discontinuation of medication. The reasons for treatment interruption or discontinuation were classified: loss of efficacy, adverse events, treatment non-adherence, manufacturing interruption.

2.6. Statistical Analyses

The quantitative variables were expressed as median (interquartile range) and the categorical variables as frequencies and percentages. Comparisons between two groups were made using the Student U test for continuous variables and the Fisher exact test for qualitative variables if the frequency was <5, otherwise the chi-squared test was used.

3. Results

3.1. Study Group

From the 248 WD patients recorded in the national registry and who were followed at the Lariboisière hospital before 2010, 62 received at least one sequence of treatment with a trientine salt. Nineteen patients were excluded because they received a zinc salt in combination with trientine over the treatment period. Thus, 43 patients were included in the study (Figure 1). Twenty-three were male (53.5%) and the age at diagnosis was 21 ± 9.3 years (min 5.6; max 46.3). Nine patients (20.9%) were diagnosed at the pre-symptomatic stage via familial screening, 19 presented with hepatic symptoms and 15 with neurological symptoms. Sixteen patients (37 %) had cirrhosis. Trientine was the first-line treatment for four patients (9.52%). Trientine was prescribed as a second-line treatment after D-penicillamine in 35 patients, zinc salts in 2 patients and D-penicillamine associated with zinc salts in 2 other patients. D-penicillamine was stopped due to WD aggravation (two cases) or due to the occurrence of adverse events in the remaining patients. The most common adverse events were renal disorders, thrombocytopenia and neutropenia, skin rash, digestive disorders and, less frequently, arthralgia, myasthenia-like syndrome and lupus-like syndrome. Zinc salts were stopped due to gastric irritation and, in one case, due to an increase in liver enzymes.

3.2. Treatment Sequences

Changes in the trientine treatment were common in this cohort. The 43 patients received 57 trientine monotherapy treatment sequences. This included 10 patients who received both TETA 4HCL and TETA 2HCL in different sequences (with a duration of more than one year); 2 patients who received only TETA 4HCl and 31 patients who received only TETA 2HCL. This corresponded to 57 trientine treatment sequences: 13 sequences with TETA 4HCL and 44 sequences with TETA 2HCL (Figure 1).

3.3. Baseline Characteristics of TETA Treatment Sequences

The mean sequence duration was significantly longer in the TETA 4HCL group, 151.7 ± 111.1 months, vs 91.1 ± 58.1 months in the TETA 2HCL group ($p = 0.011$).

Table 1 presents a comparison of the baseline parameters at the initiation of the treatment sequence in the two groups, TETA 2HCL and TETA 4HCL. The laboratory analyses were available only for a subset of the patients due to the retrospective nature of the study. However, there were no statistically significant differences between the groups relating to sex, age, laboratory values and delay in onset of treatment. Regarding the initial phenotype, more of the patients in the TETA 4HCL group had neurological signs: 62% versus 43% in the TETA 2HCL group.

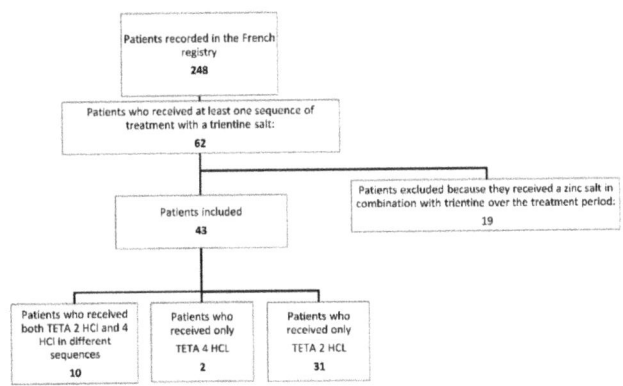

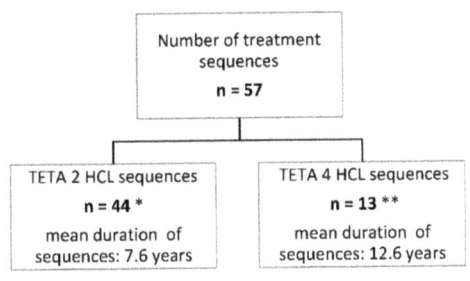

* 3 patients with two distinct TETA 2 HCL Sequences

** 1 patient with two distinct TETA 4 HCL sequencies

Figure 1. Flow-chart of patients included and treatment sequences.

Table 1. Baseline characteristics at Trientine sequence initiation.

	Trientine Treatment Sequence		p-Value
	TETA 4HCL (n = 13)	TETA 2HCL (n = 44)	
Sex ratio (male/female)	6/7	20/24	0.965
Mean age at trientine initiation (years ± SD)	28.7 ± 9.2	28.8 ± 13.6	0.979
Clinical form at sequence initiation			
Hepatic form	5/13 (38.46%)	25/44 (56.82%)	0.407
Neurological form	8/13 (61.54%)	19/44 (43.18%)	0.244
Presence of cirrhosis	4/13 (30.77%)	16/44 (36.36%)	0.710
First-line treatment	2/13 (15.38%)	2/44 (4.55%)	0.179
Delay between sequence initiation and diagnosis (years) (mean ± SD/ median/min–max)	5.3 ± 6.2/1.6/0.0–20.6	7.7 ± 10.1/3.2/0.0–36.4	0.414
Duration of treatment (months) (mean ± SD/median/min–max)	151.7 ± 111.1/138.9/22.8–391.4	91.1 ± 58.1/78.9/12.9–254.3	0.011

Table 1. Cont.

	Trientine Treatment Sequence		
	TETA 4HCL (n = 13)	TETA 2HCL (n = 44)	p-Value
ALT (IU/l)			0.936
N	9 (69.33%)	32 (72.73%)	
mean ± SD	56.3 ± 43.4	57.7 ± 43.6	
AST (IU/l)			0.727
N	9 (69.33%)	32 (72.73%)	
mean ± SD	42.9 ± 31.7	47.6 ± 36.7	
Total bilirubin (µmol/L)			0.853
N	4 (30.77%)	21 (47.73%)	
mean ± SD	16.5 ± 10.1	15.3 ± 11.6	
PT (% of normal)			0.802
N	5 (38.46%)	25 (56.82%)	
mean ± SD	86 ± 14.3	83.6 ± 20.0	
Platelets (/mm^3)			0.436
N	7 (53.85%)	29 (63.64%)	
mean ± SD	156.9 ± 30.2	182.0 ± 82.2	
Ceruloplasmin (g/L)			0.519
N	6 (46.15%)	21 (47.73%)	
mean ± SD	0.04 ± 0.03	0.03 ± 1.1	
Serum copper (µmol/L)			0.273
N	8 (61.54%)	22 (50.00%)	
mean ± SD	3.1 ± 2.3	6.0 ± 7.1	
Urine copper at start of treatment sequence (µmol/L)			0.848
N	6 (46.15%)	22 (50.00%)	
mean ± SD	5.5 ± 5.6	6.4 ± 10.8	
Urine copper at end of treatment sequence (µmol/L)			0.623
N	6 (46.15%)	39 (88.64 %)	
mean ± SD	3.9 ± 2.9	5.0 ± 5.6	

3.4. Patient Outcomes

The analysis of the evolution of hepatic and neurologic outcomes shows that the majority of the patients either improved clinically or their symptoms stabilized under the TETA treatment sequences (Table 2). The parameters relative to hepatic function, in particular serum transaminases, tended to improve (13 (29.55%)) in the TETA 2HCL group vs. 3 (23.08%) in the TETA 4HCL group), with no statistically significant differences observed between the two groups. Nevertheless, three patients worsened in the TETA 2HCL group.

Table 2. Hepatic and neurologic evolution in all patients.

	Trientine Treatment Sequence		
	TETA 4HCL (n = 13)	TETA 2HCL (n = 44)	p-Value
Hepatic outcome			0.842
Improved	3 (23.08%)	13 (29.55%)	
Unchanged	10 (76.92%)	29 (65.91%)	
Worsened	0	2 (4.55%)	
Neurologic outcome			0.172
Improved	4 (30.77%)	12 (27.27%)	
Unchanged	9 (69.23%)	31 (70.46%)	
Worsened	0	1 (2.27%)	
Mean changes of serum transaminases between the start and end of the sequence			
ALT (IU/L)	−25.3 ± 35.5	−1.2 ± 44.3	0.164
AST (IU/L)	−10 ± 22.8	−7 ± 31.5	0.802

Table 3 details the evolution between the two subgroups, based on the presence of neurological symptoms at the sequence initiation. When the hepatic symptoms were isolated at the initiation of the trientine sequence, no neurological symptoms developed. When only neurological symptoms were evident at the initiation of the treatment sequence, they improved or remained unchanged for all except for one TETA 2HCL sequence.

Table 3. Outcome in patients based on presence of neurological symptoms at the sequence initiation.

	Trientine Treatment Sequence	
Patients without Neurological Symptoms	TETA 4HCL (n = 5)	TETA 2HCL (n = 25)
Hepatic outcome		
Improved	3 (60.00%)	11 (44.00%)
Unchanged	2 (40.00%)	12 (48.00%)
Worsened	0 (0.00%)	2 (8.00%)
Neurological outcome		
Absent	5 (100.00%)	25 (100.00%)
Patients with neurological symptoms	TETA 4HCL (n = 8)	TETA 2HCL (n = 19)
Hepatic outcome		
Improved	0	2 (10.53%)
Unchanged	8 (100.00%)	17 (89.47%)
Worsened	0	0
Neurological outcome		
Improved	4 (50.00%)	12 (63.16%)
Unchanged	4 (50.00%)	6 (31.58%)
Worsened	0	1 (5.26%)

Kayser–Fleischer (KF) ring evolution was comparable in both of the treatment groups. In one sequence of the TETA 4HCL group, a slight increase in the ring was reported, without a deterioration in neurological and hepatic disease (Table 4).

Table 4. Evolution of the Kayser-Fleischer ring between sequence initiation and sequence end.

	Trientine Treatment Sequence	
	TETA 4HCL (n = 13)	TETA 2 HCL (n = 44)
Information not available	1 (7.69 %)	1 (2.27 %)
Present at treatment sequence initiation	8 (61.54%)	17 (38.63%)
At sequence end		
Increase	1 (12.50%)	0
Decrease	2 (25.00%)	8 (47.06%)
Disappearance	5 (62.50%)	8 (47.06%)
Unchanged	0	1 (5.88%)

3.5. Reasons for Discontinuation of Trientine Treatment and Adverse Effects

No adverse effects were observed during the TETA 4HCL sequences (mean duration: 12.6 years). All 13 of the TETA 4HCL sequences were stopped during the study period: 11 (85%) due to the fact that manufacturing of the hospital preparation was discontinued, 1 due to difficulties with supply and 1 due to an increase in the Kayser–Fleischer ring, without neurologic or hepatic deterioration.

The mean duration of treatment sequence was 7.6 years for TETA 2HCL. At the end of the study period, 26 (60%) of the TETA 2HCL monotherapy treatments were still ongoing. In three patients, zinc was added to TETA 2HCL due to hepatic or neurological deterioration in two cases, and as a result of an increase in liver copper without hepatic deterioration in one case. A bad adherence to TETA 2HCL was suspected in these three cases. The reasons for stopping TETA 2HCL were mainly due to adherence to medication issues (11 cases), generally linked to the requirement for cold storage. Other reasons included one case of lupus erythematosus-like syndrome in a patient with a previous diagnosis of lupus erythematosus during treatment with D-penicillamine, and one liver transplantation for suspicion of hepatocellular carcinoma. Two patients died (salivary gland neoplasm and suicide); these deaths were not considered as related to WD.

4. Discussion

Now that TETA 4HCL has received a European marketing authorization and is being marketed in Europe (as Cuprior®), this study comparing the efficacy and safety of TETA 4HCL to TETA 2HCL in everyday clinical practice is important, since many patients are still taking TETA 2HCL. Efficacy and safety are closely interrelated because any switch in treatment is usually linked to a lack of efficacy, observance issues, adverse effects or difficulties with treatment adherence.

In France, between 1970 and 2009, both of the trientine salts were available. All of the patients with WD in France are included in a national registry, allowing the possibility of conducting this retrospective study. Trientine monotherapy for more than 12 months was evaluated in 43 patients out of the 248 patients included in the WD registry in 2010, which represents a large cohort in this rare disease.

In accordance with French guidelines, trientine was mainly prescribed as a second-line treatment after D-penicillamine (81% of the patients). This switch was mainly due to the occurrence of adverse events. Adverse drug reactions are commonly reported with D-penicillamine treatment and are serious enough to lead to at least 30% of patients on D-penicillamine discontinuing the drug [10]. Four patients received zinc salts as a first-line treatment, associated or not with D-penicillamine. Discontinuation of zinc therapy, due to adverse effects such as gastrointestinal symptoms, is common in patients with WD in children, as in adults [7,8].

The study population is representative of the wide WD population, as it includes children and adult patients. The mean age at diagnosis was 20 years (range 5.6 years to 46.3 years). The majority of the patients presented with liver disease. These data are comparable to those of former studies [7,9]. Although there was non-random allocation to the treatment group, the baseline characteristics of the patients at the beginning of the sequences were relatively balanced.

The majority of the patients either improved or stabilized their symptoms under trientine. No differences in efficacy were detected when assessing the TETA 4HCL and 2HCL treatment sequences for changes in hepatic and neurological symptoms. The parameters relative to hepatic function, in particular serum transaminase levels, tended to improve in both of the groups. Many studies have demonstrated the effectiveness of TETA 2HCL, showing in addition that fewer side effects are observed than with D-penicillamine [9,11]. In this study, three patients on TETA 2HCL had hepatic or neurological deterioration and a bad adherence to treatment was highly suspected in these cases. In WD, during long-term follow-up, the most important cause of hepatic and/or neurologic worsening, leading sometimes to death, is non-adherence to WD treatment [12–15]. Up to 50% of patients are non-compliant with treatment [16,17]. The identification of the factors which compromise adherence to medication remains difficult, and findings are often contradictory. However, it is evident that the barriers to treatment dispensation or conservation should be minimized. TETA 2HCL requires refrigerated storage between 2 and 8 °C. This is certainly an important disadvantage for patients who need to take the drug several times throughout the day, while studying, working or travelling, on a daily basis for the duration of their lives.

In this study, the main reason for discontinuation of the drug was the production shutdown of one of the biochemical salts, TETA 4HCL. All 13 TETA 4HCL treatments were stopped due to cessation of manufacturing or supply difficulties, except for 1 patient whose Kayser–Fleischer rings increased. No adverse events were reported in this group following an average treatment duration of 12.5 years. In the TETA 2HCL group (n = 44), only one adverse event was reported. This was a case of lupus erythematosus-like syndrome in a patient who already had presented with penicillamine-induced lupus erythematosus-like syndrome. However, 11 treatment sequences were stopped as a result of difficulties in treatment adherence due to the refrigeration requirements (often creating problems for patients who needed to work away from home or travel) for TETA 2HCL. The published guidelines indicate that adverse effects are rarely observed with TETA 2HCL treatment: urticaria, reversible anemia and lupus-like reactions are described as the key potential side effects [2,18]. In our study, TETA 4HCL was also shown to be well tolerated, consistent with the review of Allery that describes a TETA 4HCL safety profile comparable to that of TETA 2 HCL [19].

The number of patients treated with trientine as a first-line therapy is small and does not allow for a satisfactory analysis of this sub-group. However, six other patients started trientine therapy early in the course of this lifelong disease, during the first three months following diagnosis. Trientine was introduced in these patients as a result of early adverse events associated with D-penicillamine. The clinical evolution of these patients was not different to that of the whole cohort.

This study has certain limitations, including its retrospective nature and the lack of randomization. The rarity of the disease, the fact that trientine was used in France via a compassionate use program and that manufacturing of TETA 4HCL was discontinued in 2009, explain the low number of patients included in the study. At that time, adherence was subjectively assessed during the medical examination and not with dedicated scores, such as the Morisky score [20]. However, it was possible to analyze data quite exhaustively over long periods of treatment under trientine (7.6 years for TETA 2HCL and 12.6 years for TETA 4HCL).

In conclusion, both of the trientine salts were equally effective in controlling WD. Adverse events were infrequent. In WD, the adherence to medication is a key factor for treatment success. Interruption in the TETA 2HCL therapy was frequent, linked to the requirement for cold storage. The physicians therefore have to be even more vigilant to detect non-adherence to medication as early as possible in the patients being treated with TETA 2HCL.

Author Contributions: Conceptualization, F.W. and A.P.; Data curation, F.W., D.D. and A.P.; Formal analysis, F.W., D.D., E.M., M.A.O. and A.P.; Investigation, F.W., D.D. and A.P.; Methodology, F.W., D.D. and A.P.; Project administration, F.W. and A.P.; Supervision, F.W. and A.P.; Validation, F.W. and A.P.; Writing—Original draft, F.W., D.D. and A.P.; Writing—Review and editing, F.W., D.D., E.M., M.A.O. and A.P. All authors have read and agreed to the published version of the manuscript.

Funding: This research received no external funding.

Institutional Review Board Statement: This study was approved by the Institutional Review Board of HUPNVS, Paris 7 University, AP-HP (n°1343579). An informed consent was obtained from all subjects and/or their legal guardian(s). All of the patients signed a written consent form. All methods were carried out in accordance with relevant guidelines and regulations, in accordance with the Declaration of Helsinki.

Informed Consent Statement: Written informed consent has been obtained from the patients to publish this paper in accordance with terms of the French Wilson's Disease National Registry.

Data Availability Statement: The datasets generated and/or analyzed during the current study are not publicly available due to privacy related to the French Wilson's Disease National Registry but are available from the corresponding author on reasonable request.

Conflicts of Interest: The authors declare no conflict of interest.

References

1. Poujois, A.; Woimant, F. Wilson's disease: A 2017 update. *Clin. Res. Hepatol. Gastroenterol.* **2018**, *42*, 512–520. [CrossRef] [PubMed]
2. European Association for the Study of the Liver. EASL Clinical Practice Guidelines: Wilson's disease. *J. Hepatol.* **2012**, *56*, 671–685. [CrossRef] [PubMed]
3. Masełbas, W.; Członkowska, A.; Litwin, T.; Niewada, M. Persistence with treatment for Wilson disease: A retrospective study. *BMC Neurol.* **2019**, *19*, 278. [CrossRef] [PubMed]
4. Siegemund, R.; Lößner, J.; Günther, K.; Kühn, H.J.; Bachmann, H. Mode of action of triethylenetetramine dihydrochloride on copper metabolism in Wilson's disease. *Acta Neurol. Scand.* **1991**, *83*, 364–366. [CrossRef] [PubMed]
5. Brewer, G.J. Zinc acetate for the treatment of Wilson's disease. *Expert Opin. Pharmacother.* **2001**, *2*, 1473–1477. [CrossRef] [PubMed]
6. Członkowska, A.; Litwin, T.; Karlinski, M.; Dziezyc, K.; Chabik, G.; Czerska, M. D-penicillamine versus zinc sulfate s first-line therapy for Wilson's disease. *Eur. J. Neurol.* **2014**, *21*, 599–606. [CrossRef] [PubMed]
7. Weiss, K.H.; Gotthardt, D.N.; Klemm, D.; Merle, U.; Ferenci–Foerster, D.; Schaefer, M.; Ferenci, P.; Stremmel, W. Zinc Monotherapy Is Not as Effective as Chelating Agents in Treatment of Wilson Disease. *Gastroenterology* **2011**, *140*, 1189–1198.e1. [CrossRef] [PubMed]
8. Santiago, R.; Gottrand, F.; Debray, D.; Bridoux, L.; Lachaux, A.; Morali, A.; Lapeyre, D.; Lamireau, T. Zinc Therapy for Wilson Disease in Children in French Pediatric Centers. *J. Pediatr. Gastroenterol. Nutr.* **2015**, *61*, 613–618. [CrossRef] [PubMed]
9. Weiss, K.H.; Thurik, F.; Gotthardt, D.N.; Schäfer, M.; Teufel, U.; Wiegand, F.; Merle, U.; Ferenci–Foerster, D.; Maieron, A.; Stauber, R.; et al. Efficacy and Safety of Oral Chelators in Treatment of Patients with Wilson Disease. *Clin. Gastroenterol. Hepatol.* **2013**, *11*, 1028–1035.e2. [CrossRef] [PubMed]
10. Litwin, T.; Członkowska, A.; Socha, P. Oral Chelator Treatment of Wilson Disease: D-Penicillamine. In *Clinical and Trans-Lational Perspectives on Wilson Disease*; Kerkar, N., Roberts, E.A., Eds.; Academic Press: New York, NY, USA, 2019; pp. 357–363.
11. Merle, U.; Schaefer, M.; Ferenci, P.; Stremmel, W. Clinical presentation, diagnosis and long-term outcome of Wilson's disease: A cohort study. *Gut* **2007**, *56*, 115–120. [CrossRef] [PubMed]
12. Walshe, J.M.; Dixon, A.K. Dangers of non-compliance in Wilson's disease. *Lancet* **1986**, *1*, 845–847. [CrossRef]
13. Masełbas, W.; Chabik, G.; Członkowska, A. Persistence with treatment in patients with Wilson disease. *Neurol. I Neurochir. Pol.* **2010**, *44*, 260–263. [CrossRef]
14. Weiss, K.H.; Stremmel, W. Clinical considerations for an effective medical therapy in Wilson's disease. *Ann. N. Y. Acad. Sci.* **2014**, *1315*, 81–85. [CrossRef] [PubMed]
15. Dzieżyc, K.; Karlinski, M.; Litwin, T.; Członkowska, A. Compliant treatment with anti-copper agents prevents clinically overt Wilson's disease in pre-symptomatic patients. *Eur. J. Neurol.* **2013**, *21*, 332–337. [CrossRef] [PubMed]

16. Maselbas, W.; Litwin, T.; Czlonkowska, A. Social and demographic characteristics of a Polish cohort with Wilson disease and the impact of treatment persistence. *Orphanet J. Rare Dis.* **2019**, *14*, 167. [CrossRef] [PubMed]
17. Jacquelet, E.; Beretti, J.; De-Tassigny, A.; Girardot-Tinant, N.; Wenisch, E.; Lachaux, A.; Pheulpin, M.C.; Poujois, A.; Woimant, F. Compliance with treatment in Wilson's disease: On the interest of a multidisciplinary closer follow-up. *Rev. Med. Interne* **2018**, *39*, 155–160. [CrossRef] [PubMed]
18. Socha, P.; Janczyk, W.; Dhawan, A.; Baumann, U.; D'Antiga, L.; Tanner, S.; Iorio, R.; Vajro, P.; Houwen, R.; Fischler, B.; et al. Wilson's Disease in Children: A Position Paper by the Hepatology Committee of the European Society for Paediatric Gastroenterology, Hepatology and Nutrition. *J. Pediatr. Gas-Troenterol. Nutr.* **2018**, *66*, 334–344. [CrossRef] [PubMed]
19. Allery, C. Maladie de Wilson. Place de la Trientine Dans la Stratégie Thérapeutique. Ph.D. Thesis, Université Paris Descartes, Paris, France, 2013.
20. Morisky, D.E.; Green, L.W.; Levine, D.M. Concurrent and Predictive Validity of a Self-reported Measure of Medication Adherence. *Med. Care* **1986**, *24*, 67–74. [CrossRef] [PubMed]

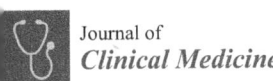

Article

Treatment of Dystonic Tremor of the Upper Limbs: A Single-Center Retrospective Study

Belén González-Herrero [1,2,*,†], Ilaria Antonella Di Vico [3,†], Erlick Pereira [1], Mark Edwards [4] and Francesca Morgante [1,5]

1. Neurosciences Research Centre, Molecular and Clinical Sciences Institute, St. George's University of London, London SW17 0RE, UK
2. Departamento de Medicina, Universidad Autónoma de Barcelona (UAB), 08193 Barcelona, Spain
3. Neurology Unit, Movement Disorders Division, Department of Neurosciences Biomedicine and Movement Sciences, University of Verona, 37134 Verona, Italy
4. Department of Clinical and Basic Neuroscience, Institute of Psychiatry, Psychology and Neuroscience, King's College London, London SE5 8AF, UK
5. Dipartimento di Medicina Clinica e Sperimentale, University of Messina, 98122 Messina, Italy
* Correspondence: bgonzale@sgul.ac.uk
† These authors contributed equally to this work.

Abstract: Tremor is part of the phenomenological spectrum of dystonia. Treatments available for tremor in dystonia are oral medications (OM), botulinum neurotoxin (BoNT), and brain surgery (deep brain stimulation or thalamotomy). There is limited knowledge regarding the outcome of different treatment options, and evidence is especially scarce for the tremor of the upper limbs occurring in people with dystonia. In this single-center retrospective study, we evaluated the outcome of different treatments in a cohort of people with upper limb dystonic tremors. Demographic, clinical, and treatment data were analyzed. Dropout rates and side effects were specifically assessed, as well as the 7-point patient-completed clinical global impression scale (p-CGI-S, 1: very much improved; 7: very much worse) as outcome measures. A total of 47 subjects (46.8% female) with dystonic tremor, tremor associated with dystonia, or task-specific tremor were included, with a median age at onset of 58 years (7–86). A total of 31 subjects were treated with OM, 31 with BoNT, and 7 with surgery. Dropout rates with OM were 74.2% due to either lack of efficacy ($n = 10$) or side effects ($n = 13$). A total of 7 patients treated with BoNT (22.6%) had mild weakness, causing dropout in 2. P-CGI-S was ≤ 3 (improvement) in 39% with OM, compared to 92% with BoNT and 100% with surgery. These findings suggest good symptom control of the tremor of the upper limb in dystonia with BoNT and surgery, with higher rates of dropout and side effects with OM. Randomized controlled studies are needed to confirm our findings and provide further insight into better selecting suitable patients for BoNT or brain surgery.

Keywords: dystonia; tremor; dystonic tremor; botulinum toxin; deep brain stimulation

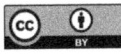

1. Introduction

Tremor is an involuntary, rhythmic, oscillatory movement of a body part [1], and it is one of the phenomenological manifestations of dystonia. Tremor in dystonia is classified into two types: dystonic tremor (Dys-T), which occurs in body parts affected by dystonia, and tremor associated with dystonia (TAD) that appears in a body part not affected by dystonia in a person with dystonia located elsewhere. Classically, tremor in dystonia (whether Dys-T or TAD) is variable in frequency and amplitude and exacerbated in specific positions. While generally a postural and kinetic tremor, it may also occur at rest and is frequently asymmetric [2,3]. Task-specific tremor (TST) is a form of action tremor that occurs only or mostly when performing a specific skilled task [4], most commonly seen during writing, called primary writing tremor (PWT). Although the pathophysiology of TST is still debated, growing data favors its dystonic nature [5,6].

There are no formal guidelines for the treatment of Dys-T, TAD, and TST. In a recent placebo-controlled, parallel-group, randomized clinical trial [7] conducted on 30 subjects with dystonic hand tremor, onabotulinum toxin A significantly improved the Fahn–Tolosa–Marin Tremor Rating Scale total score. A systematic review of the available data on the treatment of Dys-T and PWT concluded that botulinum neurotoxin (BoNT) and functional neurosurgery (deep brain stimulation, DBS, and thalamotomy by radiofrequency) might be more effective than oral medications; however, there was no data on the treatment of upper limb Dys-T with BoNT and no data at all for TAD [8]. Moreover, there are no long-term follow-up data regarding the treatment of different types of tremors in dystonia.

The present retrospective study aimed to evaluate the short and long-term clinical outcomes of people with Dys-T, TAD, and TST affecting the upper limbs and treated with oral medications, BoNT, and functional neurosurgery in a tertiary referral center for movement disorders.

2. Methods

This is a retrospective cohort study including consecutive patients diagnosed with Dys-T, TAD, or TST affecting the upper limbs at the Movement Disorders Clinic at St. George's Hospital, London, UK, between August 2016 and October 2021.

Medical records of all participants were systematically reviewed and included all documents available from two movement disorder specialists (FM and ME) at St. George's Hospital, London. Patients were excluded from the study if comprehensive medical records throughout follow-up were unavailable. We included all patients whose upper extremity tremor was classified as an idiopathic dystonic tremor and excluded individuals whose tremor was considered secondary.

Demographic and medical history data were recorded, including sex, age at the onset of tremor, duration at first assessment, follow-up duration, and family history of movement disorders.

Clinical examination was standardized and included the following aspects: assessment at resting, postural and kinetic tremor with eyes open and closed; and assessment of tremor while performing different manual tasks, including writing, using cutlery, holding a cup, typing on a keyboard and cell phone, or playing an instrument. The following clinical features were retrieved: type of tremor (Dys-T, TAD and TST), distribution (restricted to the upper limbs or present in other body districts), side of tremor, if asymmetric, presence of resting component, and predominant pattern of tremor. Patients were also asked about the daily tasks most impacted by the tremor.

Data on oral treatment included the number and type of medications prescribed, side effects, and dropout rates due to inefficacy. Inefficacy was determined when patients had been on the maximum dose for at least six months, without benefit. All patients undergoing surgical and botulinum toxin treatment were treated by the same movement disorder specialist (FM). Electromyography and/or electrical stimulation guidance was used when injecting botulinum toxin whenever clinical examination did not disclose a consistent pattern of tremor, or to inject fingers, forearm flexors, or extensors.

Incobotulinum toxin A (Merz Pharma GmbH & Co. KGaA, Frankfurt, Germany) was prepared by adding 1 or 2 mL of preservative-free saline into 100 U vials, and abobotulinum toxin A (Ipsen Biopharm limited, Wrexham, UK) by adding 2.5 mL of preservative-free saline into 500 U vials. We collected the following data on BoNT treatment: tremor duration at first injection, the number of injections received, treatment duration, injection interval, type of BoNT, the dose of BoNT at first and last injection, muscles injected, side effects, and dropout rates.

Data from patients treated with surgery included: the type of procedure (deep brain stimulation, DBS, or radiofrequency thalamotomy), type of device, age at surgery, DBS settings, and side effects.

A patient-completed Clinical Global Impression (CGI) rating scale was assessed for all patients, regardless of the treatment received. Our study included the modified patient-rated CGI-improvement (p-CGI-I) at the follow-up visits as an outcome measure. The scale measures improvement on a 7-point scale (1: Very much improved, 2: Much improved, 3: Minimally improved, 4: No change, 5: Minimally worse, 6: Much worse, 7: Very much worse) based on the perception of the patient regarding how much he or she had improved or worsened relative to a baseline state at the beginning of the intervention.

3. Statistical Analysis

Comparisons between groups were performed using Fisher's exact test for categorical variables and the U Mann–Whitney test for continuous variables. Grading scores were analyzed using the U Mann–Whitney test and the Wilcoxon signed-rank test for ordinal variables. The results were considered statistically significant at a 2-tailed $p < 0.05$. SPSS software version 28 (IBM Corp., Armonk, NY, USA) was used to perform the analysis. All data are reported as mean ± standard deviation, unless otherwise stated.

4. Results

A total of 47 patients (22 female, 46.8%) were included in the study, with a median (interquartile range, IQR) age at the first assessment of 70.9 (62.3–75.9) years and tremor duration of 8.8 (3.8–28.6) years. They were followed up for a median (IQR) of 24.8 (5.3–35.6) months.

A total of 33 patients had Dys-T (70.2%), 4 patients had TAD (8.5%), and 10 TST (21.3%). The tremor was postural or kinetic in all the patients, with 4 (8.5%) also having a rest component. The tremor was typically restricted to the upper limbs (70.2%), bilateral (66%), and asymmetric (96.8%). Complete demographic and clinical data are presented in Table 1.

Table 1. Demographic and clinical data of subjects with dystonic tremor, tremor associated with dystonia, and task-specific tremor.

	n = 47
Sex (n, %)	
Male	25 (53.4)
Female	22 (46.8)
Family history of movement disorders (n, %)	
Negative	33 (70.2)
Tremor	13 (27.7)
Parkinsonism	1 (2.1)
Age at onset, median (IQR), years	58.0 [41.5–67.7]
Age at first assessment, median (IQR), years	70.9 [62.3–75.9]
Total time follow-up, median (IQR), months	24.8 [5.3–35.6]
Tremor duration at first assessment, median (IQR), years	8.8 [3.8–28.6]
Type of tremor (n, %)	
Dystonic tremor (Dys-T)	33 (70.2)
Tremor associated with dystonia (TAD)	4 (8.5)
Task-specific tremor (TST)	10 (21.3)
Body districts involved (n, %)	
Only UL	13 (27.7)
UL + Legs	3 (6.4)
UL + Head/Neck	11 (23.4)
UL + Oromandibular	1 (2.1)
UL + Voice	4 (8.5)
Laterality (n, %)	
Monolateral	31 (66)
Bilateral	16 (34)
Asymmetric	30 (97.9)

Data are presented as numbers (n, %) for categorical variables and median (interquartile range, IQR) for continuous variables. Dys-T = dystonic tremor; TAD = tremor associated with dystonia; TST = task specific tremor; UL = upper limbs.

A total of 43 patients (91.5%) received treatment of multiple types; 4 did not, due to personal preference or mild presentation. Throughout the period of follow-up, 31 (72.1%) received oral medications, 31 (72.1%) BoNT, and 7 (16.3%) underwent surgery (6 DBS, 1 thalamotomy).

4.1. Treatment with Oral Medication

A total of 31 patients (72.1%) were treated with at least one oral medication (1.74 ± 1.1). Considering patients utilizing all oral medications together, 23 (74.2%) dropped out due to either side effects (41.9%), most commonly drowsiness and lightheadedness, or inefficacy (32.3%). Still, despite some improvement, 5 patients required combined therapy with BoNT (4, 12.9%) or surgery (1, 3.2%) to achieve satisfactory benefits. Individualized benefits and side-effect percentages resulting from the different oral medications are summarized in Figure 1.

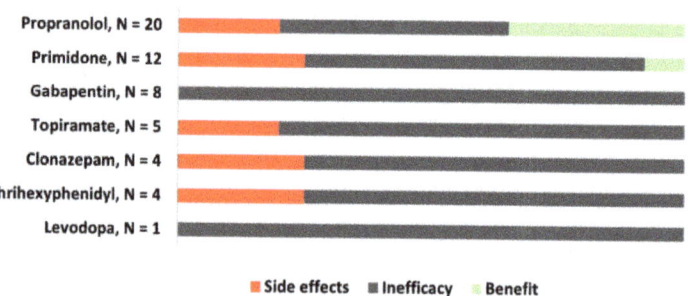

Figure 1. *Effect of oral medications for dystonic tremor of the upper limbs.* The most frequently prescribed oral medications for tremor were propranolol (64.5%), primidone (38.7%), and gabapentin (25.8%). Benefits were only reported with propranolol (35%) and primidone (8%). Topiramate, clonazepam, trihexyphenidyl, and levodopa, were either ineffective or caused side effects (topiramate in 20%, clonazepam in 25%, and trihexyphenidyl in 25%).

4.2. Treatment with BoNT

The decision to treat with BoNT was made in 31 patients (72.1%), and 19 of them had taken oral medication previously, without satisfactory outcomes. Out of 31 subjects, 26 (83.9%) were still receiving this treatment at the last follow-up. A total of 2 patients showed handgrip weakness and did not want to continue the treatment, 1 had an intercurrent stroke affecting the previously injected arm, and 2 patients were lost to the follow-up. Figure 2 reports the main tremor pattern during the execution of the manual tasks identified as goals of the BoNT treatment in each patient. These therapeutical goals included high dexterity activities (19.2%), holding a cup (65.4%), writing (34.5%), and using cutlery (19.2%).

The median (IQR) tremor duration at first injection was 8.8 (4.9–23.7) years, and the median (IQR) treatment duration with BoNT was 27.7 (4.8–34.5) months. The mean interval within injections was 4.8 ± 1.7 months. EMG and/or electrical stimulation were employed to optimize the injection in 8 subjects (25.8%).

Abobotulinum and incobotulinum toxins were similarly used (57.5% vs. 42.3%, respectively). Patients underwent, on average, 4.5 ± 3.3 injection sessions. Table 2 shows the muscles injected. The incobotulinum toxin dose was significantly higher at the last injection (68.6 ± 35.7) compared to the first injection (50.8 ± 26.1) (p = 0.03). The dose of the first (271.3 ± 196.8) and last injection (250 ± 164.1) with abobotulinum toxin was comparable (p = 0.43).

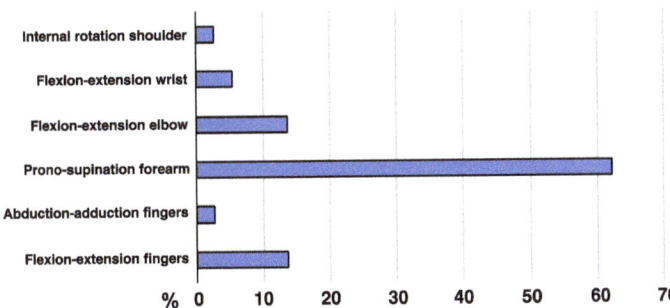

Figure 2. *Main pattern of dystonic tremor of the upper limbs.* Pronosupination was the most frequent tremor pattern observed while performing the most affected manual task.

Table 2. Type of botulinum toxin, injected muscles, and botulinum toxin dose.

		Abobotulinum Toxin/A (Units)	Incobotulinum Toxin/A (Units)
Muscles injected (*n*, %)	*n* = 31		
Pronator teres	18 (58.0)	78.0 ± 26.9	23.1 ± 9.6
Longus supinator	21 (67.7)	76.7 ± 26.7	22.8 ± 9.0
Biceps	8 (25.8)	83.7 ± 41.4	30.0 ± 10.0
Triceps	11 (35.5)	101.7 ± 28.6	20 ± 0.0
Flexor carpi radialis	3 (9.7)	20	30 ± 14.14
Flexor carpi ulnaris	3 (9.7)	55 ± 7.0	30
Extensor carpi radialis	2 (6.4)	-	30 ± 20
Teres major/minor	3 (9.7)	80 ± 40	-
Flexor superficialis digitorum	3 (9.7)	40	30 ± 0.0
Flexor profundus digitorum	3 (9.7)	-	30 ± 17.32

Data are presented as numbers (*n*, %) for categorical variables and mean ± SD for continuous variables. The most frequently injected muscles were the pronator teres, longus supinator biceps, and triceps.

A total of 7 subjects (22.6%) exhibited transitory weakness (4 with abobotulinum toxin, causing dropout in one, and 3 with incobotulinum toxin, causing dropout in one).

The duration of side effects was comparable between the two formulations of BoNT (abobotulinum toxin: 20 (IQR, 10–90) days; incobotulinum toxin: 20 (IQR, 7–60) days, U Mann–Whitney $p = 0.4$).

4.3. Treatment with Functional Neurosurgery

A total of 7 patients (14.9%) were treated with brain surgery, 6 with DBS, and 1 with unilateral radiofrequency thalamotomy in the VIM nucleus. St. Jude Medical Infinity directional DBS leads (Abbott Neuromodulation, Austin, TX, USA), spaced at 1.5 mm apart, were implanted bilaterally in all patients receiving DBS. The ventralis intermedius (VIM) nucleus of the thalamus and caudal zona incerta (cZI) were dual-targeted using classic anterior commissure, posterior commissure (ACPC) stereotactic coordinates ($x = +/-13$, $y = -4$, $z = 0$). The tips of the electrodes were positioned in the cZI (posterior subthalamic area). The rationale for deciding to use unilateral thalamotomy instead of DBS in the 1 patient was age (she was over 80 years old), and the tremor predominantly affected the right side of the body. She had some balance difficulties predating the surgery, and her expectations were gaining independence in the basic activities of daily living, such as holding cutlery and holding a stick when walking. The increased risk of bilateral DBS surgery and the unnecessary burden of attending subsequent programming sessions favored thalamotomy over DBS.

All patients treated with brain surgery had previously received treatment with oral medications, without benefit. None of them had received BoNT injections before surgery.

The average age at surgery was 70.8 ± 8.5 years, and the median (IQR) tremor duration was 23 (9–42) years. The follow-up median (IQR) time was 29.1 (14.9–47.9) months.

A total of 2 patients had chronic stimulation-induced side effects (dysarthria and balance disturbances). The patient with thalamotomy exhibited balance disturbances predating surgery, which transitorily worsened after surgery. She recovered and reached her baseline three weeks after surgery. Clinical data and DBS settings at the last follow-up are collated in Table 3.

Table 3. Subjects with dystonic tremor and task-specific tremor treated with functional neurosurgery.

Gender/Age	Type of Tremor	Age at Onset (Years)	Disease Duration at Surgery (Years)	DBS Settings	Side Effects with Current DBS Settings or after Thalamotomy
Male, 63	Dystonic Tremor	20	43	Left: 1-, case+, 60 mcs, 130 Hz, 2 mA Right: 9-, case+, 60 mcs, 130 Hz, 2.7 mA	Mild stimulation induced dysarthria and balance difficulties.
Male, 66	Dystonic Tremor	57	9	Left: 2(abc)-, case+, 60 mcs, 130 Hz, 2.6 mA Right: 9-, case+, 60 mcs, 130 Hz, 1.4 mA	None
Male, 73	Dystonic Tremor	50	23	Left 1-, 2(abc)+, 50 mcs, 170 Hz, 2.5 mA Right 9-, 10(abc)+, 60 mcs, 170 Hz, 3.0 mA	None
Male, 70	Dystonic Tremor	60	10	Left 2a-, case+, 60 mcs, 130 Hz, 4.0 mA Right 11c-, case+, 60 mcs, 130 Hz, 3.0 mA	None
Female, 60	Task-specific Tremor	56	4	Left 3c-, case+, 60 mcs, 190 Hz, 3.5 mA, Right 12-, case+, 60 mcs, 130 Hz, 2.1 mA	None
Female, 81	Dystonic Tremor	7	74	Left 1-, case+, 60 mcs, 130 Hz 3.4 mA Right 9-, case+, 30 mcs, 190 Hz, 4.0 mA	Mild stimulation induced dysarthria and balance difficulties.
Female, 82	Dystonic Tremor	50	32	Not applicable	Mild balance disturbance (present before surgery).

DBS = deep brain stimulation; mcs = microseconds; Hz = hertz; mA: milliampere. Subjects 1–6 were treated with DBS. Subject 7 was treated with a thalamotomy.

4.4. Clinical Global Improvement (CGI-I)

The patient-reported outcomes with the different therapies are represented in Figure 3. With oral medication, 40% of patients reported a p-CGI-I ≤ 3 (improvement) compared to 92% after optimized treatment with BoNT (at the last injection) and 100% after surgery. The percentage of p-CGI-I ≤ 3 was significantly higher when comparing the first and last injection of BoNT (71% vs. 92%, Fisher's exact test; $p = 0.04$). There were no significant differences in p-CGI scores in regards to botulinum toxin type (Mann–Whitney U test; $p = 0.82$) or the usage of EMG guidance ($p = 0.4$).

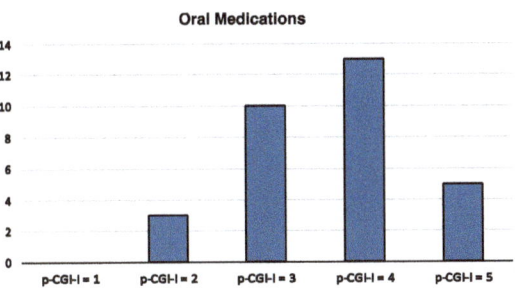

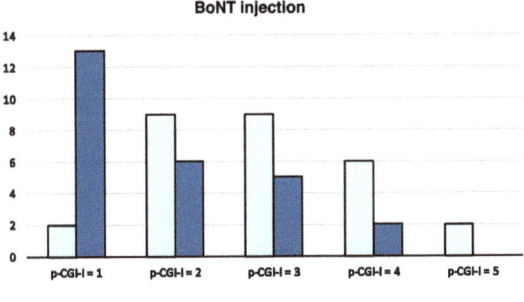

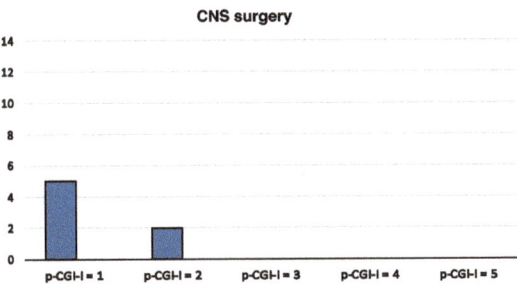

Figure 3. *Patient-based Clinical Global Improvement (p-CGI-I) as per treatment for tremor.* More patients reported improvement on the p-CGI-I with botulinum toxin (BoNT) injections and neurosurgery compared to oral medications. The percentage of p-CGI-I ≤ 3 was significantly higher when comparing the first and last injection of BoNT (74% vs. 92%, Fisher's exact test $p = 0.04$). P-CGI = 1: Very much improved, 2: Much improved, 3: Minimally improved, 4: No change, 5: Minimally worse, 6: Much worse, 7: Very much worse.

In the group of patients that received both oral medications and BoNT at any time during the entire follow-up (16, 37.2%), the pCGI-I was significantly higher with BoNT compared to oral medications (Wilcoxon Rank Squares; $p = 0.001$).

5. Discussion

There is an unmet need for evidence-based guidelines to treat tremor in dystonia [8]. The different criteria and labeling used by clinicians for isolated upper limb tremors and the lack of biomarkers to distinguish between tremor syndromes have made it difficult to draw definitive conclusions about how best to treat dystonic tremors of the upper limb.

Here, we reviewed three very different approaches to treating patients with tremor in dystonia: oral medication, BoNT, or brain surgery. While oral medication has a systemic effect, BoNT is administered by local intramuscular injections in the muscles, and deep brain stimulation or thalamotomy require brain surgery. Oral medications for tremor more commonly produce sickness, lightheadedness, or drowsiness and may be contraindicated if the patient has other comorbidities or if there is interaction with other medications; BoNT can produce bruising and weakness in the injected muscles, and brain surgery can result in a hemorrhagic stroke or a brain infection, to side effects ultimately related to the stimulation, more commonly in the target for tremor, balance, and speech disturbances.

Our study suggests that commonly used oral medications for tremor are less effective than BoNT and surgery in treating any type of tremor of the upper limbs occurring in people with dystonia and task-specific tremors. Dropout rates and side effects were higher with oral medications. BoNT appeared to be an effective and safe therapy, leading to improvement in 71% of the patients after the first injection; this percentage increased to 92% when the injection protocol was optimized at subsequent follow-up visits. In patients who received both oral medications and BoNT at any time during their follow-up, improvement based on the p-CGI-I was significantly greater with BoNT. These results are in keeping with those of Fasano et al. in their systematic review [8], in which they found BoNT to be superior to oral medication for axial dystonic tremor and task-specific tremor, as well as with the results from the placebo-controlled trial from Rajan et al. [7], in which BoNT significantly improved the outcome of 30 subjects with dystonic hand tremor.

The outcome of any tremor treatment is often assessed with validated rating scales developed for essential tremor, such as The Fahn–Tolosa–Marin [9] or the Tetras scale [10], as well as instruments measuring the quality of life, such as QUEST [11]. However, such outcome measures were not designed for subjects whose tremor occurs in the context of dystonia or for those having a purely task-specific tremor. In our study, from medical history and clinical examination, we identified the manual tasks most affected by tremor, similar to the goal attainment scale employed in spasticity studies [12]. The p-CGI was based on their satisfaction with the treatment regarding the manual task most impacted by the tremor, which was most commonly holding a cup. This also allowed us to identify the pattern of tremor (clinically or by EMG) while executing that specific action and injecting the botulinum toxin accordingly. Most frequently, there was a pronosupination of the forearm and flexion-extension at the elbow. Therefore, the most injected muscles were the supinator longus, pronator teres, biceps, and triceps (Table 2).

Previous studies using BoNT in the treatment of upper limb tremor only injected either the wrist flexors/extensors [13,14] or selected the muscles by the clinical and electrophysiological assessment of patients with arms at rest, outstretched in front of the subject, and while performing finger-to-nose action [7,15]. Injecting the wrist extensors increases the possibility of handgrip weakness [14,16], and typically, tremor in dystonia changes with different positions. This makes it imperative, in our opinion, that the selection of muscles for injection takes place in reference to specific task performance. Given our retrospective data, prospective controlled studies are warranted to test this approach in subjects with Dys-T, DAT, or TST.

Deep brain surgery was the most effective treatment for those failing first, second, and third-line oral medications for tremor. None of the patients treated with brain surgery had received BoNT. They were selected for brain surgery based on the severity of the tremor, which determined functional impairment and significant disability in the absence of exclusion criteria. Data on DBS for tremor in dystonia are scanty, with different targets proposed in addition to the globus pallidus pars interna[11], such as the VIM, ventralis oralis anterior[12], and caudal ZI[13]. Our cohort was implanted, positioning the most inferior contact in cZI/PSA, allowing for the targeting of two different structures (cZI and VIM), previously demonstrated to be effective for Dys-T [17].

Several limitations of this study should be considered. The results should be cautiously interpreted, as the data were analyzed retrospectively, and the sample number is relatively small in some analyses. Treatment decisions were based on clinical expertise and patients' preferences. Moreover, some data were not included due to incomplete reports. A standardized dystonia rating scale was not employed to formally assess tremor and dystonia symptoms. A clinical examination was not always accompanied by EMG or kinematic assessment. Lastly, the p-CGI-I is a subjective measure of improvement based on the patient's perception, which could have been supplemented by objective measures.

Despite these limitations, our data suggest that oral medications employed for essential tremor are often ineffective or not tolerated in people with dystonic tremors of the upper limbs. Botulinum toxin appears to be a safe and effective therapeutic option that warrants testing in randomized controlled trials with open-label, long-term follow-up. This seems to be particularly true if the tremor has a predominant pattern of pronosupination of the forearm or flexion-extension at the elbow when performing the most-affected manual tasks. Therefore, there is a need to develop specific rating scales for dystonic tremors that also consider essential manual tasks commonly affected. Finally, functional neurosurgery also seems to be a very effective procedure. Large randomized controlled trials are needed to confirm our findings and provide further insight into selecting patients best suited to receive BoNT, DBS, or thalamotomy.

Author Contributions: Research project—conceptualization and organization: B.G.-H., I.A.D.V. and F.M.; execution: B.G.-H. and I.A.D.V.; Statistical analysis—design and execution: B.G.-H.; review and critique: B.G.-H., I.A.D.V., E.P., M.E. and F.M.; Manuscript—writing of the first draft: B.G.-H.; review and critique: B.G.-H., I.A.D.V., E.P., M.E. and F.M. All authors have read and agreed to the published version of the manuscript.

Funding: This research received no external funding.

Institutional Review Board Statement: The study was conducted following the Declaration of Helsinki. This study is based on retrospective clinical data obtained during routine clinical care. Patients data were anonymized. This study reports on a clinical audit approved by St George's University Hospital.

Informed Consent Statement: Individualized informed consent was not required for this retrospective study as it was part of a clinical audit approved by St George's University Hospital.

Data Availability Statement: Supporting data is not publicly available.

Acknowledgments: B.G.-H. is grateful to the Alfonso Martin Escudero Foundation, Spain, for supporting her research activity.

Conflicts of Interest: E.P.: speaking honoraria from Boston Scientific; research support from NIHR, UKRI, Life after Paralysis, and the Rosetrees Trust. M.E.: grant income from NIHR and royalties from the Oxford University Press; honoraria from the International Parkinson's Disease and Movement Disorder Society and Wiley Publishing. F.M.: research support from NIHR and UKRI; speaking honoraria from Abbvie, Medtronic, Boston Scientific, Bial, and Merz; travel grants from the International Parkinson's Disease and Movement Disorder Society; advisory board fees from Merz and Boston Scientific; consultancies fees from Boston Scientific, Merz, and Bial; research support from Boston Scientific, Merz, and Global Kynetic; royalties for the book "Disorders of Movement", from Springer; member of the editorial board of Movement Disorders, Movement Disorders Clinical Practice, and the European Journal of Neurology. Sandy Maria Cartella has no disclosures to report. B.G.-H.: research support from the Alfonso Martin Escudero Foundation, Madrid, Spain. I.A.D.V.: no disclosures.

References

1. Bhatia, K.P.; Bain, P.; Bajaj, N.; Elble, R.J.; Hallett, M.; Louis, E.D.; Raethjen, J.; Stamelou, M.; Testa, C.M.; Deuschl, G.; et al. Consensus Statement on the classification of tremors. from the task force on tremor of the International Parkinson and Movement Disorder Society. *Mov. Disord.* **2018**, *33*, 75–87. [CrossRef] [PubMed]
2. Albanese, A.; Bhatia, K.; Bressman, S.B.; Delong, M.R.; Fahn, S.; Fung, V.S.; Hallett, M.; Jankovic, J.; Jinnah, H.A.; Klein, C.; et al. Phenomenology and classification of dystonia: A consensus update. *Mov. Disord.* **2013**, *28*, 863–873. [CrossRef] [PubMed]
3. Erro, R.; Rubio-Agusti, I.; Saifee, T.A.; Cordivari, C.; Ganos, C.; Batla, A.; Bhatia, K.P. Rest and other types of tremor in adult-onset primary dystonia. *J. Neurol. Neurosurg. Psychiatry* **2014**, *85*, 965–968. [CrossRef] [PubMed]
4. Bain, P.G. Task-specific tremor. *Handb. Clin. Neurol.* **2011**, *100*, 711–718. [CrossRef] [PubMed]

5. Latorre, A.; Rocchi, L.; Batla, A.; Berardelli, A.; Rothwell, J.C.; Bhatia, K.P. The Signature of Primary Writing Tremor Is Dystonic. *Mov. Disord.* **2021**, *36*, 1715–1720. [CrossRef] [PubMed]
6. Lenka, A.; Jankovic, J. Tremor Syndromes: An Updated Review. *Front. Neurol.* **2021**, *12*, 684835. [CrossRef] [PubMed]
7. Rajan, R.; Srivastava, A.K.; Anandapadmanabhan, R.; Saini, A.; Upadhyay, A.; Gupta, A.; Vishnu, V.Y.; Pandit, A.K.; Vibha, D.; Singh, M.B.; et al. Assessment of Botulinum Neurotoxin Injection for Dystonic Hand Tremor: A Randomized Clinical Trial. *JAMA Neurol.* **2021**, *78*, 302–311. [CrossRef] [PubMed]
8. Fasano, A.; Bove, F.; Lang, A.E. The treatment of dystonic tremor: A systematic review. *J. Neurol. Neurosurg. Psychiatry* **2014**, *85*, 759–769. [CrossRef] [PubMed]
9. Stacy, M.A.; Elble, R.J.; Ondo, W.G.; Wu, S.C.; Hulihan, J. Assessment of interrater and intrarater reliability of the Fahn-Tolosa-Marin Tremor Rating Scale in essential tremor. *Mov. Disord.* **2007**, *22*, 833–838. [CrossRef] [PubMed]
10. Elble, R.; Comella, C.; Fahn, S.; Hallett, M.; Jankovic, J.; Juncos, J.L.; Lewitt, P.; Lyons, K.; Ondo, W.; Pahwa, R.; et al. Reliability of a new scale for essential tremor. *Mov. Disord.* **2012**, *27*, 1567–1569. [CrossRef] [PubMed]
11. Tröster, A.I.; Pahwa, R.; Fields, J.A.; Tanner, C.M.; Lyons, K.E. Quality of life in Essential Tremor Questionnaire (QUEST): Development and initial validation. *Park. Relat. Disord.* **2005**, *11*, 367–373. [CrossRef] [PubMed]
12. Kiresuk, T.J.; Sherman, R.E. Goal attainment scaling: A general method for evaluating comprehensive community mental health programs. *Community Ment. Health J.* **1968**, *4*, 443–453. [CrossRef] [PubMed]
13. Brin, M.F.; Lyons, K.E.; Doucette, J.; Adler, C.H.; Caviness, J.N.; Comella, C.L.; Dubinsky, R.M.; Friedman, J.H.; Manyam, B.V.; Matsumoto, J.Y.; et al. A randomized, double masked, controlled trial of botulinum toxin type A in essential hand tremor. *Neurology* **2001**, *56*, 1523–1528. [CrossRef] [PubMed]
14. Jankovic, J.; Schwartz, K.; Clemence, W.; Aswad, A.; Mordaunt, J. A randomized, double-blind, placebo-controlled study to evaluate botulinum toxin type A in essential hand tremor. *Mov. Disord.* **1996**, *11*, 250–256. [CrossRef] [PubMed]
15. van der Walt, A.; Sung, S.; Spelman, T.; Marriott, M.; Kolbe, S.; Mitchell, P.; Evans, A.; Butzkueven, H. A double-blind, randomized, controlled study of botulinum toxin type A in MS-related tremor. *Neurology* **2012**, *79*, 92–99. [CrossRef] [PubMed]
16. Anandan, C.; Jankovic, J. Botulinum Toxin in Movement Disorders: An Update. *Toxins* **2021**, *13*, 42. [CrossRef] [PubMed]
17. Tsuboi, T.; Jabarkheel, Z.; Zeilman, P.R.; Barabas, M.J.; Foote, K.D.; Okun, M.S.; Wagle Shukla, A. Longitudinal follow-up with VIM thalamic deep brain stimulation for dystonic or essential tremor. *Neurology* **2020**, *94*, e1073–e1084. [CrossRef] [PubMed]

Disclaimer/Publisher's Note: The statements, opinions and data contained in all publications are solely those of the individual author(s) and contributor(s) and not of MDPI and/or the editor(s). MDPI and/or the editor(s) disclaim responsibility for any injury to people or property resulting from any ideas, methods, instructions or products referred to in the content.

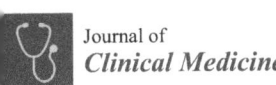

Review

Deep Brain Stimulation in the Treatment of Tardive Dyskinesia

Adrianna Szczakowska [1], Agata Gabryelska [2], Oliwia Gawlik-Kotelnicka [3] and Dominik Strzelecki [3],*

[1] Central Teaching Hospital, Medical University of Lodz, 92-213 Lodz, Poland
[2] Department of Sleep Medicine and Metabolic Disorders, Medical University of Lodz, 92-215 Lodz, Poland
[3] Department of Affective and Psychotic Disorders, Medical University of Lodz, 92-216 Lodz, Poland
* Correspondence: dominik.strzelecki@umed.lodz.pl; Tel.: +48-426757371

Abstract: Tardive dyskinesia (TD) is a phenomenon observed following the predominantly long-term use of dopamine receptor blockers (antipsychotics) widely used in psychiatry. TD is a group of involuntary, irregular hyperkinetic movements, mainly in the muscles of the face, eyelid, lips, tongue, and cheeks, and less frequently in the limbs, neck, pelvis, and trunk. In some patients, TD takes on an extremely severe form, massively disrupting functioning and, moreover, causing stigmatization and suffering. Deep brain stimulation (DBS), a method used, among others, in Parkinson's disease, is also an effective treatment for TD and often becomes a method of last resort, especially in severe, drug-resistant forms. The group of TD patients who have undergone DBS is still very limited. The procedure is relatively new in TD, so the available reliable clinical studies are few and consist mainly of case reports. Unilateral and bilateral stimulation of two sites has proven efficacy in TD treatment. Most authors describe stimulation of the globus pallidus internus (GPi); less frequent descriptions involve the subthalamic nucleus (STN). In the present paper, we provide up-to-date information on the stimulation of both mentioned brain areas. We also compare the efficacy of the two methods by comparing the two available studies that included the largest groups of patients. Although GPi stimulation is more frequently described in literature, our analysis indicates comparable results (reduction of involuntary movements) with STN DBS.

Keywords: tardive dyskinesia; schizophrenia; antipsychotics; deep brain stimulation

1. Introduction

Tardive dyskinesia (TD) is a group of symptoms characterized by irregular and involuntary movements that most commonly affect the tongue, lips, jaw, face, and sometimes the peri-orbital areas. In some cases, patients also have irregular movement of the trunk and limbs [1,2]. Tardive dyskinesia (TD) might be also present as tremor, akathisia, dystonia, chorea, tics, or as a combination of different types of abnormal movements. In addition to movement disorders (including involuntary vocalizations), TD patients may have various sensory symptoms, such as the urge to move (as in akathisia), pain, and paresthesia [3].

TD is a specific type of secondary dystonia, mainly caused by the chronic use of dopamine receptor antagonists. The onset of TD usually occurs after years of taking neuroleptics but may also appear earlier, even after several months. The risk is related, among others, to the strength of the drug binding to the dopaminergic D2 receptor. In the elderly, symptoms may become apparent after a shorter period of use of the drug, the early onset of these symptoms and their intensity may indicate features of organic brain damage [4]. Due to the need for long-term treatment, neuroleptics are the main reason for TD's appearance in clinical practice. Nevertheless, when using other antidopaminergic drugs such as antiemetics (domperidone, bromopride, and metoclopramide); antidepressants such as trazodone, amitriptyline, clomipramine, fluoxetine; and sertraline or calcium channel blockers, the risk of TD appearance, while significantly lower, should be highlighted [5].

Interestingly, tardive dyskinesia can appear both during the use and after the discontinuation of neuroleptics. The prevalence of tardive dyskinesia is estimated at 0.4–9% in patients receiving antipsychotics, while some studies indicate a more frequent occurrence of TD (20–50%) [6,7]. According to the DSM-5, TD can be diagnosed when antipsychotic-induced tardive dyskinesia follows exposure to neuroleptics for at least three months (one month in individuals aged ≥60 years) and persists for at least one month after the last dose of the drug [8]. This iatrogenic complication may persist long after drug discontinuation and might become permanent [1,6]. TD often results in disability, with mild to severe functional impairment (significantly impaired gait, speech, and swallowing) in about 10% of cases, causing a heavy burden on both patients and their caregivers [6]. In addition to physical burden and pain, tardive dyskinesia leads to social exclusion and ostracism in patients with these symptoms. The involuntary movements typical of TD are a significant burden for patients in a social context, representing one of the archetypal images of mental illness and a reason for stigmatization.

Aside from pharmacological interventions (changing the dose or the drug) or implementing TD-targeted treatment, there is a promising method that may offer new opportunities for this group of patients—deep brain stimulation (DBS). DBS is a clinical procedure in which a precisely controlled electric current is passed through electrodes surgically implanted in the brain. This method enables rapid and, more importantly, long-term improvement in motor function and quality of life (QoL) in patients with TD [1,5].

2. Etiology and Risk Factors

It is of key importance that TD has a genetic predisposition, which mediates the risk for TD development [5,9]. Nevertheless, the usage of dopamine receptor antagonists is responsible for the exposure of this predisposition [10,11]. Table 1 shows the factors associated with an increased risk of TD [12–19]. Table 2 summarizes the genetic factors that modulate the risk of TD [20–23].

Table 1. Nonmodifiable and modifiable risk factors of TD.

Nonmodifiable Factors	Modifiable Factors
Advanced age	Type of dopamine receptor blocking agents
Female sex	Duration of illness
Caucasian or African ethnicity	Dosage and length of exposure to a dopamine receptor blocker
Intellectual disability	Intermittent antipsychotic treatment
Brain damage	Anticholinergic treatment
	Smoking
Negative symptoms in schizophrenia	Alcohol and cocaine abuse/dependence
	Akathisia

The main pathogenetic mechanisms associated with the development of TD are the hypersensitivity of postsynaptic D2 receptors and their upregulation associated with their long-term blockade. This leads to changes in cortico-striatal transmission and motor symptoms [24]. The abnormalities also concern the increase in blood flow in the prefrontal cortex, the anterior cingulate gyrus, and the cerebellum, which accompany the increase in the activity of the prefrontal and premotor cortex during the appearance of involuntary movements, which may indicate a decrease in impulse selection and lead to the appearance of involuntary movements [25]. The constant blocking of D2 receptors along with D1 activation may also be important to explain the appearance of symptoms over a longer period of time and their irreversibility [26]. However, it seems that not only disorders of dopaminergic transmission are involved in the development of TD, but changes in serotonergic, glutamatergic, cholinergic, and opioid transmission may play a supportive role [27,28]. The involvement of the serotonin system in TD is indicated by studies on animal models. It was found that inhibition of serotonergic neurons with 8-OH-DPAT (8-hydroxy-

2-(dipropylamino)tetralin significantly reduces TD severity. 8-OH-DPAT is one of the first discovered agonists of the serotonergic 5-HT1A receptors. It mediates hyperpolarization and reduction of the firing rate of the postsynaptic neuron. Conversely, administration of fenfluramine or fluoxetine (both increasing the level of serotonin) suppressed the previously obtained improvement. Preclinical studies indicate that deep brain stimulation of the subthalamic nucleus (STN DBS), a technique described latter in this article, reduced the release of 5-HT in the hippocampus and prefrontal cortex, while deep brain stimulation of the EPN (entopeduncular nucleus, internal globus pallidus (GPi) equivalent in rodents) did not affect 5-HT release. Nevertheless, both STN and EPN DBS attenuate TD with equal effectiveness, despite their different effects on the 5-HT system, leading to the conclusion that the mechanism of 5-HT reduction does not determine the effectiveness of DBS in rats.

Table 2. Genes whose polymorphisms increase the risk of TD.

DRD2 and DRD3
HTR2A (5-HT2A receptors)
COMT
MnSOD
Cytochrome P450 (CYP2D6)
GSK-3ß
3′-Regulatory region of Nurr77 mRNA
SLC6A11, GABRB2, and GABRG3 related to GABAergic transmission
GRIN2A related to NMDA receptor and glutamatergic transmission
GSTM1, GSTP1, NOS3, and NQO1 involved in oxidative stress reactions
BDNF
GLI2
HSPG2

Genes DRD2 and DRD3—D2 and D3 receptor, D-dopamine; HTR2A-5—hydroxytryptamine receptor 2A, 5-HT–serotonin; COMT—catechol-O-methyl-transferase; MnSOD—manganese super dismutase; CYP2D6—cytochrome P450 2D6; GSK2ß—glycogen synthase kinase 2 beta; mRNA—messenger RNA; SLC6A11—solute carrier family 6 member 11; GABRB2—gamma-aminobutyric acid type A receptor subunit beta 2; GABRG3—gamma-aminobutyric acid type A-rho receptor subunit gamma 3; GABA—γ-aminobutyric acid; GRIN2A—glutamate ionotropic receptor NMDA type subunit 2A; NMDA—N-methyl-D-aspartate; GSTM1—glutathione S-transferase Mu 1; GSTP1—glutathione S-transferases P1; NOS3—nitric oxide synthase 3; NQO1—NAD(P)H quinone dehydrogenase 1; BDNF—brain-derived neurotrophic factor; GLI2—GLI family zinc finger 2; HSPG2—heparan sulfate proteoglycan 2.

Oxidative stress and related neuronal damage both might also participate in the etiology of TD. Antipsychotics, especially classic drugs, may be toxic by directly inhibiting complex I of the mitochondrial electron transport chain. Toxicity may also result from the increased production of free radicals and hydrogen peroxide, which are a consequence of the blockade of the D2 receptor and an increase in dopamine turnover [20,29,30]. The weakening of the antioxidant mechanisms may explain the progressive nature of the changes and their irreversibility [31–33]. In neuroimaging studies, a decrease in the caudate nucleus volume was observed in the group of patients diagnosed with schizophrenia with TD compared to those with this psychosis without dyskinesia [10,34,35].

3. Assessment Tools

The most widely used instrument to assess TD is the Abnormal Involuntary Movement Scale (AIMS). The patient performs several tasks described in the instructions. On that basis, the severity of facial and oral movements, extremity movements, trunk movements, and global judgments is scored on a 0–4 scale (up to 40 points in total) [36]. A separate evaluation concerns dental status (with an annotation yes/no). Another scale is The Burke–Fahn–Marsden Dystonia Rating Scale (BFMDRS), which consists of movement and disability subscales. This tool measures dystonia in nine body regions (incl. the eyes, mouth/speech and swallowing, neck, trunk, arms, and legs; each extremity is assessed individually) with scores ranging from 0 (lack of symptoms) to 120 [37].

4. Pharmacological Treatment

TD treatment is difficult and often leads to disappointing results, so the best method is to prevent its onset [38]. Atypical antipsychotics have a lower potential to cause TD. The drugs should be used in the lowest effective doses, particularly if TD appeared earlier or the current treatment induced its onset. When TD appears, initially, it is necessary to reduce the drug dose or, if this does not eliminate TD, switch to a drug with a lower potential for inducing TD, such as clozapine or quetiapine.

The pharmacological treatment of TD is challenging; conventionally administered pharmacotherapies are only beneficial at the initial stage, and the available data point to a lack of satisfactory outcomes in long-term use [6].

VMAT2 (vesicular monoamine transporter 2) inhibitors: tetrabenazine, valbenazine, and deutetrabenazine are the first drug group recommended for TD treatment [2]. In randomized controlled trials, valbenazine and deutetrabenazine demonstrated efficacy in ameliorating TD symptoms with a favorable benefit–risk ratio. For this reason, valbenazine and deutetrabenazine should be considered a first-line treatments for TD. While the currently available evidence suggests that tetrabenazine is another good option for TD, it is not considered a first-line drug due to greater side effects than other VMAT2 inhibitors and very few studies. Amantadine (300 mg per day) may be used when these treatments are ineffective or contraindicated. However, evidence to support the use of amantadine for TD is scarce and limited to short observations [2]. Another discussed treatment option is the short-term administration of clonazepam, but the effectiveness of this method is also limited. Furthermore, considering the acute and long-term consequences (sedation, cognitive decline, tolerance, addiction, and risk of falls, especially in the elderly), routine use of benzodiazepines is not recommended [2,6]. The use of Vitamin E does not improve TD symptoms but may prevent their worsening. When other options fail, some authors recommend pyridoxine (vitamin B6) use, but the optimal dose and treatment duration has not been established yet [2]. In focal dystonia, such as cervical dystonia, botulinum toxin injection may be applied. It is a highly effective approach, but the level of satisfaction with this treatment is low in some of the patients, and they fail to follow up for repeated injections. Therefore, the pharmacotherapeutic method should be regarded as adjuvant therapy instead of a priority choice (the dose reduction of the TD-inducing drug or change to another drug if possible) as the symptoms progress to the advanced stage [6]. The level B recommendations of the American Academy of Neurology for TD treatment indicate clonazepam, Gingko biloba extract (EGb-761), and diltiazem, while amantadine, tetrabenazine, galantamine, and eicosapentaenoic acid are level C. Other test substances, including reserpine, bromocriptine, biperiden, selegiline, vitamin E, vitamin B6, baclofen, and levetiracetam, have not received a recommendation from the academy at this stage [39]. Newer recommendations position new-generation VMAT2 inhibitors (deutetrabenazine and valbenazine) at level A of recommendation, clonazepam and Ginkgo biloba at level B, while amantadine, tetrabenazine, and GPi DBS (globus pallidus internus deep brain stimulation) are at level C [40]. The American Psychiatric Association (APA) indicates a reversible inhibitor of the VMAT2 (deutetrabenazine and valbenazine as more studied than tetrabenazine) as the first-line treatment for TD [41].

5. Deep Brain Stimulation

In recent decades, DBS has been successfully used to treat several movement disorders, including Parkinson's disease and dystonia. More recently, DBS has also been used to treat patients with tardive dyskinesia and OCD, especially in drug-resistant forms [6,7]. Monopolar (unilateral) stimulation modes are the most commonly used, although we also have descriptions of bipolar mode [42–46]. In addition to the potential for rapid and long-term improvement, the advantages of DBS include its relatively nondestructive nature, adjustability, reversibility, and the ability to perform DBS bilaterally in a single surgical session [6,47].

According to the available studies, this method is safe and minimally invasive, with no severe complications during the follow-up periods [6]. The disadvantages of the DBS technique are the requirement for continuous follow-up visits with repeated optimization of pacing parameters (it can also offer potential parameter adjustments) and the risk of hardware complications (incl. electrode displacement, battery depletion, inflammation around parts of the device) [47]. When the effectiveness of pharmacotherapeutic methods is unsatisfactory and symptoms are chronic and very severe, DBS becomes the treatment of last resort [48].

The primary criterion for inclusion in DBS is a high severity of symptoms that significantly impede function and have lasted for more than a year, with no satisfactory response to pharmacological treatment with clozapine or tetrabenazine for at least four weeks at the highest doses tolerated by the patient. Exclusion criteria are similar to those for patients with other dystonias—significant cognitive impairment, unstable mental status, severe depressive symptoms, and comorbid medical problems that may increase surgical risk; an initial brain scan before the decision on DBS applicability is recommended [45].

In addition to correct patient selection and electrode placement (more effective by image guidance or microelectrode recording implemented in leading centers), proper and time-coordinated programming of the equipment is crucial. This is important because we already have multisegment electrodes (from Abbott/St. Jude, Boston Scientific, and Medtronic), and each segment's current characteristics can be programmed separately. It complicates programming (current of different amplitude, frequency, amperage, and pulse width can be used) but certainly expands the possibilities for stimulation. Once the electrode has been placed, the adjustment of the electrical field optimizes the clinical outcome. It allows continuous monitoring of the effectiveness of the stimulation and provides an opportunity to implement modifications, but it becomes vital when the initially planned electrode placement has failed (in about 40%). The typical inaccuracy of surgical robots or stereotaxic methods is 1–2 mm. In addition, during surgery, the brain can change position by 2–4 mm, which can be minimized by a staged operation [49–58]. A similar problem arises when the electrode is displaced. Reprogramming often avoids reoperation and allows optimization of parameters if the dislocation is not critical [59,60]. It is worth adding that no clear guidelines have been developed so far, although there are recommendations regarding the programming of stimulators [61–63]. In programming, it is important to be aware of the temporal sequence of observed changes—not all symptoms respond to stimulation simultaneously. For example, during stimulation of the subthalamic nucleus in Parkinson's disease, first (in seconds) the tremor subsides, followed by rigidity (seconds–minutes), bradykinesia (minutes–hours), and axial symptoms (hours–days). These symptoms appear after the stimulation is turned off in the same order [64,65].

Previous research in TD patients has focused on the stimulation of two areas in the brain: the inner globus pallidus (GPi) and the subthalamic nucleus (STN) belonging to the basal ganglia. These nuclei belong to motor circuits, including cortico-thalamic-basal ganglia junctions, which are believed to be the morphological substrate of TD. Most projects focused on the stimulation of the GPi, the preferred target, while less is known about STN stimulation [4,6]. Nevertheless, both STN and GPi stimulation were shown to be beneficial in reducing TD [38].

5.1. Internal Globus Pallidus (GPi)

The primary target of GPi DBS is the posteroventrolateral part [46,47,66–69]. Several descriptions concern the stimulation of the posteroventromedial area [70,71]. Ventral parts of the posterior globus pallidus have a somatotopic organization associated with the motor cortex, which determines the goals of stimulation; the median part is related to the limbic cortex, while the dorsal area is associated with the prefrontal cortex [72].

Stereotactic techniques based on MRI (magnetic resonance imaging) or CT-MRI (a combination of CT and MRI techniques) help correct electrode placement [73]. The optimal electrode placement is typically within 19–22 mm lateral to the line between the anterior and posterior commissure, 4–6 mm inferior to that line, and 2–4 mm anterior to the mid-commissural point [45,46,67,71,74–79]. In one description, the electrode position corresponded to the somatotopic face area [80]. The most common practice uses microelectrode recordings (MERs) to detect discharges of neurons in the GPi and to order "noisy signals" with DBS. The most common stimulation parameters used were the voltage (amplitude) of the current (1.0–7.0 V) [43,67], frequency (60–185 Hz) [42,69,78,81], and pulse width (60–450 µs) [42,45,78,81–83]. A detailed list of electrodes used, voltages, location, and effectiveness of the treatments can be found in the study by Morigaki et al. [84]. With several exceptions of bipolar modes [42–46], other reports concern monopolar stimulations.

Much of the literature was single-patient reports [43,47,68,70,73–75,77,78,80,82,85–89], small groups of 2–4 people [46,48,67,69,71,79,90,91], or slightly larger groups [42,45,76,81,83,92–95], and 19 patients comprised the largest cohort [38] (Table 3).

Table 3. Basic parameters and outcomes from GPi DBS studies.

Author [Reference]	Localization	Mono-/Bipolar (N, When >1)	Scale (% of Improvement)/Follow Up (Months)
Pouclet-Courtemanche [38]	PV-GPi	M	AIMS (63)/12–132
Sako [42]	PV-GPi	M/B (5)	BFMDRS-M (58–100), BFMDRS-D (67–100)/3–49
Nandi [43]	PV-GPi	B	BFMDRS-M (28), BFMDRS-D (39), AIMS (42)/ 12
Gruber [45]	PVL-GPi	M/B (8)	BFMDRS-M (64-100), BFMDRS-D (25–100), AIMS (33–100)/26–80
Capelle [46]	PVL-GPi	B (4)	BFMDRS-M (70–91), BFMDRS-D (50–100)/16–36
Kim [47]	PVL-GPi	M	BFMDRS-M (97), BFMDRS-D (100)/20
Sobstyl [48]	PVL-GPi	B (2)	BFMDRS-M (69–78), BFMDRS-D (56–73)/12–24
Franzini [67]	PVL-GPi	M (2)	BFMDRS-M (86–88)/12
Kovacs [68]	PVL-GPi	?	BFMDRS-M (97), BFMDRS-D (96)/12
Starr [69]	PVL-GPi	? (4)	BFMDRS-M (6–100)/9–27
Trottenberg [70]	PV-GPi	M	BFMDRS-M (73), AIMS (54)/6
Hälbig [71]	PVM-GPi	M (2)	BFMDRS-M (77–93)/?
Spindler [73]	GPi	M	AIMS (67)/<60
Magariños-Ascone [74]	GPi	?	BFMDRS-M (48), BFMDRS-D (44)/12
Eltahawy [75]	PV-GPi	M	BFMDRS-M (60)/18
Trottenberg [76]	PVM-GPi	M (5)	BFMDRS-M (75–98), BFMDRS-D (80–100)/6
Katsakiori [77]	GPi	M	BFMDRS-M (94), BFMDRS-D (84)/12
Kefalopoulou [78]	GPi	M	BFMDRS-M (91), AIMS (77)/6
Krause [79]	GPi	M (3)	BFMDRS-M (−1–0), no benefit/≤36
Kosel [80]	GPi	M	BFMDRS-M (35)/18
Shaikh [81]	GPi	M (8)	BFMDRS-M (67–100)/6–60
Schrader [82]	GPi	M	AIMS (63)/ 5
Egidi [83]	GPi	M	BFMDRS-M (47), BFMDRS-D (55)/?
Pretto [85]	GPi	B	BFMDRS (~90)/6

Table 3. Cont.

Author [Reference]	Localization	Mono-/Bipolar (N, When >1)	Scale (% of Improvement)/Follow Up (Months)
Boulogne [86]	PVL-GPi	M	AIMS (79)/120
Trinh [87]	GPi	?	BFMDRS-M (90), BFMDRS-D (87)/18
Puri [88]	GPi	?	AIMS (55)/6
Ogata [89]	PL-GPi	B	BFMDRS-M (69), BFMDRS-D (64), AIMS (94)/7
Woo [90]	PV-GPi	M (3)	BFMDRS-M (54–100)/3–120
Cohen [91]	GPi	M (2)	BFMDRS-M (63–88), BFMDRS-D (53–100)/7–13
Damier [92]	PVL-GPi	M (10)	AIMS (33–78)/6
Chang [93]	PV-GPi	M	BFMDRS-M (71), BFMDRS-D (48), AIMS (77)/27–76
Krause [94]	GPi	B (7)	BFMDRS-M (90), BFMDRS-D (79), AIMS (73)/63–171
Koyama [95]	GPi	B (12)	BFMDRS (78)/6–186

GPi—internal globus pallidus; DBS—deep brain stimulation; PV—posteroventral, PVL—posteroventral lateral; PVM—posteroventral medial; PL—posterolateral; AIMS—Abnormal Involuntary Movement Scale; BFMDRS-M—Burke–Fahn–Marsden Dystonia Rating Scale, movement subscale; BFMDRS-D—Burke–Fahn–Marsden Dystonia Rating Scale, disability subscale; BFMDRS—Burke–Fahn–Marsden Dystonia Rating Scale, total score; ?—data not provided.

5.1.1. Motor Effects of GPi DBS

The reported efficacy (reduction in dystonia scores) ranges from 28% to 100%, with most reports showing ≧60% improvement, with a follow-up period of up to 11 years [38]. Improvement is described as stable even after 4-year follow up. In addition to improvement in symptoms, most investigators consistently report a significantly favorable change in the quality of life and daily functioning. Nevertheless, there are also descriptions of no overall change in this area [45,96].

Clinical responses appear either during the surgical procedure and the first activation of stimulation or in the first days after turning on the equipment [45,46,67,68,70,76,86,91]. If clinical responses are observed shortly after switching on the device, we can precisely program the equipment at the outset; in other cases, patient adjustments are carried out at follow-up visits or via the Internet, more recently [97]. The manufacturer recommends the lowest sufficient stimulator settings, combining optimal performance with less load and then longer battery life or less frequent recharging.

Changes in the treatment of choreiform dyskinesia are noted earlier, tonic postural dystonia responds later, symptoms improve gradually, and changes are observed after weeks or even months of stimulation [44,46,75,86,91–93]. In fixed dystonias, the efficacy of GPi DBS is lower [42,45,67,81].

5.1.2. Side Effects of GPi DBS

Despite its invasiveness, DBS is characterized by a low number of complications and is considered a safe, effective, and well-tolerated method [4]. The frequency of all side effects reaches 9%. Observations of nonmotor effects are very rare. DBS may induce transient affective states (mild to moderate depressive syndrome in most cases); the authors also emphasized some increase in suicidal risk [73,98]. However, at longer follow up, there was an improvement in mood, which could also be explained by relief from the burden of motor symptoms, disability, or social impact [38,45,76,80,99]. In one study, six months after treatment, one patient had a brief psychotic episode, and another patient had symptomatic improvement allowing the discontinuation of antipsychotic drugs [76]. Contrary to the first reports, the negative influence of continuous pallidal (GPi) DBS on cognitive functions has not been confirmed [38,45,71], while one study notes improvement [99].

The procedure of implanting the electrode (in both locations, GPi and STN) is associated with the possibility of incorrect placement or electrode displacement, infections, pain associated with the connection cable, intracranial hemorrhage, and seizure. Gait and balance disturbances contributing to falls have also been observed. These disturbances were transient and resolved after the optimization of DBS parameters [38]. The GPi is involved in speech fluency; thus, slowing, halting, and imprecise oral articulation and reduced voicing control are common symptoms during DBS in this area. Bilateral DBS induces more speech difficulties [100]. Dysarthria occurs in almost 30% of patients; severe cases may require speech therapy [38]. Despite the complications being infrequent, the risk–benefit ratio always needs to be weighed. DBS becomes the last resort in patients with severe TD when symptoms are severe, functioning is significantly impaired, and other treatment options are insufficient. Table 4 shows the most common side effects, along with the structures whose stimulation is responsible for their appearance.

Table 4. Side effects of GPi DBS and the areas whose stimulation is responsible for these symptoms.

Side Effect	Brain Area
Mood and cognitive symptoms	Ventral part of GPi
Motor side effects (corticospinal and corticobulbar side, i.e., tonic muscle contractions)	Posterior part of GPi/capsular fibers
Phosphenes (seeing light without light entering the eye)	Ventral/optic tract
Low threshold for capsular side effects (i.e., muscle contractions)	Medial GPi
Speech impairment	Internal capsule, medial and posterior to GPi

GPi—globus pallidus internus.

5.2. Subthalamic Nucleus (STN)

The subthalamic nucleus (STN), belonging to the basal ganglia, was the first neurosurgical target in the treatment of dystonia (thalamotomy), but data about STN DBS in treating TD are still scarce. Less frequent use is, among others, related to psychiatric complications (depression, suicidality, mania, and impulse-control problems) observed during DBS of this brain structure in patients with Parkinson's disease. The best control of motor symptoms is provided by stimulation of the sensorimotor (dorsolateral) area of the STN [101].

5.2.1. Motor Symptoms of STN DBS

So far, only a limited number of cases of STN DBS for TD have been reported. In addition to the Deng study, which we will discuss later [6], Zhang et al. published a description of a series of nine patients treated with STN DBS for secondary dystonia (two with tardive dystonia) [102]. In one case, the dystonia following neuroleptic treatment improved by 92% in the BFMDRS 3 months after stimulator implementation. Long-term observation of one of those patients with severe TD dystonic symptoms initially is described by Meng et al.; the patient had no neurological symptoms after 144 months (6 and 12 years after the operation BFMDRS total score was 0) [4]. Another study (12 patients with primary dystonia and 2 with TD) using STN DBS showed improvement ranging from 76 to 100% in the BFMDRS [103]. One patient underwent DBS electrode placement in the left and right STN with a near-complete resolution of tremors [104] (data summarized in Table 5).

Table 5. Basic parameters and outcomes from STN DBS studies.

Author [Reference]	Localization	Mono-/Bipolar (N, When >1)	Scale (% of Improvement) /Follow Up (Months)
Deng [6]	STN	B (10)	BFMDRS (88), AIMS (94)/12–105
Zhang [102]	STN	B (2)	BFMDRS (>90)/3–36
Sun [103]	STN	B (2)	AIMS (63) BFMDRS (>77)/6–42
Kashyap [104]	STN	B	?, "near-complete resolution of tremors"/24

STN—subthalamic nucleus; DBS—deep brain stimulation; BFMDRS—Burke-Fahn-Marsden Dystonia Rating Scale, total score; AIMS—Abnormal Involuntary Movement Scale; ?—data not provided.

5.2.2. Side Effects of STN DBS

The anatomical location of the STN is very close to several functionally significant areas. Therefore, the induced side effects are also associated with stimulating adjacent nuclei and nerve tracts. Table 6 presents the most common side effects with the postulated structures responsible for their appearance. Due to the lack of detailed descriptions regarding TD, the table lists observations during STN DBS in Parkinson's disease.

Table 6. Side effects and the brain area surrounding STN, which stimulation may be responsible for the appearance of symptoms.

Side Effect	Brain Area
Spastic muscle contraction	Internal capsule
Uni- or bilateral gaze deviation	Fibers stemming from the frontal eye field running in the internal capsule, fibers of the third nerve (inferomedial to the STN and within the red nucleus), sympathetic fibers within the zona incerta or STN
Autonomic symptoms	Hypothalamus and red nucleus
Paresthesia	Medial lemniscus
Speech impairment	Internal capsule, the pallidal and cerebello-thalamic fiber tracts medial and dorsal of the STN, medial left-sided STN stimulation in right-handed patients, higher left STN voltage
Depression	Substantia nigra
Mania	Medial and ventral areas of STN
Impulse control disorder	Ventromedial and limbic areas of STN, SNr, medial forebrain bundle
Cognitive problems	Ventral and medial parts of STN, perforation of the caudate nucleus during surgery

STN—subthalamic nucleus, SNr—substantia nigra pars reticulata.

5.3. Internal Globus Pallidus (GPi) and Subthalamic Nucleus (STN) DBS Comparison

Authors suggest better results for STN DBS using lower stimulation parameters than in GPi DBS, but no studies compared the effects of DBS in the two areas. In the following section, we will compare the results of two studies of the GPi and STN involving the largest groups of TD patients.

The largest study evaluating the efficacy of GPi DBS is by Pouclet-Courtemanche et al. It originally included 19 patients, while 18 reached a 6-month follow up, 14 participants were assessed at long-term follow up (6–11 years) [38]. Meanwhile, Deng et al. analyzed STN DBS results in a group of 10 patients, with all included evaluations at 6 months and long-term follow up (12–105 months) [6]. The aforementioned time points were common for both studies among other follow-up lengths. Furthermore, the mutual form of assessment of motor symptoms was only the AIMS. We compared the effectiveness of DBS at the different sites using a two-sample z-test for proportions. In the case of the study by Pouclet-Courtemanche et al., no median/mean data for the AIMS score were available at all time points. Regardless, the calculation of proportions was possible based on the graph analysis presenting a change in the AIMS score at the different follow ups. For the 6-month follow-up time point, the proposition was 0.49 ($n = 18$) and 0.15 ($n = 10$) for the GPi DBS and the STN DBS, respectively. In the comparison, the difference did not reach statistical significance with $p = 0.079$, mostly due to the small sample sizes in both studies, as the trend is visible (Figure 1). We did perform a statistical analysis of a long-term follow up due to a disparity in the observation period, which could affect the result.

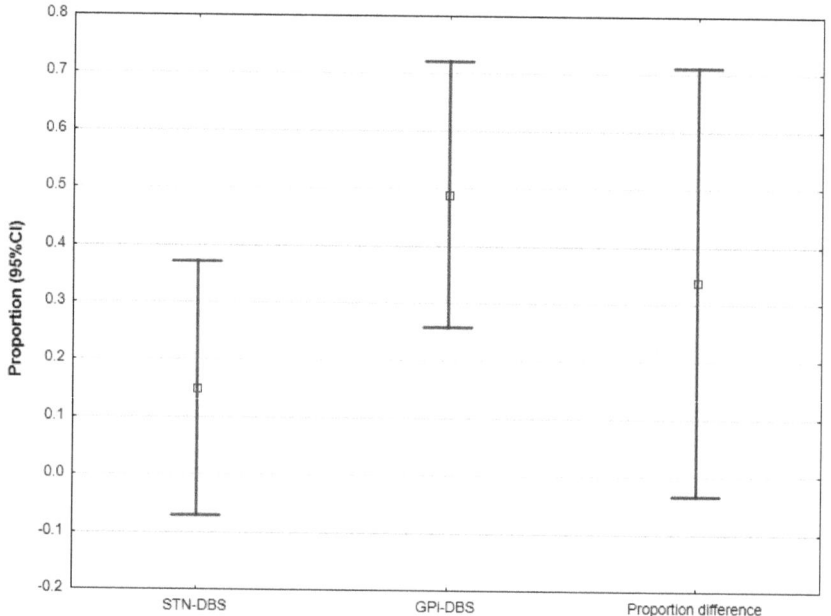

Figure 1. Proportion comparison of AIMS score (initial evaluation to 6-months follow up) between STN DBS and GPi DBS. AIMS—Abnormal Involuntary Movement Scale, DBS—deep brain stimulation, GPi—internal globus pallidus, STN—subthalamic nucleus.

6. Discussion

Deep brain stimulation (DBS) is an established treatment for patients with tardive dyskinesia when pharmacological therapy alone does not provide sufficient relief or is associated with disabling side effects. With this method, patients achieve satisfactory results in both the short and long term, with a relatively small number of complications. As we previously mentioned, the main sites with proven efficacy of stimulation are the subthalamic nucleus (STN) and internal globus pallidus (GPi). Although the GPi remains the standard stimulation target, our comparison in small groups shows at least comparable efficacy of STN and GPi DBS, including 6-month follow up. Similar conclusions come from comparisons of the two methods in PD [105]. However, further research is needed to confirm this conclusion, also because the trend may indicate an advantage for STN DBS. DBS studies in PD allow some conclusions that may also apply to the treatment of TD with this method. The advantage of GPi stimulation lies in the possibility of effective use of the electrode unilaterally and somewhat easier optimization of current parameter programming. On the other hand, some researchers report that STN DBS may be less likely to cause adverse symptoms in mood, cognitive function, gait, and speech [106]. The GPi is occasionally indicated as the preferred target in treating oral TD and dystonia, while STN DBS could be considered an effective and safe procedure in patients with predominant tardive Parkinsonism and/or tardive tremor [104].

In contrast, studies by Sun et al. indicate some advantages of STN DBS stimulation in dystonias, including TD. According to these authors, symptomatic improvement begins immediately after stimulation, which allows for a quick selection of the best stimulation parameters. The stimulation parameters used for the GPi are higher than those used during STN DBS, resulting in longer battery life for STN DBS (longer intervals between charges). According to the authors, STN DBS results in better symptomatic control than GPi DBS in dystonia patients (compared to data obtained by other teams) [103].

To broaden knowledge and outline plans for necessary research, it is worth looking at solutions employed in DBS procedures in patients with other health problems. DBS is a method that has been implemented for years in various conditions such as dystonia, Parkinson's disease, and obsessive–compulsive disorder. This method is also recommended for patients with severe and treatment-resistant forms of the disease. It is noteworthy that the STN is the standard site of stimulation in PD [107]. According to the symptomatic profile of PD, preferences include alternative targets, e.g., the thalamic ventral intermediate nucleus (VIM) or the GPi. Recent research in this area has focused on the search for other sites of stimulation such as the posterior subthalamic area (PSA) or the caudal zona incerta (cZi). The PSA is located ventrally to the VIM, between the red nucleus and the STN. PSA DBS is not significantly different from VIM DBS in suppressing tremor, but clinical benefit from PSA DBS is attained at lower stimulation amplitudes [108]. Furthermore, several open-label studies have shown a good effect in the reduction of PD symptoms with DBS in the caudal zona incerta (cZi) [109].

While both TD and PD treatment have the same standard stimulation sites, it is worth investigating other experimental stimulation sites in TD treatment, such as the PSA or the cZi, or finding new targets. Treatment of refractory TD with DBS is not a low-cost method, requiring an experienced neurosurgical team and precise instrumentation. It is also not a life-saving method, but, if we want to have a full range of possible medical procedures that may expand our understanding of the brain (we consider it crucial), this research must be continued and intensified. The latest technical achievements in the field of construction of stimulators and electrodes, e.g., modeling the shape of the impact field, as well as the results of new studies focused on the paths connecting the gray matter of various brain regions allow us to expect discoveries in research using DBS, hopefully also in TD.

Author Contributions: Conceptualization, D.S.; methodology, D.S.; validation, D.S.; formal analysis, A.S., A.G. and D.S.; investigation, A.G. and D.S.; resources, D.S.; data curation, A.G. and D.S.; writing—original draft preparation, A.S., A.G. and D.S.; writing—review and editing, A.G., O.G.-K. and D.S.; visualization, A.G. and D.S.; supervision, D.S.; project administration, D.S.; funding acquisition, D.S. All authors have read and agreed to the published version of the manuscript.

Funding: This research received no external funding.

Institutional Review Board Statement: Not applicable.

Informed Consent Statement: Not applicable.

Data Availability Statement: Not applicable.

Conflicts of Interest: The authors declare no conflict of interest.

References

1. Creed, M.C.; Hamani, C.; Bridgman, A.; Fletcher, P.J.; Nobrega, J.N. Contribution of decreased serotonin release to the antidyskinetic effects of deep brain stimulation in a rodent model of tardive dyskinesia: Comparison of the subthalamic and entopeduncular nuclei. *J. Neurosci.* **2012**, *32*, 9574–9581. [CrossRef] [PubMed]
2. Ricciardi, L.; Pringsheim, T.; Barnes, T.R.E.; Martino, D.; Gardner, D.; Remington, G.; Addington, D.; Morgante, F.; Poole, N.; Carson, A.; et al. Treatment Recommendations for Tardive Dyskinesia. *Can. J. Psychiatry* **2019**, *64*, 388–399. [CrossRef] [PubMed]

3. Waln, O.; Jankovic, J. An update on tardive dyskinesia: From phenomenology to treatment. *Tremor Other Hyperkinetic Mov.* **2013**, *3*, tre-03-161-4138-1. [CrossRef]
4. Meng, D.W.; Liu, H.G.; Yang, A.C.; Zhang, K.; Zhang, J.G. Long-term effects of subthalamic nucleus deep brain stimulation in tardive dystonia. *Chin. Med. J.* **2016**, *129*, 1257–1258. [CrossRef] [PubMed]
5. Frei, K. Tardive dyskinesia: Who gets it and why. *Park. Relat. Disord.* **2019**, *59*, 151–154. [CrossRef]
6. Deng, Z.D.; Li, D.Y.; Zhang, C.C.; Pan, Y.X.; Zhang, J.; Jin, H.; Zeljec, K.; Zhan, S.K.; Sun, B.M. Long-term follow-up of bilateral subthalamic deep brain stimulation for refractory tardive dystonia. *Park. Relat. Disord.* **2017**, *41*, 58–65. [CrossRef]
7. Carroll, B.; Irwin, D.E. Health care resource utilization and costs for patients with tardive dyskinesia. *J. Manag. Care Spec. Pharm.* **2019**, *25*, 810–816. [CrossRef]
8. Citrome, L.; Isaacson, S.H.; Larson, D.; Kremens, D. Tardive dyskinesia in older persons taking antipsychotics. *Neuropsychiatry Dis. Treat.* **2021**, *17*, 3127–3134. [CrossRef]
9. Lerner, V.; Miodownik, C. Motor symptoms of schizophrenia: Is tardive dyskinesia a symptom or side effect? A modern treatment. *Curr. Psychiatry Rep.* **2011**, *13*, 295–304. [CrossRef]
10. Sarró, S.; Pomarol-Clotet, E.; Canales-Rodríguez, E.J.; Salvador, R.; Gomar, J.J.; Ortiz-Gil, J.; Landín-Romero, R.; Vila-Rodríguez, F.; Blanch, J.; McKenna, P.J. Structural brain changes associated with tardive dyskinesia in schizophrenia. *Br. J. Psychiatry* **2013**, *203*, 51–57. [CrossRef]
11. Whitty, P.F.; Owoeye, O.; Waddington, J.L. Neurological signs and involuntary movements in schizophrenia: Intrinsic to and informative on systems pathobiology. *Schizophr. Bull.* **2009**, *35*, 415–424. [CrossRef]
12. Zhang, J.P.; Malhotra, A.K. Pharmacogenetics and antipsychotics: Therapeutic efficacy and side effects prediction. *Expert Opin. Drug Metab. Toxicol.* **2011**, *7*, 9–37. [CrossRef] [PubMed]
13. Lee, H.J.; Kang, S.G. Genetics of tardive dyskinesia. In *International Review of Neurobiology*; Elsevier: Amsterdam, The Netherlands, 2011; Volume 98.
14. Thelma, B.K.; Srivastava, V.; Tiwari, A.K. Genetic underpinnings of tardive dyskinesia: Passing the baton to pharmacogenetics. *Pharmacogenomics* **2008**, *9*, 1285–1306. [CrossRef] [PubMed]
15. Bakker, P.R.; Van Harten, P.N.; Van Os, J. Antipsychotic-induced tardive dyskinesia and polymorphic variations in COMT, DRD2, CYP1A2 and MnSOD genes: A meta-analysis of pharmacogenetic interactions. *Mol. Psychiatry* **2008**, *13*, 544–556. [CrossRef] [PubMed]
16. Åberg, K.; Adkins, D.E.; Bukszár, J.; Webb, B.T.; Caroff, S.N.; Miller, D.D.; Sebat, J.; Stroup, S.; Fanous, A.H.; Vladimirov, V.I.; et al. Genomewide Association Study of Movement-Related Adverse Antipsychotic Effects. *Biol. Psychiatry* **2010**, *67*, 279–282. [CrossRef] [PubMed]
17. Inada, T.; Koga, M.; Ishiguro, H.; Horiuchi, Y.; Syu, A.; Yoshio, T.; Takahashi, N.; Ozaki, N.; Arinami, T. Pathway-based association analysis of genome-wide screening data suggest that genes associated with the γ-aminobutyric acid receptor signaling pathway are involved in neuroleptic-induced, treatment-resistant tardive dyskinesia. *Pharm. Genom.* **2008**, *18*, 317–323. [CrossRef]
18. Greenbaum, L.; Alkelai, A.; Rigbi, A.; Kohn, Y.; Lerer, B. Evidence for association of the *GLI2* gene with tardive dyskinesia in patients with chronic schizophrenia. *Mov. Disord.* **2010**, *25*, 2809–2817. [CrossRef]
19. Syu, A.; Ishiguro, H.; Inada, T.; Horiuchi, Y.; Tanaka, S.; Ishikawa, M.; Arai, M.; Itokawa, M.; Niizato, K.; Iritani, S.; et al. Association of the HSPG2 gene with neuroleptic-induced tardive dyskinesia. *Neuropsychopharmacology* **2010**, *35*, 1155–1164. [CrossRef]
20. Aquino, C.C.H.; Lang, A.E. Tardive dyskinesia syndromes: Current concepts. *Park. Relat. Disord.* **2014**, *20*, S113–S117. [CrossRef]
21. Ferentinos, P.; Dikeos, D. Genetic correlates of medical comorbidity associated with schizophrenia and treatment with antipsychotics. *Curr. Opin. Psychiatry* **2012**, *25*, 381–390. [CrossRef]
22. Souza, R.P.; Remington, G.; Chowdhury, N.I.; Lau, M.K.; Voineskos, A.N.; Lieberman, J.A.; Meltzer, H.Y.; Kennedy, J.L. Association study of the GSK-3B gene with tardive dyskinesia in European Caucasians. *Eur. Neuropsychopharmacol.* **2010**, *20*, 688–694. [CrossRef]
23. Ethier, I.; Kagechika, H.; Shudo, K.; Rouillard, C.; Lévesque, D. Docosahexaenoic acid reduces haloperidol-induced dyskinesias in mice: Involvement of Nur77 and retinoid receptors. *Biol. Psychiatry* **2004**, *56*, 522–526. [CrossRef] [PubMed]
24. Teo, J.T.; Edwards, M.J.; Bhatia, K. Tardive dyskinesia is caused by maladaptive synaptic plasticity: A hypothesis. *Mov. Disord.* **2012**, *27*, 1205–1215. [CrossRef] [PubMed]
25. Thobois, S.; Poisson, A.; Damier, P. Surgery for tardive dyskinesia. In *International Review of Neurobiology*; Elsevier: Amsterdam, The Netherlands, 2011; Volume 98.
26. Trugman, J.M.; Leadbetter, R.; Zalis, M.E.; Burgdorf, R.O.; Wooten, G.F. Treatment of severe axial tardive dystonia with clozapine: Case report and hypothesis. *Mov. Disord.* **1994**, *9*, 441–446. [CrossRef] [PubMed]
27. Tsai, G.; Goff, D.C.; Chang, R.W.; Flood, J.; Baer, L.; Coyle, J.T. Markers of glutamatergic neurotransmission and oxidative stress associated with tardive dyskinesia. *Am. J. Psychiatry* **1998**, *155*, 1207–1213. [CrossRef]
28. Lu, R.B.; Ko, H.C.; Lin, W.L.; Lin, Y.T.; Ho, S.L. CSF neurochemical study of tardive dyskinesia. *Biol. Psychiatry* **1989**, *25*, 717–724.
29. Hori, H.; Ohmori, O.; Shinkai, T.; Kojima, H.; Okano, C.; Suzuki, T.; Nakamura, J. Manganese superoxide dismutase gene polymorphism and schizophrenia: Relation to tardive dyskinesia. *Neuropsychopharmacology* **2000**, *23*, 170–177. [CrossRef]

30. Cloud, L.J.; Zutshi, D.; Factor, S.A. Tardive Dyskinesia: Therapeutic Options for an Increasingly Common Disorder. *Neurotherapeutics* **2014**, *11*, 166–176. [CrossRef]
31. Cho, C.H.; Lee, H.J. Oxidative stress and tardive dyskinesia: Pharmacogenetic evidence. *Prog. Neuro-Psychopharmacol. Biol. Psychiatry* **2013**, *46*, 207–213. [CrossRef]
32. Elkashef, A.M.; Wyatt, R.J. Tardive dyskinesia: Possible involvement of free radicals and treatment with vitamin E. *Schizophr. Bull.* **1999**, *25*, 731–740. [CrossRef]
33. Sachdev, P.; Saharov, T.; Cathcart, S. The preventative role of antioxidants (selegiline and vitamin E) in a rat model of tardive dyskinesia. *Biol. Psychiatry* **1999**, *46*, 1672–1681. [CrossRef]
34. Bartels, M.; Themelis, J. Computerized tomography in tardive dyskinesia—Evidence of structural abnormalities in the basal ganglia system. *Archiv Für Psychiatrie UND Nervenkrankheiten Vereinigt MIT Zeitschrift Für Die Gesamte Neurologie UND Psychiatrie* **1983**, *233*, 371–379. [CrossRef]
35. Mion, C.C.; Andreasen, N.C.; Arndt, S.; Swayze, V.W.; Cohen, G.A. MRI abnormalities in tardive dyskinesia. *Psychiatry Res. Neuroimaging* **1991**, *40*, 157–166. [CrossRef]
36. Guy, W.; Ban, T.A.; Wilson, W.H. The prevalence of abnormal involuntary movements among chronic schizophrenic. *Int. Clin. Psychopharmacol.* **1986**, *1*, 134–144. [CrossRef] [PubMed]
37. Burke, R.E.; Fahn, S.; Marsden, C.D.; Bressman, S.B.; Moskowitz, C.; Friedman, J. Validity and reliability of a rating scale for the primary torsion dystonias. *Neurology* **1985**, *35*, 73. [CrossRef] [PubMed]
38. Pouclet-Courtemanche, H.; Rouaud, T.; Thobois, S.; Nguyen, J.M.; Brefel-Courbon, C.; Chereau, I.; Cuny, E.; Derost, P.; Eusebio, A.; Guehl, D.; et al. Long-term efficacy and tolerability of bilateral pallidal stimulation to treat tardive dyskinesia. *Neurology* **2016**, *86*, 651–659. [CrossRef] [PubMed]
39. Bhidayasiri, R.; Fahn, S.; Weiner, W.J.; Gronseth, G.S.; Sullivan, K.L.; Zesiewicz, T.A. Evidence-based guideline: Treatment of tardive syndromes: Report of the Guideline Development Subcommittee of the American Academy of Neurology. *Neurology* **2013**, *81*, 463–469. [CrossRef]
40. Bhidayasiri, R.; Jitkritsadakul, O.; Friedman, J.H.; Fahn, S. Updating the recommendations for treatment of tardive syndromes: A systematic review of new evidence and practical treatment algorithm. *J. Neurol. Sci.* **2018**, *389*, 67–75. [CrossRef]
41. American Psychiatric Association. *The American Psychiatric Association Practice Guideline for the Treatment of Patients with Schizophrenia*; American Psychiatric Association: Washington, DC, USA, 2020.
42. Sako, W.; Goto, S.; Shimazu, H.; Murase, N.; Matsuzaki, K.; Tamura, T.; Mure, H.; Tomogane, Y.; Arita, N.; Yoshikawa, H.; et al. Bilateral deep brain stimulation of the globus pallidus internus in tardive dystonia. *Mov. Disord.* **2008**, *23*, 1929–1931. [CrossRef]
43. Nandi, D.; Parkin, S.; Scott, R.; Winter, J.L.; Joint, C.; Gregory, R.; Stein, J.; Aziz, T.Z. Camptocormia treated with bilateral pallidal stimulation: Case report. *Neurosurg. Focus* **2002**, *97*, 461–466.
44. Yianni, J.; Bain, P.; Giladi, N.; Auca, M.; Gregory, R.; Joint, C.; Nandi, D.; Stein, J.; Scott, R.; Aziz, T. Globus pallidus internus deep brain stimulation for dystonic conditions: A prospective audit. *Mov. Disord.* **2003**, *18*, 436–442. [CrossRef] [PubMed]
45. Gruber, D.; Trottenberg, T.; Kivi, A.; Schoenecker, T.; Kopp, U.A.; Hoffmann, K.T.; Schneider, G.H.; Kühn, A.A.; Kupsch, A. Long-term effects of pallidal deep brain stimulation in tardive dystonia. *Neurology* **2009**, *73*, 53–58. [CrossRef] [PubMed]
46. Capelle, H.H.; Blahak, C.; Schrader, C.; Baezner, H.; Kinfe, T.M.; Herzog, J.; Dengler, R.; Krauss, J.K. Chronic deep brain stimulation in patients with tardive dystonia without a history of major psychosis. *Mov. Disord.* **2010**, *25*, 1477–1481. [CrossRef] [PubMed]
47. Kim, J.P.; Chang, W.S.; Chang, J.W. Treatment of secondary dystonia with a combined stereotactic procedure: Long-term surgical outcomes. *Acta Neurochir.* **2011**, *153*, 2319–2328. [CrossRef] [PubMed]
48. Sobstyl, M.; Ząbek, M.; Mossakowski, Z.; Zaczyński, A. Deep brain stimulation of the internal globus pallidus for disabling haloperidol-induced tardive dystonia. Report of two cases. *Neurol. Neurochir. Pol.* **2016**, *50*, 258–261. [CrossRef]
49. Mobin, F.; De Salles, A.A.F.; Behnke, E.J.; Frysinger, R. Correlation between MRI-based stereotactic thalamic deep brain stimulation electrode placement, macroelectrode stimulation and clinical response to tremor control. *Stereotact. Funct. Neurosurg.* **1999**, *72*, 225–232. [CrossRef] [PubMed]
50. Patel, N.K.; Plaha, P.; O'Sullivan, K.; McCarter, R.; Heywood, P.; Gill, S.S. MRI directed bilateral stimulation of the subthalamic nucleus in patients with Parkinson's disease. *J. Neurol. Neurosurg. Psychiatry* **2003**, *74*, 1631–1637. [CrossRef]
51. Burchiel, K.J.; McCartney, S.; Lee, A.; Raslan, A.M. Accuracy of deep brain stimulation electrode placement using intraoperative computed tomography without microelectrode recording. *J. Neurosurg.* **2013**, *119*, 301–306. [CrossRef]
52. Von Langsdorff, D.; Paquis, P.; Fontaine, D. In vivo measurement of the frame-based application accuracy of the Neuromate neurosurgical robot. *J. Neurosurg.* **2015**, *122*, 191–194. [CrossRef]
53. Lefranc, M.; Capel, C.; Pruvot, A.S.; Fichten, A.; Desenclos, C.; Toussaint, P.; Le Gars, D.; Peltier, J. The impact of the reference imaging modality, registration method and intraoperative flat-panel computed tomography on the accuracy of the ROSA® stereotactic robot. *Stereotact. Funct. Neurosurg.* **2014**, *92*, 242–250. [CrossRef]
54. D'haese, P.F.; Pallavaram, S.; Konrad, P.E.; Neimat, J.; Fitzpatrick, J.M.; Dawant, B.M. Clinical accuracy of a customized stereotactic platform for deep brain stimulation after accounting for brain shift. *Stereotact. Funct. Neurosurg.* **2010**, *88*, 81–87. [CrossRef]

55. Bjartmarz, H.; Rehncrona, S. Comparison of accuracy and precision between frame-based and frameless stereotactic navigation for deep brain stimulation electrode implantation. *Stereotact. Funct. Neurosurg.* **2007**, *85*, 235–242. [CrossRef] [PubMed]
56. Winkler, D.; Tittgemeyer, M.; Schwarz, J.; Preul, C.; Strecker, K.; Meixensberger, J. The first evaluation of brain shift during functional neurosurgery by deformation field analysis. *J. Neurol. Neurosurg. Psychiatry* **2005**, *76*, 1161–1163. [CrossRef] [PubMed]
57. Khan, M.F.; Mewes, K.; Gross, R.E.; Škrinjar, O. Assessment of brain shift related to deep brain stimulation surgery. *Stereotact. Funct. Neurosurg.* **2007**, *86*, 44–53. [CrossRef] [PubMed]
58. Hunsche, S.; Sauner, D.; Maarouf, M.; Poggenborg, J.; Lackner, K.; Sturm, V.; Treuer, H. Intraoperative X-ray detection and MRI-based quantification of brain shift effects subsequent to implantation of the first electrode in bilateral implantation of deep brain stimulation electrodes. *Stereotact. Funct. Neurosurg.* **2009**, *87*, 322–329. [CrossRef]
59. Okun, M.S.; Tagliati, M.; Pourfar, M.; Fernandez, H.H.; Rodriguez, R.L.; Alterman, R.L.; Foote, K.D. Management of Referred Deep Brain Stimulation Failures. *Arch. Neurol.* **2005**, *62*, 1250–1255. [CrossRef] [PubMed]
60. Moro, E.; Poon, Y.Y.W.; Lozano, A.M.; Saint-Cyr, J.A.; Lang, A.E. Subthalamic nucleus stimulation: Improvements in outcome with reprogramming. *Arch. Neurol.* **2006**, *63*, 1266–1272. [CrossRef] [PubMed]
61. Volkmann, J.; Herzog, J.; Kopper, F.; Geuschl, G. Introduction to the programming of deep brain stimulators. *Mov. Disord.* **2002**, *17*, S181–S187. [CrossRef]
62. Volkmann, J.; Moro, E.; Pahwa, R. Basic algorithms for the programming of deep brain stimulation in Parkinson's disease. *Mov. Disord.* **2006**, *21*, S284–S289. [CrossRef]
63. Bronstein, J.M.; Tagliati, M.; Alterman, R.L.; Lozano, A.M.; Volkmann, J.; Stefani, A.; Horak, F.B.; Okun, M.S.; Foote, K.D.; Krack, P.; et al. Deep brain stimulation for Parkinson disease an expert consensus and review of key issues. *Arch. Neurol.* **2011**, *68*, 165. [CrossRef]
64. Temperli, P.; Ghika, J.; Villemure, J.G.; Burkhard, P.R.; Bogousslavsky, J.; Vingerhoets, F.J.G. How do parkinsonian signs return after discontinuation of subthalamic DBS? *Neurology* **2003**, *60*, 78–81. [CrossRef] [PubMed]
65. Levin, J.; Krafczyk, S.; Valkovič, P.; Eggert, T.; Claassen, J.; Bötzel, K. Objective measurement of muscle rigidity in Parkinsonian patients treated with subthalamic stimulation. *Mov. Disord.* **2009**, *24*, 57–63. [CrossRef]
66. Thobois, S.; Ballanger, B.; Xie-Brustolin, J.; Damier, P.; Durif, F.; Azulay, J.P.; Derost, P.; Witjas, T.; Raoul, S.; Le Bars, D.; et al. Globus pallidus stimulation reduces frontal hyperactivity in tardive dystonia. *J. Cereb. Blood Flow Metab.* **2008**, *28*, 1127–1138. [CrossRef] [PubMed]
67. Franzini, A.; Marras, C.; Ferroli, P.; Zorzi, G.; Bugiani, O.; Romito, L.; Broggi, G. Long-term high-frequency bilateral pallidal stimulation for neuroleptic-induced tardive dystonia: Report of two cases. *J. Neurosurg.* **2005**, *102*, 721–725. [CrossRef] [PubMed]
68. Kovacs, N.; Balas, I.; Janszky, J.; Simon, M.; Fekete, S.; Komoly, S. Status dystonicus in tardive dystonia successfully treated by bilateral deep brain stimulation. *Clin. Neurol. Neurosurg.* **2011**, *113*, 808–809. [CrossRef] [PubMed]
69. Starr, P.A.; Turner, R.S.; Rau, G.; Lindsey, N.; Heath, S.; Volz, M.; Ostrem, J.L.; Marks, W.J. Microelectrode-guided implantation of deep brain stimulators into the globus pallidus internus for dystonia: Techniques, electrode locations, and outcomes. *J. Neurosurg.* **2006**, *104*, 488–501. [CrossRef]
70. Trottenberg, T.; Paul, G.; Meissner, W.; Maier-Hauff, K.; Taschner, C.; Kupsch, A. Pallidal and thalamic neurostimulation in severe tardive dystonia. *J. Neurol. Neurosurg. Psychiatry* **2001**, *70*, 557–559. [CrossRef]
71. Hälbig, T.D.; Gruber, D.; Kopp, U.A.; Schneider, G.H.; Trottenberg, T.; Kupsch, A. Pallidal stimulation in dystonia: Effects on cognition, mood, and quality of life. *J. Neurol. Neurosurg. Psychiatry* **2005**, *76*, 1713–1716. [CrossRef]
72. Nambu, A. Somatotopic organization of the primate basal ganglia. *Front. Neuroanat.* **2011**, *5*, 26. [CrossRef]
73. Spindler, M.A.; Galifianakis, N.B.; Wilkinson, J.R.; Duda, J.E. Globus pallidus interna deep brain stimulation for tardive dyskinesia: Case report and review of the literature. *Park. Relat. Disord.* **2013**, *19*, 141–147. [CrossRef]
74. Magariños-Ascone, C.M.; Regidor, I.; Gómez-Galán, M.; Cabañes-Martínez, L.; Figueiras-Méndez, R. Deep brain stimulation in the globus pallidus to treat dystonia: Electrophysiological characteristics and 2 years' follow-up in 10 patients. *Neuroscience* **2008**, *152*, 558–571. [CrossRef]
75. Eltahawy, H.A.; Feinstein, A.; Khan, F.; Saint-Cyr, J.; Lang, A.E.; Lozano, A.M. Bilateral globus pallidus internus deep brain stimulation in tardive dyskinesia: A case report. *Mov. Disord.* **2004**, *19*, 969–972. [CrossRef] [PubMed]
76. Trottenberg, T.; Volkmann, J.; Deuschl, G.; Kühn, A.A.; Schneider, G.H.; Müller, J.; Alesch, F.; Kupsch, A. Treatment of severe tardive dystonia with pallidal deep brain stimulation. *Neurology* **2005**, *64*, 344–346. [CrossRef]
77. Katsakiori, P.F.; Kefalopoulou, Z.; Markaki, E.; Paschali, A.; Ellul, J.; Kagadis, G.C.; Chroni, E.; Constantoyannis, C. Deep brain stimulation for secondary dystonia: Results in 8 patients. *Acta Neurochir.* **2009**, *151*, 473–478. [CrossRef] [PubMed]
78. Kefalopoulou, Z.; Paschali, A.; Markaki, E.; Vassilakos, P.; Ellul, J.; Constantoyannis, C. A double-blind study on a patient with tardive dyskinesia treated with pallidal deep brain stimulation. *Acta Neurol. Scand.* **2009**, *119*, 269–273. [CrossRef] [PubMed]
79. Krause, M.; Fogel, W.; Kloss, M.; Rasche, D.; Volkmann, J.; Tronnier, V. Pallidal stimulation for dystonia. *Neurosurgery* **2004**, *55*, 1361–1370. [CrossRef]
80. Kosel, M.; Sturm, V.; Frick, C.; Lenartz, D.; Zeidler, G.; Brodesser, D.; Schlaepfer, T.E. Mood improvement after deep brain stimulation of the internal globus pallidus for tardive dyskinesia in a patient suffering from major depression. *J. Psychiatry Res.* **2007**, *41*, 801–803. [CrossRef]

81. Shaikh, A.G.; Mewes, K.; DeLong, M.R.; Gross, R.E.; Triche, S.D.; Jinnah, H.A.; Boulis, N.; Willie, J.T.; Freeman, A.; Alexander, G.E.; et al. Temporal profile of improvement of tardive dystonia after globus pallidus deep brain stimulation. *Park. Relat. Disord.* **2015**, *21*, 116–119. [CrossRef]
82. Schrader, C.; Peschel, T.; Petermeyer, M.; Dengler, R.; Hellwig, D. Unilateral deep brain stimulation of the internal globus pallidus alleviates tardive dyskinesia. *Mov. Disord.* **2004**, *19*, 583–585. [CrossRef] [PubMed]
83. Egidi, M.; Franzini, A.; Marras, C.; Cavallo, M.; Mondani, M.; Lavano, A.; Romanelli, P.; Castana, L.; Lanotte, M.; Farneti, M. A survey of Italian cases of dystonia treated by deep brain stimulation. *J. Neurosurg. Sci.* **2007**, *51*, 153.
84. Morigaki, R.; Mure, H.; Kaji, R.; Nagahiro, S.; Goto, S. Therapeutic perspective on tardive syndrome with special reference to deep brain stimulation. *Front. Psychiatry* **2016**, *7*, 207. [CrossRef] [PubMed]
85. Pretto, T.E.; Dalvi, A.; Kang, U.J.; Penn, R.D. A prospective blinded evaluation of deep brain stimulation for the treatment of secondary dystonia and primary torticollis syndromes. *J. Neurosurg.* **2008**, *109*, 405–409. [CrossRef] [PubMed]
86. Boulogne, S.; Danaila, T.; Polo, G.; Broussolle, E.; Thobois, S. Relapse of tardive dystonia after globus pallidus deep-brain stimulation discontinuation. *J. Neurol.* **2014**, *261*, 1636–1637. [CrossRef] [PubMed]
87. Trinh, B.; Ha, A.D.; Mahant, N.; Kim, S.D.; Owler, B.; Fung, V.S.C. Dramatic improvement of truncal tardive dystonia following globus pallidus pars interna deep brain stimulation. *J. Clin. Neurosci.* **2014**, *21*, 515–517. [CrossRef] [PubMed]
88. Puri, M.; Albassam, A.; Silver, B. Deep brain stimulation in the treatment of tardive dyskinesia. *Psychiatr. Ann.* **2014**, *44*, 123–125. [CrossRef]
89. Ogata, E.; Ogura, M.; Nishibayashi, H.; Sasaki, T.; Kakishita, K.; Nakao, N. GPi-DBS for tardive dystonia: A case report. *Jpn. J. Neurosurg.* **2014**, *23*, 348–353. [CrossRef]
90. Woo, P.Y.M.; Chan, D.T.M.; Zhu, X.L.; Yeung, J.H.M.; Chan, A.Y.Y.; Au, A.C.W.; Cheng, K.M.; Lau, K.Y.; Wing, Y.K.; Mok, V.C.T.; et al. Pallidal deep brain stimulation: An effective treatment in chinese patients with tardive dystonia. *Hong Kong Med. J.* **2014**, *20*, 455–459. [CrossRef]
91. Cohen, O.S.; Hassin-Baer, S.; Spiegelmann, R. Deep brain stimulation of the internal globus pallidus for refractory tardive dystonia. *Park. Relat. Disord.* **2007**, *13*, 541–544. [CrossRef]
92. Damier, P.; Thobois, S.; Witjas, T.; Cuny, E.; Derost, P.; Raoul, S.; Mertens, P.; Peragut, J.C.; Lemaire, J.J.; Burbaud, P.; et al. Bilateral deep brain stimulation of the globus pallidus to treat tardive dyskinesia. *Arch. Gen. Psychiatry* **2007**, *64*, 170–176. [CrossRef]
93. Chang, E.F.; Schrock, L.E.; Starr, P.A.; Ostrem, J.L. Long-term benefit sustained after bilateral pallidal deep brain stimulation in patients with refractory tardive dystonia. *Stereotact. Funct. Neurosurg.* **2010**, *88*, 304–310. [CrossRef]
94. Krause, P.; Kroneberg, D.; Gruber, D.; Koch, K.; Schneider, G.H.; Kühn, A.A. Long-term effects of pallidal deep brain stimulation in tardive dystonia: A follow-up of 5–14 years. *J. Neurol.* **2022**, *269*, 3563–3568. [CrossRef] [PubMed]
95. Koyama, H.; Mure, H.; Morigaki, R.; Miyamoto, R.; Miyake, K.; Matsuda, T.; Fujita, K.; Izumi, Y.; Kaji, R.; Goto, S.; et al. Long-term follow-up of 12 patients treated with bilateral pallidal stimulation for tardive dystonia. *Life* **2021**, *11*, 477. [CrossRef] [PubMed]
96. Mentzel, C.L.; Tenback, D.E.; Tijssen, M.A.J.; Visser-Vandewalle, V.E.R.M.; Van Harten, P.N. Efficacy and safety of deep brain stimulation in patients with medication-induced tardive dyskinesia and/or dystonia: A systematic review. *J. Clin. Psychiatry* **2012**, *73*, 1434–1438. [CrossRef] [PubMed]
97. Krauss, J.K.; Lipsman, N.; Aziz, T.; Boutet, A.; Brown, P.; Chang, J.W.; Davidson, B.; Grill, W.M.; Hariz, M.I.; Horn, A.; et al. Technology of deep brain stimulation: Current status and future directions. *Nat. Rev. Neurol.* **2021**, *17*, 75–87. [CrossRef]
98. Foncke, E.M.J.; Schuurman, P.R.; Speelman, J.D. Suicide after deep brain stimulation of the internal globus pallidus for dystonia. *Neurology* **2006**, *66*, 142–143. [CrossRef]
99. de Gusmao, C.M.; Pollak, L.E.; Sharma, N. Neuropsychological and psychiatric outcome of GPi-deep brain stimulation in dystonia. *Brain Stimul.* **2017**, *10*, 994–996. [CrossRef]
100. Chiu, S.Y.; Tsuboi, T.; Hegland, K.W.; Herndon, N.E.; Shukla, A.W.; Patterson, A.; Almeida, L.; Foote, K.D.; Okun, M.S.; Ramirez-Zamora, A. Dysarthria and Speech Intelligibility following Parkinson's Disease Globus Pallidus Internus Deep Brain Stimulation. *J. Park. Dis.* **2020**, *10*, 1493–1502. [CrossRef]
101. Zhang, F.; Wang, F.; Li, W.; Wang, N.; Han, C.; Fan, S.; Li, P.; Xu, L.; Zhang, J.; Meng, F. Relationship between electrode position of deep brain stimulation and motor symptoms of Parkinson's disease. *BMC Neurol.* **2021**, *21*, 847. [CrossRef] [PubMed]
102. Zhang, J.; Zhang, K.; Wang, Z.; Ge, M.; Ma, Y. Deep brain stimulation in the treatment of secondary dystonia. *Chin. Med. J.* **2006**, *119*, 2069–2074. [CrossRef]
103. Sun, B.; Chen, S.; Zhan, S.; Le, W.; Krahl, S.E. Subthalamic nucleus stimulation for primary dystonia and tardive dystonia. *Acta Neurochir. Suppl.* **2007**, *97*, 207–214. [CrossRef] [PubMed]
104. Kashyap, S.; Ceponiene, R.; Savla, P.; Bernstein, J.; Ghanchi, H.; Ananda, A. Resolution of tardive tremor after bilateral subthalamic nucleus deep brain stimulation placement. *Surg. Neurol. Int.* **2020**, *11*, 444. [CrossRef] [PubMed]
105. Celiker, O.; Demir, G.; Kocaoglu, M.; Altug, F.; Acar, F. Comparison of subthalamic nucleus vs. globus pallidus interna deep brain stimulation in terms of gait and balance; A two year follow-up study. *Turk. Neurosurg.* **2019**, *29*, 355–361. [CrossRef] [PubMed]
106. Au, K.L.K.; Wong, J.K.; Tsuboi, T.; Eisinger, R.S.; Moore, K.; Lopes, J.L.M.L.J.; Holland, M.T.; Holanda, V.M.; Peng-Chen, Z.; Patterson, A.; et al. Globus Pallidus Internus (GPi) Deep Brain Stimulation for Parkinson's Disease: Expert Review and Commentary. *Neurol. Ther.* **2021**, *10*, 7–30. [CrossRef] [PubMed]
107. Karl, J.A.; Ouyang, B.; Goetz, S.; Metman, L.V. A Novel DBS Paradigm for Axial Features in Parkinson's Disease: A Randomized Crossover Study. *Mov. Disord.* **2020**, *35*, 1369–1378. [CrossRef]

108. Barbe, M.T.; Reker, P.; Hamacher, S.; Franklin, J.; Kraus, D.; Dembek, T.A.; Becker, J.; Steffen, J.K.; Allert, N.; Wirths, J.; et al. DBS of the PSA and the VIM in essential tremor. *Neurology* **2018**, *91*, e543–e550. [CrossRef]
109. Blomstedt, P.; Persson, R.S.; Hariz, G.M.; Linder, J.; Fredricks, A.; Häggström, B.; Philipsson, J.; Forsgren, L.; Hariz, M. Deep brain stimulation in the caudal zona incerta versus best medical treatment in patients with Parkinson's disease: A randomised blinded evaluation. *J. Neurol. Neurosurg. Psychiatry* **2018**, *89*, 710–716. [CrossRef]

Disclaimer/Publisher's Note: The statements, opinions and data contained in all publications are solely those of the individual author(s) and contributor(s) and not of MDPI and/or the editor(s). MDPI and/or the editor(s) disclaim responsibility for any injury to people or property resulting from any ideas, methods, instructions or products referred to in the content.

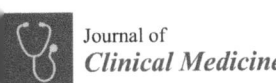

Article

Treatment Changes and Prognoses in Patients with Incident Drug-Induced Parkinsonism Using a Korean Nationwide Healthcare Claims Database

Siin Kim [1,2] and Hae Sun Suh [1,2,3,*]

[1] College of Pharmacy, Kyung Hee University, Seoul 02447, Republic of Korea; siin@khu.ac.kr
[2] Institute of Regulatory Innovation through Science, Kyung Hee University, Seoul 02447, Republic of Korea
[3] Department of Regulatory Science, Graduate School, Kyung Hee University, Seoul 02447, Republic of Korea
* Correspondence: haesun.suh@khu.ac.kr

Abstract: This retrospective cohort study assessed treatment changes and prognoses after incident drug-induced parkinsonism (DIP). We used the National Health Insurance Service's National Sample Cohort database in South Korea. We selected patients diagnosed with incident DIP and given prescriptions to take offending drugs (antipsychotics, gastrointestinal (GI) motility drugs, or flunarizine) for a period of time that overlapped with the time of DIP diagnosis during 2004–2013. The proportion of patients experiencing each type of treatment change and prognosis was assessed for 2 years after DIP diagnosis. We identified 272 patients with incident DIP (51.9% of patients were aged ≥ 60 years and 62.5% of them were women). Switching (38.4%) and reinitiation (28.8%) were the most common modifications in GI motility drug users, whereas dose adjustment (39.8%) and switching (23.0%) were common in antipsychotic users. The proportion of persistent users was higher among antipsychotic users (7.1%) than that among GI motility drug users (2.1%). Regarding prognosis, 26.9% of patients experienced DIP recurrence or persistence, the rate being the highest in persistent users and the lowest in patients who discontinued the drug. Among patients with incident DIP diagnoses, the patterns of treatment change and prognosis differed across the types of offending drugs. Over 25% of patients experienced DIP recurrence or persistence, highlighting the need for an effective strategy to prevent DIP.

Keywords: antipsychotics; drug-induced parkinsonism; metoclopramide; parkinsonism; prognosis; treatment pattern

Citation: Kim, S.; Suh, H.S. Treatment Changes and Prognoses in Patients with Incident Drug-Induced Parkinsonism Using a Korean Nationwide Healthcare Claims Database. *J. Clin. Med.* **2023**, *12*, 2860. https://doi.org/10.3390/jcm12082860

Academic Editor: Lazzaro di Biase

Received: 15 March 2023
Revised: 7 April 2023
Accepted: 12 April 2023
Published: 13 April 2023

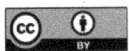

Copyright: © 2023 by the authors. Licensee MDPI, Basel, Switzerland. This article is an open access article distributed under the terms and conditions of the Creative Commons Attribution (CC BY) license (https://creativecommons.org/licenses/by/4.0/).

1. Introduction

Drug-induced parkinsonism (DIP) is a parkinsonian syndrome induced by medications that inhibit dopamine function in the brain categorized as secondary parkinsonism [1,2]. Compared with Parkinson's disease, DIP is characterized by acute, symmetrical, and reversible symptoms [3]. However, it is difficult to completely distinguish the two diseases in clinical practice, leading to misdiagnosis and inappropriate management [4].

Antipsychotics, gastrointestinal (GI) motility drugs, dopamine depleters, and calcium channel blockers are well-known offending drugs which pose a high risk of developing DIP [1–3,5]. Although typical antipsychotics have been known to pose a high risk of developing DIP, atypical antipsychotics and GI motility drugs, especially levosulpiride and metoclopramide, also have a risk level comparable to that of typical antipsychotics [6].

As DIP is generally under-recognized in clinical settings, its true incidence may be much higher [7,8]. Nevertheless, DIP is the second most common cause of parkinsonism after Parkinson's disease [9]. In South Korea, the incidence of DIP increased from 2012 to 2015, reaching 13.9 per 100,000 person-years, with a particularly high incidence among middle-aged individuals [10]. A retrospective study using nationwide hospital-based data in China reported a higher comorbidity burden and hospitalization expenses among patients with secondary parkinsonism than that among patients with Parkinson's disease, suggesting the considerable economic burden of secondary parkinsonism [11]. As one of the main adverse drug reactions related to antipsychotics, DIP can result in decreased health-related quality of life and working memory performance in patients with schizophrenia [12,13]. In these patients, DIP is associated with increased healthcare resource utilization (e.g., hospitalization and emergency room visits) and higher costs of care, and can hinder the optimal treatment with antipsychotics [14,15]. Moreover, patients with DIP had a significantly increased risk of developing Parkinson's disease, which can add the burden of managing of Parkinson's disease for patients with DIP [16].

Avoiding offending drugs is the most effective way of preventing or treating DIP [1,8]. DIP is generally resolved within 4 months if patients stop taking the offending drugs [17]. However, some patients may be unable to avoid taking offending drugs, as the expected clinical benefits may outweigh the risk of DIP [8]. Furthermore, some patients may experience persistent symptoms even after the discontinuation of the offending drugs [8,17]. Considering the growing number of patients being prescribed offending drugs, the effective management of DIP is essential to minimize the societal and economic burden of adverse drug reactions [18]. To seek an effective strategy to manage DIP, it is important to understand the current treatment patterns and prognoses in patients with DIP. However, the evidence for the management status of DIP is very scant, and the evidence reported so far is based on old data or a limited patient group [17,19].

Therefore, this study aimed to explore the status of treatment changes and prognoses after the occurrence of incident DIP using a representative Korean national claims database. We followed-up on patients who had experienced incident DIP for 2 years, and assessed the treatment changes and prognoses associated with three major types of offending drugs: antipsychotics, GI motility drugs, and flunarizine.

2. Materials and Methods

2.1. Study Design and Data Source

We conducted a retrospective cohort study using the National Health Insurance Service's National Sample Cohort (NHIS-NSC; NHIS-2018-2-238) database of South Korea from 1 January 2002 to 31 December 2015. The NHIS provides single-payer coverage to the entirety of Korea's population through the National Health Insurance program (97%) and Medical Aid program (3%) [20]. The National Health Insurance program covers employees and self-employed individuals, while the Medical Aid program is administered by the Korean government as a public assistance scheme that safeguards the basic livelihood of individuals with low incomes by offering healthcare services. The NHIS-NSC database comprises longitudinal information on demographic characteristics, diagnoses, healthcare service uses, and healthcare costs among a representative sample (approximately 1 million citizens) from the general Korean population [21]. This study was exempt from a review from the Institutional Review Board (IRB) of Pusan National University (PNU IRB/2016_29_HR).

2.2. Selection of Incident DIP Cases

We identified individuals diagnosed with DIP (International Classification of Diseases, Tenth Revision (ICD-10) codes G21.1 (other drug-induced secondary parkinsonism) or G25.1 (drug-induced tremor)) as the primary or secondary diagnosis between 1 January 2004 and 31 December 2013 (Figure 1). The earliest date of DIP diagnosis was defined as the index date. At least one outpatient prescription for the offending drug was required to be for a time period that overlapped the index date. Offending drugs included typical and atypical antipsychotics (amisulpride, aripiprazole, chlorpromazine, clozapine, haloperidol, olanzapine, paliperidone, perphenazine, pimozide, quetiapine, risperidone, sulpiride, and ziprasidone), GI motility drugs (clebopride, domperidone, itopride, levosulpiride, metoclopramide, and mosapride), and flunarizine, which were available in South Korea during the study period. To identify incident DIP cases, patients with DIP diagnoses preceding the index date by up to two years were excluded from the study.

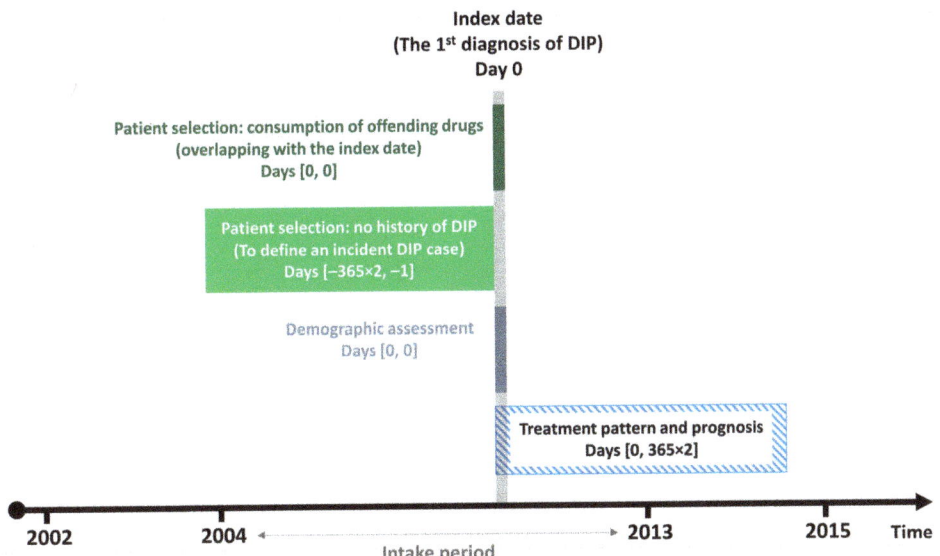

Figure 1. Study design scheme. Abbreviations: DIP, drug-induced parkinsonism.

2.3. Outcome Measures

To explore the treatment changes in the consumption of offending drugs and prognoses of DIP, individuals with incident DIP were followed-up for 2 years from the index date. The first treatment change for each patient was defined based on the pattern in which the offending drugs were prescribed (Table 1). The types of treatment changes included discontinuation, dose adjustment, persistent use, reinitiation, and switching to other offending drugs. Each treatment change was mutually exclusive. A continued use of offending drugs was defined as having consecutive prescriptions with a gap period of ≤60 days. Replacing drugs with drugs from the same therapeutic class (i.e., antipsychotics, GI motility drugs, and flunarizine) was considered switching, while replacing drugs with drugs from other therapeutic classes was considered temporary discontinuation. For example, replacing metoclopramide with domperidone was considered an act of switching to other offending drugs, while replacing metoclopramide with nizatidine (histamine type 2 receptor antagonists) was considered an act of temporary discontinuation. As a switch to other offending drugs was required to occur within consecutive prescriptions, a switch after a temporary discontinuation was regarded as reinitiation in this study.

Table 1. Definitions of treatment change and prognosis after incident drug-induced parkinsonism.

Category	Definition
Treatment change in consumption of offending drugs	
Discontinuation	Absence of new prescription for more than 60 days
Dose adjustment	Altering the dose of the offending drugs
Persistent use	Continued use of the offending drug without any temporary discontinuation, dose adjustment, or switching
Reinitiation	Restarting the discontinued drug, or switching within a therapeutic class after temporary discontinuation
Switching to other offending drugs	Altering drugs within a therapeutic class

Table 1. *Cont.*

Category	Definition
Prognosis of DIP	
Persisting DIP	Continuation of DIP diagnosis
Recurrence of DIP	Occurrence of DIP diagnosis after a remittance
Remittance of DIP	Absence of new diagnosis of DIP over 4 months

Abbreviations: DIP, drug-induced parkinsonism.

The first prognosis for each patient was defined based on the pattern of DIP diagnosis, and categorized into persisting DIP, DIP recurrence, and DIP remittance. An episode of DIP was considered a remittance if no further DIP was diagnosed over 4 months based on the published literature [8,17]. In other words, consecutive prescriptions with a DIP diagnosis within 4 months were considered part of the same episode of DIP.

We estimated the proportion of patients with each type of treatment change and prognosis. The proportion was calculated among all patients with incident DIP and for each therapeutic class (i.e., antipsychotics, GI motility drugs, and flunarizine). We estimated the time from the index date to the first treatment change, DIP remittance, and DIP recurrence. The time to event was analyzed in patients who experienced each type of event. For example, we estimated the time to remittance in patients who had previously experienced remittance during the follow-up period. Additionally, the proportion of patients with each type of prognosis was categorized by the type of treatment change to compare the proportion of DIP remittance across the types of treatment change.

We assessed the baseline characteristics of the study population, including demographic characteristics (age, sex, type of health insurance, income deciles, and presence of disability) as of the index date, clinical characteristics (Charlson comorbidity index (CCI) within 1 year and Parkinson's disease within 2 years) before the index date, and the type of offending drugs on the index date [22]. The definition of Parkinson's disease was established by utilizing ICD-10 code G20 (Parkinson's disease) for either the primary or secondary diagnosis.

2.4. Statistical Analysis

The baseline characteristics of patients with incident DIP and all outcome variables were analyzed descriptively as means, standard deviations, medians, and interquartile ranges (IQRs) for continuous variables, or as proportions for categorical variables. All analyses were performed using SAS Enterprise Guide version 7.1 (SAS Institute Inc., Cary, NC, USA).

3. Results

3.1. Baseline Characteristics of the Study Population

We identified 1252 patients diagnosed with DIP between 1 January 2004 and 31 December 2013, and 42 patients were excluded because of the presence of a history of DIP diagnosis within two years from the index date. Among them, 272 patients who were prescribed offending drugs to be taken for a period that overlapped the index date were selected as the study population. Approximately half of the selected patients were aged $\geq$ 60 years, and 62.5% were women (Table 2). The proportion of National Medical Aid beneficiaries among the study population was 7.4%, which was higher than that among the total NHIS-NSC population (2–3%). Parkinson's disease was diagnosed in 15.4% of the study population. Most patients (95.2%) received GI motility drugs or antipsychotics as the offending drugs.

Table 2. Baseline characteristics of patients with drug-induced parkinsonism.

Characteristics	DIP Patients (n = 272)
Age (years)	
0–19	10 (3.7%)
20–29	28 (10.3%)
30–39	25 (9.2%)
40–49	31 (11.4%)
50–59	37 (13.6%)
60–69	53 (19.5%)
70–79	68 (25%)
80+	20 (7.4%)
Sex	
Male	102 (37.5%)
Female	170 (62.5%)
Type of health insurance	
National Health Insurance program	252 (92.6%)
National Medical Aid program	20 (7.4%)
Income deciles [1]	
0	21 (7.7%)
1	20 (7.4%)
2	15 (5.5%)
3	18 (6.6%)
4	23 (8.5%)
5	17 (6.3%)
6	23 (8.5%)
7	25 (9.2%)
8	19 (7.0%)
9	36 (13.2%)
10	55 (20.2%)
Disability	
No disability	225 (82.7%)
Mild disability	32 (11.8%)
Severe disability	15 (5.5%)
Comorbidities	
Charlson comorbidity index, mean (SD)	2.2 (2.3)
Parkinson's disease	42 (15.4%)
Offending drugs	
Antipsychotics	146 (53.7%)
GI motility drugs	113 (41.5%)
Flunarizine	13 (4.8%)

Abbreviations: DIP, drug-induced parkinsonism; GI, gastrointestinal; SD, standard deviation. [1] Income deciles were defined based on health insurance contributions. The values 0 and 10 denote the lowest and highest deciles, respectively.

3.2. Treatment Patterns after Incident DIP Diagnosis

Among all the patients, the most common modification after the occurrence of incident drug-induced parkinsonism (DIPs) was switching to other offending drugs (30.2%), followed by dose adjustment (26.1%), reinitiation (21.3%), and discontinuation (18.0%) (Figure 2). Notably, 4.4% of patients consistently received offending drugs. Of the patients who discontinued offending drugs, 69.4% discontinued taking these drugs right after DIP occurrence. More than half of the patients who reinitiated offending drugs chose another drug within the same therapeutic class (56.9%), while 32.8% restarted the same drug at the same dose. Male patients had a higher proportion of discontinuation (20.3% vs. 16.5%) and a lower proportion of reinitiation (19.6% vs. 22.4%) and dose adjustment (24.5% vs. 27.1%) compared to female patients.

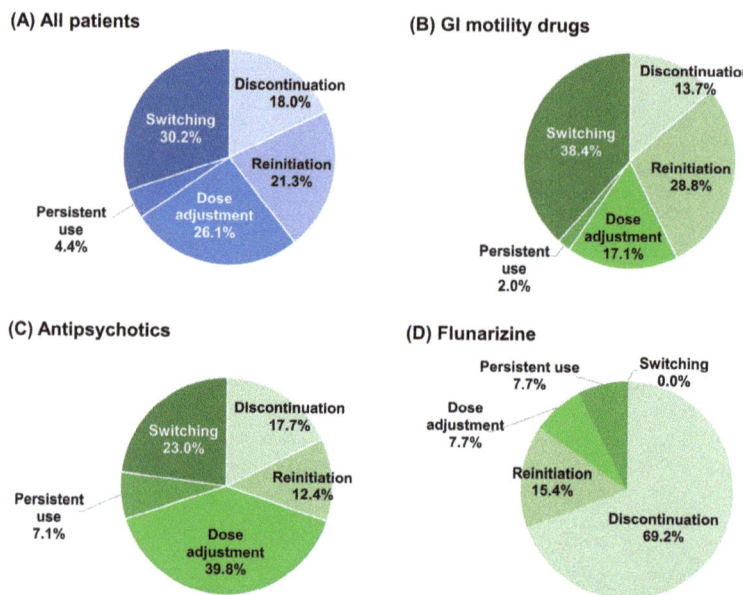

Figure 2. Treatment patterns after the occurrence of incident drug-induced parkinsonism. Abbreviations: GI, gastrointestinal.

Treatment patterns differed according to the type of drug used. Most patients taking GI motility drugs switched to other GI motility drugs (38.4%) or reinitiated drugs after temporary discontinuation (28.8%). Among the patients who reinitiated drugs, 61.9% initiated other kinds of GI motility drugs, while 38.1% initiated the same drug with or without dose adjustment (11.9% and 26.2%, respectively). Patients taking antipsychotics mostly adjusted the dose of antipsychotics (39.8%) or switched to other antipsychotics (23.0%). The proportion of patients who persistently used offending drugs was higher in antipsychotic users (7.1%) than in GI motility drug users (2.0%). Most patients taking flunarizine discontinued the drug (69.2%).

The median time to the first treatment modification was 42.0 days (an IQR of 17.0 to 166.0 days and a mean of 113.3 days), 61.0 days (an IQR of 22.0 to 191.0 days and a mean of 125.2 days), 31.0 days (an IQR of 14.0 to 97.0 days and a mean of 101.9 days), and 25.0 days (an IQR of 10.5 to 153.5 days and a mean of 70.8 days) in all patients, GI motility drugs users, antipsychotics users, and flunarizine users, respectively. Among the patients whose drugs had ever been discontinued during the follow-up period (either temporarily or permanently), the median time to discontinuation was 90.0 days (an IQR of 26.0 to 229.0 days and a mean of 154.8 days), 88.5 days (an IQR of 21.0 to 182.0 days and a mean of 143.4 days), 88.5 days (an IQR of 36.0 to 326.5 days and a mean of 180.6 days), and 149.0 days (an IQR of 56.0 to 158.0 days and a mean of 108.4 days) in all patients, GI motility drug users, antipsychotic users, and flunarizine users, respectively.

3.3. Prognosis after Incident DIPs

DIP remittance occurred in more than 70% of all patients, from 61.5% of the flunarizine users to 77.4% of the GI motility drug users (Figure 3). However, approximately 25% of the patients had recurrent or persistent DIP. Male patients had a higher proportion of recurrent (17.6% vs. 13.5%) and persistent (13.7% vs. 10.6%) DIP compared to female patients.

The median time to remittance was 4.0 days (an IQR of 0.0 to 85.0 days and a mean of 70.3 days), 0.0 days (an IQR of 0.0 to 69.0 days and a mean of 62.6 days), 35.5 days (an IQR of 0.0 to 98.0 days and a mean of 86.4 days), and 0.0 days (an IQR of 0.0 to 4.5 days and a mean of 23.1 days) in all patients, GI motility drug users, antipsychotic users, and flunarizine users, respectively. Among the patients who had recurrent DIP, the median time to recurrence was 376.0 days (an IQR of 230.0 to 542.0 days and a mean of 399.8 days), 500.0 days (an IQR of 300.0 to 630.0 days and a mean of 462.1 days), 324.0 days (an IQR of 219.0 to 439.0 days and a mean of 354.5 days), and 210.0 days (an IQR of 209.0 to 427.0 days and a mean of 338.2 days) in all patients, GI motility drug users, antipsychotic users, and flunarizine users, respectively.

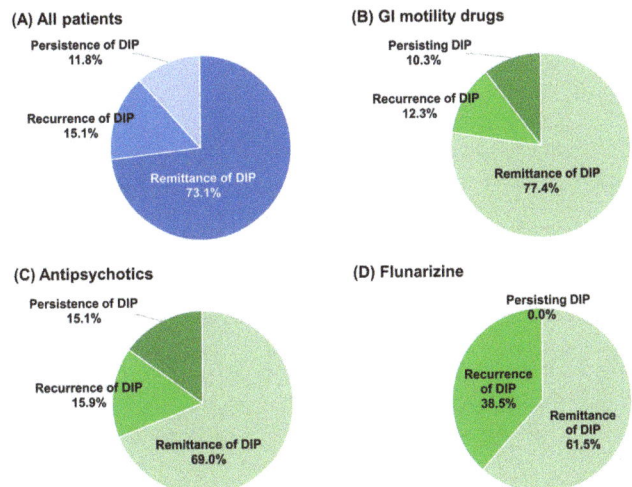

Figure 3. Prognosis after incident drug-induced parkinsonism. Abbreviations: DIP, drug-induced parkinsonism; GI, gastrointestinal.

Figure 4 shows the prognosis for each type of treatment pattern. Among the patients who discontinued the offending drugs, over 80% also showed DIP remittance. However, patients with other patterns had a lower proportion of remittance, especially those who persistently used the offending drugs (50.0%). Among patients who reinitiated offending drugs, patients who chose another drug within the same therapeutic class (75.8%) showed a higher proportion of remittance compared to patients who restarted the same drug at the same dose (63.2%).

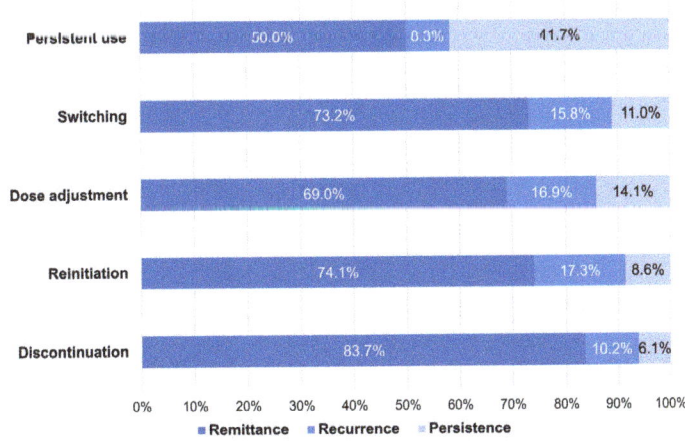

Figure 4. Prognosis by treatment patterns after incident drug-induced parkinsonism.

4. Discussion

This retrospective cohort study explored the treatment changes and prognosis status in patients who had experienced incident DIP in South Korea using a representative national claims database. Among 272 patients with incident DIP, the majority received GI motility drugs or antipsychotics as offending drugs. The patterns of treatment change differed across the types of offending drugs. Patients taking GI motility drugs mostly switched to other GI motility drugs or reinitiated the drugs after temporary discontinuation, while patients taking antipsychotics mostly adjusted the dose of antipsychotics or switched to other antipsychotics. The proportion of persistent users was higher among antipsychotic users than among GI motility drug users. Regarding prognosis, approximately a quarter of patients experienced DIP recurrence or persistence, the occurrence of which was lower in patients who had discontinued the offending drugs than it was in those with other treatment patterns.

This study investigated treatment changes and prognoses among patients with DIP using large, nationwide, and population-based real-world data. Because all citizens in South Korea are covered under either the National Health Insurance program or the Medical Aid program, the NHIS-NSC database could represent the entire Korean population [20]. Herein, we tried to identify patients with definite DIP by defining incident DIP case as an event with a diagnosis code of G21.1 or G25.1, and when the period for which offending drugs were prescribed overlapped with the time of DIP diagnosis. This definition was based on the views of Korean neurologists; therefore, it may reflect the features of the disease in clinical practice [10]. Based on these strengths, we anticipate that our findings may offer valuable insights into predicting DIP in patients prescribed high-risk drugs. Consequently, this could aid in personalized treatment selection for these patients.

In a study using hospital-based data in South Korea, 48% of patients diagnosed with levosulpiride-induced parkinsonism experienced persistent or recurrent parkinsonism even after the withdrawal of levosulpiride [23]. In our study, GI motility drug users showed a lower proportion of DIP recurrence or persistence (22.6%). This estimate is much lower than that of the previous study, considering that the proportion in our study was estimated regardless of the withdrawal of GI motility drugs. The difference might have resulted from the features of the data source because the previous study used data from a large teaching hospital that generally takes care of more severely ill patients compared to those attended to in various hospital settings included in the nationwide data. In addition, levosulpiride entails a high risk of DIP among the GI motility drugs, suggesting its potential impact on the prognosis of DIP [1,6].

Treatment options are lacking for patients experiencing DIP [24]. Although anticholinergic agents or amantadine may alleviate extrapyramidal symptoms, their efficacy has not been established in a large study, and the evidence is conflicting [24–26]. Therefore, discontinuing the offending drug may be the best choice if possible [27]. For patients who cannot stop the drug immediately, dose adjustment or switching could be an alternative approach [24]. Appropriate strategies may differ according to the type of offending drug. Given that GI motility drugs are generally used in the short-term and that several alternatives are available for the management of functional dyspepsia, discontinuation or switching to other classes (e.g., histamine type 2 receptor antagonists and proton pump inhibitors) could be considered an effective strategy [28]. Conversely, discontinuing antipsychotics may be unfeasible when considering the risk of exacerbating psychotic symptoms. In this case, dose adjustment or switching to antipsychotics that have a lower propensity to cause DIP would be better approaches than discontinuation [24]. In our previous study, itopride and quetiapine were found to exhibit a comparatively low likelihood of inducing DIP within the respective categories of GI motility drugs and antipsychotics [6]. Nevertheless, the selection of treatment should be based on a thorough assessment of clinical patient features, including the severity of the disease, the presence of comorbidities, concurrent medication usage, and the susceptibility to specific types of adverse events.

Considering the limited evidence on the treatment of DIP, prevention should be the first-line strategy to manage DIP and optimize treatment outcomes in patients prescribed high-risk drugs. Future studies are needed to assess the risk of developing DIP based on patient and drug characteristics. Moreover, our research revealed that approximately a quarter of patients experienced DIP recurrence or persistence. This underscores the importance of healthcare providers monitoring patients with DIP for symptom remission. In order to prevent the recurrence of DIP, healthcare providers should employ effective strategies that take into account the clinical benefits of utilizing drugs, as well as the potential harm of DIP based on individual patient characteristics.

To properly assess the burden of DIP, it is important to understand its association with the risk of developing Parkinson's disease. A recent study analyzing nationwide healthcare claims data in South Korea found that patients with DIP had a significantly increased risk of developing Parkinson's disease [16]. This suggests that DIP may be a strong risk factor for the progression of preexisting subclinical parkinsonism to Parkinson's disease. To fully understand the relationship between DIP and Parkinson's disease, it would be beneficial to investigate the association between DIP prognosis and the likelihood of developing Parkinson's disease. This analysis was not feasible in the present study due to the limited number of DIP patients and the short-term follow-up period. Further studies using a larger database encompassing the entire DIP patient population with an extended follow-up period are necessary.

The findings of this study should be interpreted with caution because of the following limitations: The diagnosis codes for defining DIP may not fully capture all patients with DIP. Because we only used the codes explicitly indicating "drug-induced" symptoms, we could not explore the treatment changes and prognoses in some patients with diagnosis codes related to parkinsonism but not specific to DIP or ion those who were undiagnosed. Nevertheless, we attempted to identify patients with definite DIP, considering that parkinsonism not specific to DIP may not be distinguishable from the early signs of idiopathic Parkinson's disease. We assessed treatment changes and prognoses during the same follow-up period; therefore, the prognosis might have preceded the treatment changes in some cases. However, we assessed the time to treatment changes and prognoses, and the results partly confirm that treatment changes preceded prognoses in most patients. Our findings are limited to GI motility drugs and antipsychotics that are approved in South Korea and may not be generalizable to other drugs in these categories. In particular, certain GI motility drugs such as metoclopramide and domperidone have varying indications and approval statuses across different countries; therefore, the findings regarding GI motility drugs should be interpreted with caution depending on the context. Furthermore, it is noteworthy that the number of DIP patients included in this study is limited, which is due in part to the utilization of the Sample Cohort database, which comprises only approximately 2% of the Korean population. It should be acknowledged that DIP is frequently under-recognized in clinical settings, and the utilization of data collected from the entire population may provide additional insights into the treatment patterns and prognosis of DIP patients. Nevertheless, the Sample Cohort database employed in this study was constructed through a representative sampling process, thereby ensuring the generalizability of our research findings. Lastly, it should be noted that the percentage of patients undergoing treatment changes and prognosis, which was defined based solely on prescription information, may have been subject to either overestimation or underestimation. This is because healthcare claims data lack information on medication adherence, symptoms, and laboratory test results. Despite these limitations, our study offers valuable insights into the current state of DIP management in the real world and highlights areas of unmet need in DIP care. Based on our findings, future research utilizing a larger database with a longer follow-up period is necessary to investigate effective strategies for managing DIP.

5. Conclusions

Overall, DIP patients who were taking GI motility drugs primarily switched to alternative GI motility drugs or resumed their medication after temporary discontinuation. Conversely, those who were taking antipsychotics typically adjusted their dosage or switched to alternative antipsychotic medication. Approximately a quarter of patients experienced DIP recurrence or persistence, which were more prevalent in antipsychotic users than in those taking GI motility drugs. To enhance treatment outcomes, it is imperative to assess the risk of developing DIP in patients who are prescribed GI motility drugs or antipsychotics. Additionally, healthcare providers should monitor patients experiencing DIP for symptom remittance and employ effective strategies to prevent its recurrence.

Author Contributions: Conceptualization, S.K. and H.S.S.; methodology, S.K. and H.S.S.; software, S.K.; validation, S.K.; formal analysis, S.K.; investigation, S.K. and H.S.S.; resources, H.S.S.; data curation, S.K.; writing—original draft preparation, S.K.; writing—review and editing, H.S.S.; visualization, S.K.; supervision, H.S.S.; project administration, H.S.S.; funding acquisition, H.S.S. All authors have read and agreed to the published version of the manuscript.

Funding: This research was funded by the National Research Foundation of Korea (NRF) grant funded by the Korean government (Ministry of Science and ICT) (grant number: NRF-2020R1F1A1069526) and the Ministry of Food and Drug Safety in 2022 (grant number: 21153MFDS601).

Institutional Review Board Statement: The study was conducted in accordance with the Declaration of Helsinki, and approved by the Institutional Review Board of Pusan National University (PNU IRB/2016_29_HR; 23 March 2016).

Informed Consent Statement: Patient consent was waived due to the retrospective study design and anonymity of the NHIS database.

Data Availability Statement: Not applicable.

Acknowledgments: This study used NHIS-NSC data (NHIS-2018-2-238) provided by the National Health Insurance Service (NHIS). The author(s) declare no conflicts of interest with NHIS.

Conflicts of Interest: The authors declare no conflict of interest.

References

1. López-Sendón, J.; Mena, M.A.; de Yébenes, J.G. Drug-induced parkinsonism. *Expert Opin. Drug Saf.* **2013**, *12*, 487–496. [CrossRef] [PubMed]
2. Shin, H.-W.; Chung, S.J. Drug-induced parkinsonism. *J. Clin. Neurol.* **2012**, *8*, 15–21. [CrossRef] [PubMed]
3. López-Sendón, J.L.; Mena, M.A.; García de Yébenes, J. Drug-Induced Parkinsonism in the Elderly. *Drugs Aging* **2012**, *29*, 105–118. [CrossRef] [PubMed]
4. Brigo, F.; Erro, R.; Marangi, A.; Bhatia, K.; Tinazzi, M. Differentiating drug-induced parkinsonism from Parkinson's disease: An update on non-motor symptoms and investigations. *Parkinsonism Relat. Disord.* **2014**, *20*, 808–814. [CrossRef]
5. Mena, M.A.; de Yébenes, J.G. Drug-induced parkinsonism. *Expert Opin. Drug Saf.* **2006**, *5*, 759–771. [CrossRef]
6. Kim, S.; Cheon, S.-M.; Suh, H.S. Association between drug exposure and occurrence of parkinsonism in Korea: A population-based case-control study. *Ann. Pharmacother.* **2019**, *53*, 1102–1110. [CrossRef]
7. Esper, C.D.; Factor, S.A. Failure of recognition of drug-induced parkinsonism in the elderly. *Mov. Disord.* **2008**, *23*, 401–404. [CrossRef]
8. Thanvi, B.; Treadwell, S. Drug induced parkinsonism: A common cause of parkinsonism in older people. *Postgrad. Med. J.* **2009**, *85*, 322–326. [CrossRef]
9. Barbosa, M.T.; Caramelli, P.; Maia, D.P.; Cunningham, M.C.Q.; Guerra, H.L.; Lima-Costa, M.F.; Cardoso, F. Parkinsonism and Parkinson's disease in the elderly: A community-based survey in Brazil (the Bambuí study). *Mov. Disord.* **2006**, *21*, 800–808. [CrossRef]
10. Han, S.; Kim, S.; Kim, H.; Shin, H.-W.; Na, K.-S.; Suh, H.S. Prevalence and incidence of Parkinson's disease and drug-induced parkinsonism in Korea. *BMC Public Health* **2019**, *19*, 1328. [CrossRef]
11. Wang, X.; Zeng, F.; Jin, W.-S.; Zhu, C.; Wang, Q.-H.; Bu, X.-L.; Luo, H.-B.; Zou, H.-Q.; Pu, J.; Zhou, Z.-H. Comorbidity burden of patients with Parkinson's disease and Parkinsonism between 2003 and 2012: A multicentre, nationwide, retrospective study in China. *Sci. Rep.* **2017**, *7*, 1671. [CrossRef] [PubMed]
12. Rekhi, G.; Tay, J.; Lee, J. Impact of drug-induced Parkinsonism and tardive dyskinesia on health-related quality of life in schizophrenia. *J. Psychopharmacol.* **2022**, *36*, 183–190. [CrossRef] [PubMed]

13. Potvin, S.; Aubin, G.; Stip, E. Antipsychotic-induced parkinsonism is associated with working memory deficits in schizophrenia-spectrum disorders. *Eur. Arch. Psychiatry Clin. Neurosci.* **2015**, *265*, 147–154. [CrossRef] [PubMed]
14. Brown, S.; Downes, E.; Welch, S.; Turner, A. A severe case of paliperidone palmitate-induced Parkinsonism leading to prolonged hospitalization: Opportunities for improvement. *Fed. Pract.* **2017**, *34*, 24.
15. Abouzaid, S.; Tian, H.; Zhou, H.; Kahler, K.H.; Harris, M.; Kim, E. Economic burden associated with extrapyramidal symptoms in a medicaid population with schizophrenia. *Community Ment. Health J.* **2014**, *50*, 51–58. [CrossRef]
16. Jeong, S.; Cho, H.; Kim, Y.J.; Ma, H.-I.; Jang, S. Drug-induced Parkinsonism: A strong predictor of idiopathic Parkinson's disease. *PLoS ONE* **2021**, *16*, e0247354. [CrossRef]
17. Alvarez, M.V.G.; Evidente, V.G.H. Understanding drug-induced parkinsonism: Separating pearls from oy-sters. *Neurology* **2008**, *70*, e32–e34. [CrossRef]
18. Factor, S.A.; Burkhard, P.R.; Caroff, S.; Friedman, J.H.; Marras, C.; Tinazzi, M.; Comella, C.L. Recent developments in drug-induced movement disorders: A mixed picture. *Lancet Neurol.* **2019**, *18*, 880–890. [CrossRef]
19. Llau, M.; Nguyen, L.; Senard, J.; Rascol, O.; Montastruc, J. Drug-induced parkinsonian syndromes: A 10-year experience at a regional center of pharmaco-vigilance. *Rev. Neurol.* **1994**, *150*, 757–762.
20. Song, S.O.; Jung, C.H.; Song, Y.D.; Park, C.-Y.; Kwon, H.-S.; Cha, B.S.; Park, J.-Y.; Lee, K.-U.; Ko, K.S.; Lee, B.-W. Background and data configuration process of a nationwide population-based study using the korean national health insurance system. *Diabetes Metab. J.* **2014**, *38*, 395–403. [CrossRef]
21. Lee, J.; Lee, J.S.; Park, S.-H.; Shin, S.A.; Kim, K. Cohort Profile: The National Health Insurance Service–National Sample Cohort (NHIS-NSC), South Korea. *Int. J. Epidemiol.* **2016**, *46*, e15. [CrossRef] [PubMed]
22. Quan, H.; Sundararajan, V.; Halfon, P.; Fong, A.; Burnand, B.; Luthi, J.-C.; Saunders, L.D.; Beck, C.A.; Feasby, T.E.; Ghali, W.A. Coding algorithms for defining comorbidities in ICD-9-CM and ICD-10 administrative data. *Med. Care* **2005**, *43*, 1130–1139. [CrossRef] [PubMed]
23. Shin, H.W.; Kim, M.J.; Kim, J.S.; Lee, M.C.; Chung, S.J. Levosulpiride-induced movement disorders. *Mov. Disord.* **2009**, *24*, 2249–2253. [CrossRef] [PubMed]
24. Wisidagama, S.; Selladurai, A.; Wu, P.; Isetta, M.; Serra-Mestres, J. Recognition and management of antipsychotic-induced Parkinsonism in older adults: A narrative review. *Medicines* **2021**, *8*, 24. [CrossRef] [PubMed]
25. Estevez-Fraga, C.; Zeun, P.; López-Sendón Moreno, J.L. Current methods for the treatment and prevention of drug-induced parkinsonism and tardive dyskinesia in the elderly. *Drugs Aging* **2018**, *35*, 959–971. [CrossRef] [PubMed]
26. Hardie, R.; Lees, A. Neuroleptic-induced Parkinson's syndrome: Clinical features and results of treatment with levodopa. *J. Neurol. Neurosurg. Psychiatry* **1988**, *51*, 850–854. [CrossRef]
27. Blanchet, P.J.; Kivenko, V. Drug-induced parkinsonism: Diagnosis and management. *J. Park. Restless Legs Syndr.* **2016**, *6*, 83–91. [CrossRef]
28. Oh, J.H.; Kwon, J.G.; Jung, H.-K.; Tae, C.H.; Song, K.H.; Kang, S.J.; Kim, S.E.; Jung, K.; Kim, J.S.; Park, J.K. Clinical practice guidelines for the treatment of functional dyspepsia in Korea. *Korean J. Med.* **2021**, *96*, 116–138. [CrossRef]

Disclaimer/Publisher's Note: The statements, opinions and data contained in all publications are solely those of the individual author(s) and contributor(s) and not of MDPI and/or the editor(s). MDPI and/or the editor(s) disclaim responsibility for any injury to people or property resulting from any ideas, methods, instructions or products referred to in the content.

MDPI
St. Alban-Anlage 66
4052 Basel
Switzerland
www.mdpi.com

Journal of Clinical Medicine Editorial Office
E-mail: jcm@mdpi.com
www.mdpi.com/journal/jcm

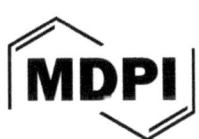

Disclaimer/Publisher's Note: The statements, opinions and data contained in all publications are solely those of the individual author(s) and contributor(s) and not of MDPI and/or the editor(s). MDPI and/or the editor(s) disclaim responsibility for any injury to people or property resulting from any ideas, methods, instructions or products referred to in the content.

www.ingramcontent.com/pod-product-compliance
Lightning Source LLC
LaVergne TN
LVHW070658100526
838202LV00013B/993